LEAVES OF LIFE
Select Medicinal Plants from Guyana With Healing Properties
Volume 1

Kazembe Bediako MPS, MSTOM

Published by Khianga Publishing

Book cover designed by Enensa Amen of Graphika Group

Interior design by Khianga Publishing

First Printing 2012

Library of Congress Cataloging-in-Publication Data

p. cm.

Kazembe Bediako: Leaves of Life - 1st ed. (Soft Cover)

ISBN 978-0-9845715-3-6

1. Phytochemicals Plants. 2. Medicinal plants - Guyana. 3. Materia Medica.

4. Ethno Botantical. 5. Phytosciences. 6. Herbal Remedies 7. Ethnobotanical Therapeutics

Non-Fiction 1 Title: Leaves of Life

Library of Congress Catalog Card Number: 2010906865

Important Warning

This book contains general information about medicinal plants and their uses. It is intended as a scientific overview and not as a medical handbook for treatment. Several medical plants described in this book have toxic ingredients and many cause severe allergic reactions or serious poisoning. Neither the author nor the publisher can be held responsible for claims arising from the mistaken identity of plants or their appropriate use. Do not attempt self-diagnosis or self-treatment. Always consult a medical professional or qualified practitioner.

The author and publisher specifically disclaim any responsibility for any liability, loss or risk, personal or otherwise, which is incurred as a consequence, directly or indirectly, of the use and application of any of the contents of this book.

Table of Contents

Acknowledgements

I would like to thank my mother, Mrs. Inez Hodge, my father, the late Wilfred O. Hodge and my grandmother, the late Mrs. Alberta Harding, for making this book possible. My children, Amkhetnu, Basta, Khat Sa Ra and Autqem Neter deserve special thanks for watching over my shoulder as I worked.

Special thanks to my brothers and sisters for all their spiritual support, Errol, Egland, Leon, Michael, Basil, Eardley, Ingham, Ralph, Hazel and Desiree. For my nieces and nephews Oshanda, Idesta, Carleen, Taisha, Shekeima, Jude, Eli, Errol, Erland and Ewin.

My wonderful wife Ausara Senuas who has grown with me as we weave a rich and interesting life together. Thank you for being instrumental in making sure everything came together at the proper time.

There are literally hundreds of people whom I have had conversations with throughout the years. I am especially indebted to friends who continuously provide me with tidbits and stories as they pass my way.

Anetch Hrak! Tuau, special thanks to my spiritual teacher, Shekhem Ur Shekhem, Ra Un Nefer Amen 1, for being the example of living the Ankh En Maat and reminding us of the greatness of our culture and ourselves.

Herb Song.[1]

One day I meet a old woman selling, and I wanted something to eat.
I thought I could put a little bit in she way, but I take back when I did meet.
I thought she had bananas, orange or pear, nothing that I need,
I asked the old woman what she was selling, she said she was selling weed.
She had she coat tie up over she waist, and was stepping along with grace,
She had a pair of old dogs on her feet, and was waddling down the street.
Just then she start to name the different weed, and was really more than glad,
I can't remember all she call, but these were a few she had.
She had the Manpeabber, Womanpeabber, Tan-tan, Fall-back and Lemon-grass,
Minnie-root, Gully-Root, Granny-back-bone, Bitter-tally, Lime-leaf and Caroon,
Coolie-bitters, Cariella-bush, Flat-earth and de Iron-weed, Sweet-bloom, Foul-tongue
and the Wild-daisies Sweet-sage and even to you.
She had de Cat-mint, de Pepper-mint, Soldier-rod, Pastee-lena and de Cow-foot bush,
Milk-weed, Fit-weed, Bird-vine, de Bishop-cap-bush and de Rock-balsam,
Surinam bitters, de Wild-green-tree, Three-fingers and the Wurum-bush,
A worm grass, Z-grass, Man-grass, Carron~crow, Snake-bitters and also Tezzan.
She had de Cassava-mama, Okra-babba, Jacob la1adder, mixed with Finegona,
lob-tea, Peter-parslee, John-Belly-parslee and the White Clary,
Bill-bush, Wild-cane, Duck~weed, Aniseed, War-bitters and Wild-grey-root.
She even had down to a certain bush Barbados call Puss-in-Boots.
When I hear the names she call, I went down, can't even talk.
She start to call from Camp Street corner, never stop till she reach Orange Walk.
The woman had me so surprise, I didn't know what to do
Till a girl come along, one cuff in me eyes, and I didn't know who was who.
Sweet-broom, Sweet-sage and the Lemon-grass, I hear them good making tea,
When I hear Dutch-grass, and the Wild-daisy am good to cool the body.
Yes the Woman-tongue was even listed, calling out at the time,
She only had a little Congo eye, but the other one now left blind.
She had Tansa-bitters, Pumgranate-bark, Congo-cane, de Pear-leaf, de young Bizziebizzie,
Young Grape-vine, Back-pain, Stinging-nettle, Do-ra-me bush and de Broad-leaf thyme,
De Mimosa-leaf with the Evergreen-seed, Bitter-fence, bitter just like gall,
Doctor Doodles squashy bitters, and the Anamus grass, Snake-bitters and dat wasn't even all.
She had de Bitter-gumma, Porta-demma, Congo-lalla and the Creva-cot broom,
Stavilla, Wild-samatoo, Sour-sop leaf, and the Half-of-it weed,
Cool de-body, Sweet-mint, Porter-bush, White Clary and de Xmas bush,
Cat-tongue, and even the Monkey-ladder, and this the rest you may need.
She had de Pap-bush, Elder-bush, de Black-pepper bush, French-to-you and de
Cure-for-all, Sapodilla, Tamarind leaf, Money bush, and de Soldier-parsley,
Pumpkin-blossom, with the Double-do-me, and Congo-pumps in galore,
Physic-nut, and even the Lily-root root is the list of her every day soup.

---

[1] Morton, Julia F. *Atlas of Medical Plants of Middle America: Bahamas to Yucatan.* Springfield, Illinois: Charles C. Thomas Publisher, 1981; 1262. Reproduced by permission from Bayley, Iris. *The Bush Teas of Barbados*, Taylor's Version, (Journal of the Barbados Museum and Historical Society, Vol. XVI, No.3, May 1949).

Introduction

Leaves of Life, Volume1: Single Herbs, cites the enormous importance of the natural world of plants at a time when plant resources are decreasing at a rapid rate. No other time in history have human beings placed such importance on the natural world of plants. Conservative estimates state that there are about 250,000 species of higher plants on this planet.[2] The National Cancer Institute (NCI), over a period of 30 years, screened more than 32,000 higher plant species for their ability to inhibit various tumors.[3] While industrialized countries during the last hundred years have gradually reduced the use of plant remedies and medicinal plants are threatened by extinction through exploitation of natural vegetation. Guyana, which lies at the point where the Caribbean meets South America on its North Atlantic seaboard, consists of eighty percent rainforest and is home to one of the richest regions of the world with expanses of untouched neotropical forests and different species of plants found nowhere else on earth.[4]

Plants have fed the world and cured its ills since time immemorial. About 80% of the world depends on herbal-based alternative systems of medicine.[5] Consumer demand for natural medicines is higher than ever before. Both in Europe and in the United States consumers spend at least $4 billion a year on herbal medicinal products.[6] Many of these plants are researched to develop scientific evidence based rational herbal therapies. Much is not yet known regarding the vast pharmacology of herbal remedies. Less than ten percent of all plant species have been subjected to investigations of secondary metabolites and their effects.[7] The Chinese pharmacopeia depends on the 5,757 plants listed in the *Encyclopedia of Traditional Chinese Medicinal Substances.*[8] The Indian Ayurveda pharmacopeia boasts between 1,000[9] and 2,000 medicinal plants[10] while the total number of medicinal herbs in the world is about 70,000. [11] The German compendium *Arzneidrogenprojile* contains the profiles of about 200 commonly used medicinal herbs.[12]

Plants produce a wide variety of chemical compounds called phytochemicals. There was a big upsurge in the popularity of complementary and alternative medicine (CAM) in the United States in the 1990s. A survey showed the use of herbal medicines increased from 2.5% in 1990 to 12.1% in 1997. The usage of CAM is generally more frequent among women and people in the 35 to 49 age groups. In the western United States research results showed that the prevalence of herbal use among ethnically diverse primary care patients varies, ranging from thirty percent among primary care patients residing in urban setting on

---

[2] Chadwick, Derek J., and Joan Mash. *Bioactive Compounds from Plants: A Wiley-Interscience Publication.* Chichester [etc.: John Wiley & Sons, 1990; 5.

[3] Ibid., 3.

[4] Leeuwenberg, A.J.M. *Medicinal and Poisonous Plants of the Tropics.* Wagenlngen: Center for Agricultural Publishing and Documentation, 1987; 26.

[5] Daniel, M. *Medicinal Plants: Chemistry and Properties.* New Hampshire: Science Publishers, 2006; 17.

[6] Duke, James A. *CRC Handbook of Medicinal Herbs.* Boca Raton, FL: CRC, 1985; 459.

[7] Leeuwenberg, A.J.M. *Medicinal and Poisonous Plants of the Tropics.* Wagenlngen: Center for Agricultural Publishing and Documentation, 1987; 9.

[8] Daniel, M. *Medicinal Plants: Chemistry and Properties.* New Hampshire: Science Publishers, 2006; 17.

[9] Ahmad Iqbal, Aqil Farrukh and Owais Mohammad. *Modern Phytomedicine: Turning Medical Plants into Drugs.* Germany: Wiley-Vch Verlag Gmbh & Co. KGaA, 2006; 64.

[10] Daniel, M. *Medicinal Plants: Chemistry and Properties.* New Hampshire: Science Publishers, 2006; 17.

[11] Leeuwenberg, A.J.M. *Medicinal and Poisonous Plants of the Tropics.* Wagenlngen: Center for Agricultural Publishing and Documentation, 1987; 9.

[12] Gehrmann, Beatrice, Wolf-Gerald Koch, Tschirch Claus O., and Brinkmann, Helmut, *Medicinal Herbs: A Compendium.* New York: The Haworth Herbal, 2005; ix.

the West coast to seventy seven percent among primary care patients residing in the largest United States/Mexico border city. Herbal use is common (36%) among urban multi-ethnic primary care patients, but has a wide variability among ethnic groups. Hispanic and Asian groups reported the highest rates of herbal use (50%), and African Americans reported the lowest (22%) rates.[13]

The Efficacy of Herbs Compared to Drugs

Herbs are often considered to be safer, gentler, and of lower cost than conventional pharmaceutical drugs. Herbs are safer than modern-day synthetic or lab-produced drugs because they are naturally rich in both biologically active and inert substances. Many of these nutrients have strong antioxidant, detoxicant, scavenging, and dual-functioning properties, which a great number of people do not realize. Herbs do not act like chemical drugs but more closely resemble the orthomolecular substances of vitamins, minerals and enzymes that naturally exist in our bodies. There are those who argue that medicinal herbs usually do not give immediate reactions and are not the first choice to treat severe, life threatening diseases. However, herbs have been used as the primary choice of treatment for thousands of years in Africa, Asia and the Americas. The effects or herbs are subtle and gradual. They tend to fill the needs of one's system as a whole. The herbal properties balance the positive and the negative, gradually bringing the entire body to a natural state.

Advantages of natural (herbal) medicines are that they are mild in action, lack side effects at normal dosage, and are relatively inexpensive compared to most synthetic drugs. In addition, crude preparations of herbal medicines, when taken orally, have interesting benefits. With oral consumption, the release of active ingredients into the bloodstream is relatively slow. The low concentrated release of the medication provides for a sustained dosage, which is a possible explanation for the minimal side effects experienced from herbal preparations. The body is not subjected to a sudden surge of chemicals. Instead, the herb is introduced to the body's system slowly and gently.

Leaves of Life (LOL) presents an ecological perspective of health and disease as it examines the interrelationships among environmental, cultural, social, and physiological factors. It incorporates the traditional pharmaceutical practices with modern medicine, and presents a compendium of over a hundred medicinal plants from Guyana and their usage. Plants have aided us in the fight against diseases. The remedy *quinine* from the cinchona bark eradicated the disease malaria; *morphia* remains perhaps the most effective pain killer; *mahuang (*Ephedra vulgaris*)* for treatment of asthma (ephedrine is the active alkaloid component); *emetine*, the most effective controller of amebic dysentery; *rauwolfia* used in the treatment of high blood pressure (the alkaloid reserpine being the active principle) introduced the much abused concept of tranquillizers; the heart drug *digitalis* from the purple foxglove and *curare* remains one of the most valuable handmaidens of modern anesthesia, not to mention *penicillin*.[14]

Traditional Healers – The Obeah Practitioners and the Local Spiritualist

Leaves of Life offers a holistic perspective on the time tested use of medicinal plants as practiced by *Obeah* healers and spiritualists, the renowned group of African centered, skilled healers and herbalists in Guyana. *Leaves of Life* reveals the age old tradition of administering hundreds of medicinal plants to cure the sick. Some ridicule them for their astrological beliefs such as insisting on harvesting their herbs at a certain time

---

[13] Ahmad, Iqbal, Farrukh Aqil, and Mohammad Owais. *Modern Phytomedicine: Turning Medical Plants into Drugs*. Weinheim: Wiley-VCH, 2006; 343.

[14] Thomson M.D., William A. R. *Herbs that Heal*. New York: Scribner, 1976; 12.

of day or a certain period of the moon. But about eighty percent of the rural population in Guyana still depends on traditional healers such as the *Obeah* men and women for their knowledge of herbs. Most of these herbal remedies sold in the local markets to people in search of cures, are nature's equivalent of aspirin, penicillin, quinine and others still yet to be discovered by modern medicine. In applying myrtle leaves to a sore tooth, the *Obeah* healers are doing the same as a dentist applying *eugenol* oil to a sore tooth. In both cases, the toothache immediately disappears, writes Duke.[15] It took a long time to learn the bitter principle from quinine bark can cure malaria and it would take even longer for medical research to show that the calcium consumed with *coca leaves* in Bolivia, or with *betel* in Burma might prevent or alleviate osteoporosis.

Brekhman in his book, *Man and Biologically Active Substances, claims* that ginseng and Siberian ginseng have broad-spectrum adaptogenic, prophylactic and therapeutic actions.[16] Ginseng and Siberian ginseng contain ingredients found in the human body. These herbal substances are consistent tonics because they can raise levels of physiological adaptation and prevention activities within the body. Brekhman believes this is because the herbs arc able to accelerate (biosynthesis of proteins and nucleic acids). The general tonic restorative remedies listed in Chapters 5 and 6 are typical, naturally occurring, biologically active substances for prevention.

Many medicinal herbs appear to impact homeostatic control mechanisms. They are called "dual activities," because they aid in the normalization or balancing many of the body's processes. For example, to combat hypertension, ginseng root will have a calming effect. To combat hypostate, or feeling of tiredness, the same herb will have an energizing tonic effect on the body's system, all much to the bafflement of conventional Western pharmacologists.[17]

The Obeah healers treat diseases which the local population view as an adversity imposed upon them by outside forces they do not comprehend and are expected to perform rites, ritual and magic to aid in physical and mental illness. They understood the importance of a holistic approach to illness long before this received attention in modern medicine. They deliver a more integrated approach to medicine and emphasize the prevention, as well as the cure, to diseases. Their role is closely aligned to mystic practices and magic and is often more concerned with the spirit than with the body. The Obeah men and women argue that it is the spirit that governs the body and to take care of the spirit is to take care of the body. It can be further argued that all herbs address some emotional component. Ra Un Nefer Amen reiterates this point when he writes, “the key to healing resides in the divine spirit of man.”[18]

It is common for the *Obeah* men and women to say that they chose a plant possessing a spirit stronger than the disease spirit, and the soul of the medicine is not manifested before the Obeah men and women have chanted certain hekau[19] or words of power over the plant. Among the compendium of herbs is a category where certain barks are used to drive away evil. Before removal of the bark, however, the offering of gifts must propitiate the spirit of the tree. The key to deciphering what these gifts are is embedded in the Kamitic cosmology. The Kamitic sages outline this aspect of gift giving or sacrifice as the rendering up of a negative conditioning. This is the equivalent of saying leave a gift on the altar, or in the case at the base of the tree. In other words, it is again saying give it up to God. Healing is in the spirit. Ra Un Nefer Amen cites that “the Ancient Egyptians, and the other by the Taoist Sages of China put this approach in place. For

---

[15] Duke, James A. *CRC Handbook of Medicinal Herbs*. Boca Raton, FL: CRC, 1985; 98.

[16] Ibid., 98.

[17] Ibid., 98.

[18] Amen, Ra Un Nefer. *Healing is in the Spirit*. Brooklyn: Khamit Media Trans Vision, Inc. 2010; 7.

[19] Ibid., 7.

many reasons, the great contributions of these people to the advancement of knowledge and the wellbeing of the world have gone largely unnoticed in the case of the Ancient Egyptians and unappreciated and minimally understood in the case of the Taoist Sages.[20]

Doctrine of Signatures

The *doctrine of signatures* further gives an examination of the ethnobotanical practices of these *Obeah* traditional healers and how they classify diseases and herbs. They have unique perspectives on the causes of diseases and how the human body functions. All this is interwoven into an underlying cognitive and symbolic system that holds together the diversity of the beliefs, techniques and practices.

According to the *doctrine of signatures*, a holistic approach to classifying herbs, nature has provided a plant for every disease and has indicated by an obvious sign for which disease or which part of the body each drug plant is to be used. Thus the shape of a plant or of one of its components may suggest a cure. If the herb has an appearance of an eye, brain, arm, head, foot or hand, this would serve as a reference to gain further insight into the actual action of the herb. For example, a walnut, which has the shape of a brain, is used for diseases affecting the brain. Plants with red flowers are used in blood disorders and those with yellow flowers are used in jaundice like the Dandelion and Agrimony. Saxifrages, which grow on rocks and break them up, would be useful for stones in the bladder. Plants with white latex are used to increase milk production and those with big swollen fruits to favor fertility. For instance, the flower of the Scullcap used for insomnia resembles the shape of the human skull. The blue flower of the Eyebright with its yellow center suggests the human eye and is used to treat tired eyes. The flowers of many of the herbs which purify the blood are red in color, e.g. the Scarlet Pimpernel, the Burdock and the Red Clover. The medicinal value of Nettles is indicated by its sting and is used to stimulate the circulation. Plants with a particularly unpleasant smell like the stinking Arrach is used for foul ulcers. The bark of the Willow cures rheumatism brought on by damp and the tree grows in wet places. Lungwort, because of its spotted leaves, is used for diseased lungs.

However, the most important concept of the doctrine of signatures is the integration of magical properties of herbs in effecting the mind, body and spirit. The same herb that removes physical toxins from the body, also removes psychic toxins from the spirit.

Herb-based Alternative Systems of Medicine

Herbal medicine is now globally accepted as a valid alternative system of therapy. About 80% of people living in developing countries are almost completely dependent on traditional medical practices for their primary health care needs. Higher plants are known to be the main source of drug therapy in traditional medicine.[21] It is further claimed that 64% of the total population of the world utilizes plants as drugs, i.e. 3.2 billion people.[22] Approximately, 119 plant based derived chemical compounds of known structure and derived from ninety species of plants are currently used as drugs or as biodynamic agents that affect human health.[23]

---

[20] Ibid., 10.
[21] Chadwick, Derek J., and Joan Mash. *Bioactive Compounds from Plants: A Wiley-Interscience Publication.* Chichester [etc.: John Wiley & Sons, 1990; 3.
[22] Ibid., 3.
[23] Ibid., 3.

Nearly one-third of Americans engage in alternative medicine practices. 25% of all prescriptions dispensed from community pharmacies contained active principles that were extracted from higher plants. In 1980, consumers in the United States paid more than 8 billion dollars for prescriptions containing active principles obtained from higher plants.[24] Therefore, the potential for interactions with conventional medicine exists.

Health is influenced by religion, society and environment. The World Health Organization (WHO) defines health as not only the absence of disease and malnutrition but also the positive wellbeing of the person. Ra Un Nefer Amen writes "all functions of the body, mind and spirit—and in all departments of nature are composed and regulated by two interdependent and seemingly opposite factors."[25] In the West, we call these structures positive and negative currents. In medical terms, it is known as anabolism (yin) and catabolism (yang). Anabolism corresponds to all the supportive nutrients and structural substances (blood, water, hormones, nutrients, etc.). Catabolism (yang) corresponds to the forces (electricity, magnetism, etc.) through which activity takes place. Diseases therefore arise as the result of the underlying malfunctions of the organs or imbalance of the yin and yang of the body, anabolic and catabolic.

Activity (yang) requires nutrition (fuel/yin) and the transformation and mobilization of yin agents require force (yang). An additional correspondence is heat (yang), which facilitates activity, and cold (relative less heat), which facilitates the formation and function of yin. To rest, the body must cool down, while to act, it must heat up. Thinking is facilitated by coolness and communication by warmth, etc. The electromagnetic energy in life's vital force is called Qi, which activates all organ functions and chemical processes of the body. Ra Un Nefer Amen states this best in his summary:

> "Nothing happens without energy. All activities in our being, every thought that we have, every breath that we take, are carried out by our life force. The Ancient Egyptians referred to it as Ra-the Spirit/life-force (not the "Sun God,") and the Taoist Sages referred to it as Qi. We will later see that the Egyptians and the Chinese have as much knowledge about man's life force as the present day scientists have about biology, biochemistry, physics, etc. If we want to understand the energy that is in charge of all activities in our being it is to our advantage to reclaim the vast ocean of knowledge on the subject that was developed by these ancient people during a span of several thousands of years of investigation and practice."[26]

The Obeah man uses a combination of herbs and ritual to restore balance in the body, mind and spirit. Specifically, the herbs are used to assist in removing the stagnation that prevents the healing to fully take place. Healing can only take place when the underlying condition that causes the disturbance in the life force is removed. Establishing and maintaining the balance between the general yin and yang of the body, mind and spirit is the goal of healing, according to traditional Chinese medicine (TCM). Health is the balance of all yin and yang functions. It is ultimately manifested in happiness, which is the balanced interplay of peace (yin) and pleasure (yang).

This is in contrast to the allopathic system of medicine in which the diseases are identified first and then the healing therapies are applied. When one system or organ of the body is affected, all other systems of the body are similarly affected (For example, an infection in the stomach weakens the circulatory, urino-genital, respiratory system and even affects the psyche of the patient). The body becomes weak, immunity declines and this paves the way for secondary infections. But normally a remedy in the form of a laxative is meant only for the alimentary canal and does not take care of the other affected systems. Therefore, even when a patient is cured of a stomach problem, he or she remains weak. In contrast, with a traditional herbal

[24] Ibid., 4.

[25] Amen, Ra Un Nefer. *Healing is in the Spirit*. Brooklyn: Khamit Media Trans Vision, Inc. 2010; 10.

[26] Ibid., 10,11.

formula, a number of plants are involved in the formula that reflect the multitude of components, including a large amount of metabolites, are available to the body to repair the systems. That is the reason why a person becomes healthy and remains so after herbal treatment.

The Story Behind the Wonder Drugs

The aim of *Leaves of Life* is to assist the layperson in self-healing through the use and preparation of herbs by providing important information on the medicinal and traditional uses of herbs from Guyana in a succinct easy-to-use form. In Guyana, the knowledge of the uses of these medicinal plants is traditionally passed down from generation to generation by word of mouth. Both in its philosophy and its practical application toward healing, *Obeah,* as an African healing system, has a great deal to offer Western Medicine. There are still large numbers of medicinal plants which remain undocumented and uncharacterized. Every day new plant sources of medicine are also being discovered.[27] The advent of pharmaceutical chemistry during the early twentieth century brought with it the ability to synthesize an enormous variety of medicinal drug molecules and allowed the treatment of previously incurable and/or life-threatening diseases. It is estimated that Americans consume more than 40 billion tablets a year.[28] Nearly $500 million is spent on over-the-counter drugs containing aspirin each year.[29] However, synthetic drugs have been plagued by unwanted toxic side effects. The emergence of new infectious diseases, the proliferation of disorders such as cancer, and growing multidrug resistance in pathogenic microorganisms have prompted renewed interest in the discovery of potential drug molecules from medicinal plants.

Starting in the nineteenth century, the science era and the evolution of modern medicine began. William Withering, the English physician, in 1783 advocated for the use of digitalis. In 1807, the German pharmacist, Serturner chemically isolated the alkaloid morphine from opium. This was the first active ingredient ever isolated from opium for pain management.[30] In 1828, Wohler, another German chemist, published his synthesis of urea from ammonia cyanate. He was the first chemist to make organic urea through a chemical reaction without the kidneys.[31] As a result, Wohler laid the foundation for the elimination of routine dependency upon natural botanical and mineral substances.

With little delay, many organic chemists in Germany became famous for producing new drugs in the laboratories and became the "new drug creators." More than a million new chemical entities were created at the prodigious rate of nearly 30,000 each year.[32] Suddenly, there was an abundance of new dyes, perfumes, flavoring agents, vitamins and synthetic chemical drugs, all supposedly accomplished for the benefit of humanity. In 1838, Piria, a German chemist discovered salicin, a chemical isolated from white willow which was found to be a powerful pain reliever, fever reducing, and anti-inflammatory agent.[33] The "wonder-drug" era began in the twentieth century. Paul Ehrlich first synthesized sulfanilamide in 1966. [34] Gerhard Domagk discovered the anti-infectant sulfanilamide, prontosil, initially using its

---

[27] Ahmad, Iqbal, Farrukh Aqil, and Mohammad Owais. *Modern Phytomedicine: Turning Medical Plants into Drugs*. Weinheim: Wiley-VCH, 2006; 252.
[28] Hou, Joseph P., and Youyu Jin. *The Healing Power of Chinese Herbs and Medicinal Recipes*. New York: Haworth Integrative Healing, 2005; 2.
[29] Ibid., 2.
[30] Ibid., 2.
[31] Ibid., 3.
[32] Ibid., 3.
[33] Ibid., 3.
[34] Ibid., 3.

properties against streptococca infections in mice.[35] The Sulfanilamide drugs exhibit a wide antibacterial spectrum for fighting infectious diseases; sulfamerazine, sulffamethazine, and sulfaisoxazol have been most frequently prescribed, primarily because of their low toxicity and broad spectrum benefits. However, serious toxic reactions can occur after a period including cyanosis, leukopenia, granulocytopenia, hemolytic anemia, and serious kidney damage.

The development of modern psycholyptic drugs resulted in the production of tranquilizers. The most popular anti-anxiety tranquillers were made with chlordiazepoxide, which was developed in 1954.[36] The trade names are Librium, Novopoxide and Ativan. During the 1960s, another series of anti-depressant drugs were made with diazepam, under the trade names of Valium and Vivol. [37]All benzediazepines and diazepam drugs essentially have the same action in the brain. Some calm its activity and alleviate anxiety, insomnia, epilepsy, muscle spasms and mental and mood disorders. Disadvantages of antianxiety drugs are that their continued use can cause physical and mental dependence, tolerance and addition. The other noted side effects are confusion, stumbling, memory loss, drowsiness, lightheadedness, hangover effect, increased aggression, weight gain and impaired ability to drive or operate machinery.[38]

In 1924, K.K. Chen, an outstanding Chinese pharmacologist at Beijing Union Medical College, introduced the studies of isolated ephedrine alkaloid from the bark of the ephedra, botanically known as Ephedra Sinica.[39] His research influenced the exploration of the pharmacology and therapeutic uses of ephedrine, and the research of homologs and analogs of epinephrine, a natural hormone found in the body. Chen's report initiated a significant movement among chemists around the world to search for new stimulants. Subsequently, new synthetic drugs including amphetamines, phenylephedrines, isoprotenenol, and other sympathomimetic amines were born.[40] This group of drugs is widely used in the treatment of depression, nasal congestion, asthma and blocked arteries.

In 1929, Fleming discovered penicillin, which was possibly the single most valuable discovery in modern medicine and which spawned an entire class of antibiotics for the treatment of infectious disease. Later, many classes of antibiotics were produced by various strains of *Penicillium Nototum* and *P. Chrysogenum*. A highly potent strain of fungi was eventually isolated that was called *Penicillin G*. Attempts to increase the penicillin yield from a mold culture by the addition of various chemical intermediates also led to the discovery of many new types of penicillin. By this method, thirty-six new penicillins were soon isolated.[41] Broad-spectrum peniciilins, for oral use, were successfully manufactured by different pharmaceutical companies. The ampicillin series and cephalosporin group, the "second-generation" antibiotics, were synthesized in laboratories. Doctors joyfully referred to these antibiotics as "wonder drugs" or "miracle drugs.[42]

As a result of the availability of these wonder or miracle drugs, Western medicine underwent a significant medical revolution. After World War II, in particular, development of new synthetic drugs progressed at a rapid pace by all pharmaceutical companies in numerous countries. In addition to antibiotics, new vitamins,

---

[35] Ibid., 3.
[36] Hou, Joseph P., and Youyu Jin. *The Healing Power of Chinese Herbs and Medicinal Recipes*. New York: Haworth Integrative Healing, 2005; 3.
[37] Ibid., 3.
[38] Ibid., 3.
[39] Ibid., 3.
[40] Ibid., 4.
[41] Ibid., 4.
[42] Ibid., 4.

steroids, cortisones, and other anti-inflammatory, drugs were developed. Doctors and researchers predicted there could be an end to infectious diseases in the world by the 1980s.[43]

Despite more than fifty years of experience working with these modern synthetic drugs and despite millions upon millions of dollars spent on their development, there still remains a dark side to all that has been done. Many of these chemical amalgamations have been doing as much harm as good. One example of this dilemma is aspirin. If the prescribed dosage of aspirin is too high, or the drug is used continuously, the patient may develop sensation of ringing in the ears or slight deafness.[44] Overdoses of aspirin car cause headache, dizziness, gastric irritation and peptic ulcer. Basically, the drug becomes counterproductive. In addition, some patients cannot tolerate aspirin at all, at any dosage level. A second example is cortisone. Notable side effects of cortisone medication and corticosteroids used for easing pain and arthritis are degeneration of joint cartilage, deposits of fat and weigh gain, male impotence, fluid retention, insomnia, depression and reduced resistance to infections. *No synthetic drug is without some side effect, particularly when used on a continuous basis.*

The side effects and toxicity of drugs are cumulative, ranging from mild to severe, and can affect every part of the body, particularly the nervous system, liver and kidneys. Because or overuse of potential drugs in many Western societies, more people are suffering from allergies, headaches, migraines, fatigue, depression, weight gain, and kidney failure, in companion with people who live in Asia and Africa. There is a more simplistic solution to these problems through herbal medicine which is an ever-present alternative.

Medicinal herbs have been used since antiquity by cultures all over the world. Approximately 20,000 plant species are now used for medicinal purposes around the world.[45] There are an estimated 200,000 to 500,000 higher plants and 200,000 or more lower plants on the earth with about 90% of the world's flora not subjected to any form of scientific phytochemical or biological screening study.[46] Yet the plant kingdom yields approximately 250% or more of tile drugs used in prescription medicines today.[47] Crude plant drugs became used as aqueous or alcoholic extracts and chemical work resulting in the isolation of their active principles began in the 19th Century. The World Health Organization (WHO) estimates that at least 80% of the world population relies on traditional (herbal) medicines for its primary health care needs.[48]

Phytocompounds Found in Plants

Plants have become increasingly important as a source of biologically active natural products. Phytosciences combine the use of medicinal plants and their bioactive phytocompounds with scientific knowledge and tries to determine whether plants commonly used in traditional medicine can provide cures against devastating diseases and, if so, what their mechanisms of action are. A single metabolome, the sum total of primary and secondary metabolite of a plant, contains from 4,000 to 10,000 compounds. The total

---

[43] Ibid., 4.
[44] Ibid., 5.
[45] Nigg, Herbert N., and David S. Seigler. *Phytochemical Resources for Medicine and Agriculture*. New York: Plenum, 1992; 77.
[46] Ibid., 76.
[47] Chadwick, Derek J., and Joan Mash. *Bioactive Compounds from Plants: A Wiley-Interscience Publication*. Chichester [etc.: John Wiley & Sons, 1990; 22.
[48] Hou, Joseph P., and Youyu Jin. *The Healing Power of Chinese Herbs and Medicinal Recipes*. New York: Haworth Integrative Healing, 2005; 3.

number of compounds present in the plant kingdom is about 200,000.[49] It is estimated that twenty five percent of all medicines contain plant derivatives and plant components have been used as the starting material for many semi-synthetic drugs.[50] All these compounds are used by plants for various purposes such as nutrition, maintenance, reproduction and healing. The active chemical compounds in medicinal plants and phytomedicines are known as secondary metabolites. Among the bioactive phytocompounds found in medicinal plants are alkaloids, glycosides, essential oils, organic acids (not including amino acids), tannin, amino acids, protein and enzymes, sugars, wax and lipid, resin, inorganic components and pigments.

Alkaloids comprise the largest class of secondary plant substances, at present numbering more than 7,000. The term 'alkaloid' means 'alkali-like substance'. A typical alkaloid is a basic plant product possessing a nitrogen-containing heterocyclic ring system and exhibiting marked pharmacological activity. Alkaloids are colorless bitter tasting crystals of organic compounds of plant that contain nitrogen. Few alkaloids such as berberine is yellow in color, and nicotine is a liquid. Most of the alkaloids have very strong actions. Arecoline is anthelmintic and has flaccid paralysis action on tapeworm.[51] Dichroine is anti-malarial.[52] Berberine is antibacterial and anti-inflammatory.[53] Aconitine is an analgesic used for local anesthetic.[54] Corydalis B is a sedative and analgesic.[55] Atropine can relieve the spasms of the smooth muscles and inhibit the secretion of glands.[56] Scopolamine has inhibitory action on the adrenal cortex.[57] Rhynchophylline can lower the blood pressure.[58] Pseudoephedrine is anti-asthmatic.[59] Vinblastine and camptothecine are anti-tumor.[60]

The glycosides yield one or more sugars (glycone) and one or more other compounds (aglycones). The glycosides are usually bitter, colorless, odorless, neutral crystals. The flavonoid glycoside is yellowish in color and the atachine can be red, blue or purple in color.[61] Most of the glycosides are soluble in water or ethyl alcohol. Enzymes usually exist together with the glycosides in the cells. When the glycosides react with the weak acid or enzymes, they are hydrolyzed into glycone and aglycones. The aglycones can reduce the solubility in water and thus the therapeutic effects are reduced. The aglycones can be one of the following compounds, flavonoid, anthraquinone, essential oil, phenol, ketone, steroid, aldehyde, triterpenes and alcohol.[62]

---

[49] Daniel, M. *Medicinal Plants: Chemistry and Properties*. Enfield, NH: Science, 2006; 6.
[50] Ahmad, Iqbal, Farrukh Aqil, and Mohammad Owais. *Modern Phytomedicine: Turning Medical Plants into Drugs.* Weinheim: Wiley-VCH, 2006; 343.
[51] Yeun Him-che. *Handbook of Chinese Herbs: Chinese Materia Media.* Los Angeles: Institute of Chinese Medicine, 1996; 26.
[52] Ibid., 26.
[53] Ibid., 26.
[54] Ibid., 26.
[55] Ibid., 26.
[56] Ibid., 26.
[57] Ibid., 26.
[58] Ibid., 26.
[59] Ibid., 26.
[60] Ibid., 26.
[61] Ibid., 26.
[62] Ibid., 26.

Essential oil is volatile at room temperature and can be easily extracted by distillation. It may form crystals on cooling, such as camphor.[63] Most of them have a fragrant odor, and some have a pungent taste. Essential oil is soluble in ethyl alcohol, fatty oil and other organic solvents. Eugenol and methyleugenol are analgesic, anesthetic, antiseptic, and preservative.[64] Menthol and menthone are analgesic and anti-inflammatory.[65] Camphor is cardiac tonic.[66] Cineole and camphor oil can inhibit the bacterial growth. Houttuynia oil is anti-bacterial and anti-inflammatory.[67] Rutin oil and piperitone are expectorant, and antitussive and anti-·asthmatic.[68] Angelic oil is analgesic. Bupleurum oil is antipyretic.[69] Cardamon oil is a carminative.[70]

Organic acids (not including amino acids) can combine with sodium, potassium and calcium into organic salts; or combine with alkaloids into salts. The organic acids are soluble in ethyl alcohol, acetone, ether, and chloroform. The degree of solubility in water varies. The content of organic acids is higher in the immature fruits.

Citric acid is an anti-coagulant.[71] Benzoic acid is a preservative and expectorant.[72] Salicylic acid is antipyretic and analgesic.[73] Oleanolic acid is diuretic and cardiotonic.[74] Ascorbic acid is hemostatic and can lower blood lipid level[75] Succinic acid is antitussive and anti-asthmatic.

Tannin is a powder of irregular shape, with acrid taste and astringent nature. It is soluble in water, ethyl alcohol and ethyl acetate. It can combine with protein, mucous, alkaloid salt and heavy metallic salt into sediment. It can be oxidized into brownish red sediment on exposure to air or with alkaline solvent. It may turn blue or blue-green with ferric salt. Tannin is divided into condensed tannin and hydrolytic tannin. The condensed tannin cannot be hydrolyzed, but its solvent can react with weak acid on boiling to form tannic red. The hydrolytic tannin can be hydrolyzed by enzyme or weak acid into simple substance. Since tannin is astringent in nature, it is used for burns, bleeding, diarrhea, inflammation, and bacterial infections.[76] It can also be used to neutralize the toxicity produced by alkaloid and heavy metals. The condensed tannin has very little toxic effect on the liver, so its medicinal use is greater than the hydrolytic tannin.

An Amino acid is an organic substance containing nitrogen found widely in the plants. Its molecule contains amino and hydroxy groups. It is a colorless crystal. It is soluble in water and little in organic solvents. The amino acid found in pumpkin seed is used for tapeworm and blood fluke. Asparagine is antitussive and anti-asthmatic.[77]

---

[63] Ibid., 27.
[64] Ibid., 27.
[65] Ibid., 27.
[66] Ibid., 27.
[67] Ibid., 27.
[68] Ibid., 27.
[69] Ibid., 27.
[70] Ibid., 27.
[71] Ibid., 28.
[72] Ibid., 28.
[73] Ibid., 28.
[74] Ibid., 28.
[75] Ibid., 28.
[76] Ibid., 28.
[77] Ibid., 28.

Protein is made up of amino acids. Most protein are soluble in water, only a few are soluble in weak ethyl alcohol. Protein is not stable. Its nature can be changed by coagulation on exposure to heat or ultra violet light. The catalyst enzymes are protein and are found inside the body cells. Amylase helps the digestion of starch. Trichosanthin is used to induce labor at the secondary stage of pregnancy. Concanavalin is effective against cancer.[78]

Sugars are divided into simple, oligosaccharide and polysaccharide. The simple sugars are soluble in ethyl alcohol, e.g. glucose, fructose and rhamnose. The oligosaccharide are not soluble in ethyl alcohol, (e.g. saccharose, maltose, stachyose). The polysaccharide are gum, starch, inulin, mucous, pectin, lignin, and cellulose. Starch is not soluble in cold water or organic solvent; but if boiled in water, it becomes a sticky paste. Inulin is soluble in water, but not in organic solvent. Gum, mucous and pectin are the mucin component in plant and they form a smooth mucous solution in water. Lignin and cellulose are not soluble in water nor organic solvent. The percentage of sugars in the plant may be up to 50 -80% in weight. Polysaccharide can be used for medicinal preparation. b-Pachyman from poria, glucan from polyporus and the sugars from mushroom and bamboos can inhibit cancer cells.[79] Laminarin is used for atherosclerosis.[80]

A Lipid is a combination of fatty acid and glycerol. Vegetable oil is the liquid form of lipid at room temperature. Fat is the solid or semi solid form of lipid at room temperature. The suberin and corneal layers of a plant are also lipoid substances, and have no medicinal use. Wax is a solid form of lipid at room temperature, found on the surface layer of a plant. Fatty oils are yellow in color and usually have special odor. They are soluble in ether, chloroform and other essential oil. They can be hydrolyzed by lipase, and can be oxidized easily. About 50% of lipid is found in the seeds.[81] They are used as emollients. Some are stimulatory purgatives, such as castor oil, croton oil, almond oil, sesame seed oil, hemp seed oil.[82] Coix seed oil can be used to fight against cancer cells.[83] Chaulmoogra oil is used for leprosy.[84] Brucea oil is used for vegetation.[85] Wax and lipid can also be used as materials for ointment, paste, suppository, or for injection oil.

Resin is a metabolite of the plant and exists together with gum, organic acids and essential oil. Resin exist in a soft solid form that is flexible in shape. It becomes very soft on heating and then liquify. It is not soluble in water, but soluble in ethyl alcohol and other organic solvents. If the resin of the plant is mixed with gum, it is called gum resin. If the resin is mixed with essential oil, it is called oleoresin (e.g. turpentine). If the resin is mixed with both gum and essential oil, it is called oleoresin gum (e.g. myrrh, asafoetida). [86]

The inorganic components of plants are potassium, calcium, magnesium and iodine. They are usually combined with other organic substances. They can be found as crystals of different shapes, such as calcium oxalate crystals in rhubarb. They are usually soluble in water and not in organic solvents.

---

[78] Ibid., 29.
[79] Ibid., 29.
[80] Ibid., 29.
[81] Ibid., 28.
[82] Ibid., 28.
[83] Ibid., 28.
[84] Ibid., 28.
[85] Ibid., 29.
[86] Ibid., 30.

The pigments found in plants include the chlorophylls, Carotenoids, flavonoids and betalains.[87] The terpenoids include the quad terpene (e.g. carotene) and diterpene (e.g. crocetin). The anthraquinone is usually yellow or orange crystals and is generally purgative in action (e.g. rhein and emodin). The chlorophyll and terpenoids are soluble in ethyl alcohol and ethyl acetate, but not in water.

1. Chlorophylls: The chlorophylls are oil-soluble. Chlorophyll is a pigment in green plants for the transfer of light energy to a chemistry receptor. The light that is absorbed provides the energy for photosynthesis. A green leaf absorbs blue light (430 nm) and red light (660 nm). The soluble salts or the fresh leaves rich in chlorophyll can be applied externally for inflammation and granulation.

2. Carotenoids: Like the chlorophylls, the carotenoids are not water soluble. They absorb violet and blue light between 400 and 500 nm; and they reflect red, orange, yellow, brown and the green avocado fruit color. They give color to carrot roots, tomato fruit and many other yellow flowers. Carotenoids are revealed in autumn leaves after the chlorophyll has disappeared. B-carotene is the most important of carotenes.[88]

3. Flavinoids: These water-soluble pigments accumulate in cell vacuoles. They absorb ultraviolet wavelengths of light. Anthocyanin are found in most fruits and flowers.[89] These red, purple, and blue reflecting pigments are seen in apples, fuchsia flower and geranium flower. Flavins appear as yellow or ivory colored flowers. Some flavin, such as riboflavin (vitamin B2), act as co-factors in enzyme reactions, in the bending of plants toward light (phototropic response).[90]

4. Betalains: These pigments are water soluble, and found in the vacuoles of cells. Betacyanin appears as blue-violet to red and is found in beet roots and red cactus flowers. Betaxanthin pigments reflect yellow, orange and orange-red.[91]

ORGANIZATION OF CHAPTERS

For each medicinal plant profiled in *Leaves of Life, Volume1: Single Herbs,* the following information is provided.

Nomenclature:

The naming convention used in this book is that of the Guyana Creole, local/folk names followed by the pharmaceutical, botanical and/or other known names. It is difficult to identify most of the selected plants, solely on the basis of their local/folk common names because the names sometimes vary from region to region. Sometimes different local names were used for the same plant located in different regions in Guyana. In order to meet this challenge in nomenclature, not only were the scientific names (Plant Family) necessary, but photographs are also included in the plant profiles. The most commonly used vernacular names are given in several languages, together with well known botanical synonyms.

[87] Ibid., 30.
[88] Ibid., 30.
[89] Ibid., 30.
[90] Ibid., 30.
[91] Ibid., 30.

Region Where Grown:

Plant locations are based on collections made in Guyana by the Smithsonian's Biological Diversity of the Guianas Program.[92] Plant identifications do not reflect a complete inventory of Guyana's regions, as sampling has been focused on the country's interior.

I. Barima/Waini
II. Pomeroon/Supenaam
III. Essequibo/West Demerara
IV. Demerara/Mahaica
V. Mahaica/Berbice
VI. E. Berbice/Corentyne
VII. Cuyuni/Mazaruni
VIII. Potaro/Siparuni
IX. Takutu/Upper Essequibo
X. Upper Demerara/Berbice

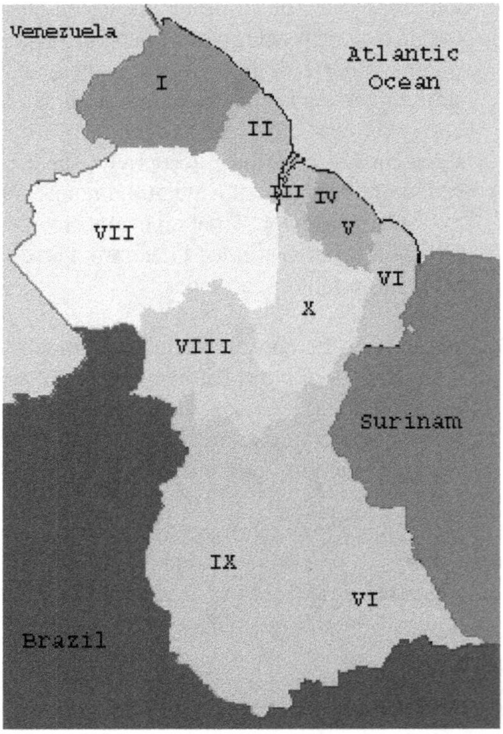

Category:

The category corresponds to the chapter titles in chronological order.

1. Chapter 1 Diaphoretics (Producing Perspiration): Febrifungal/Anti-viral

Diaphoretic plants are used for relieving infections in the upper respiratory tract and acute infectious diseases by causing an increase of perspiration by stimulation of the sweat glands. There are changes in the contraction and dilation of the blood vessels in the brain and mucous membrane of the skin and respiratory tract. Plants such as *Elephant Foot, Lemon Grass, Morompo* and *Ginger* can adjust the blood flow to the brain and mucosa of the respiratory tract through the process of perspiration. Other plants such as *Soldier's Rod* can dilate the periphereal capillaries and increase the blood circulation in the skin. Symptoms include fever, headache and aversion to cold. Most of the plants of this group are anti-bacterial in nature.

2. Chapter 2 Purgatives/Carthatics (Purging the Bowels)

These plants stimulate the bowel by inducing increased peristalsis and bowel movement. Some plants such as *Buttercup* and *Ziba Grass* contain anthracene glycosides and polyhydroxyanthroquinones from bacterial action in the large bowel. *Buttercup* and *Senna* contain rhein, emodin and aloe-emodin. They can inhibit the growth of streptococcus and shigella. Some plants contain sodium sulfate considered to be a saline cathartics. Because mirabilitum contains sodium it is advisable for patients with edema.

Others plants such as *Stinging Nettle* can stimulate the peristalsis of the intestines. The *Castor oil* plant contains croton oil. The croton oil contains "croton resin" which is reputed to be the most potent carthartic.

---

[92] Kelloff C. L. and V. A. Funk. *Preliminary Checklist of the Plants of the Kaiteur National Park, Guyana.* Washington, DC: Smithsonian Institute, 1997; 1.

It can increase the peristalsis action of the intestine and the reabsorption of the small intestine. It's action is very drastic with diarrhea, tenesmus and abdominal cramps.

3. Chapter 3 Antipyretics or Febrifugals (Prevent/Reduce Fever)

The plants in this category are usually cold or cool in nature. They are used to alleviate heat symptoms such as blood shot eyes, bleeding, constipation, amber urine, delirium, mania, abscess, inflammation. The antipyretic plants such as *Wild Coffee* can lower the body temperature while the anti-hypertensive plants can lower the blood pressure. The sedative plants also have sedative action. The Antipyretics are divided into the following major groups: (a) plants that can eliminate heat and fire, (b) plants that can eliminate heat by cooling the blood, (c) plants that can eliminate heat and toxin, and (d) plants that eliminate heat, dampness and moisture.

4. Chapter 4 Antitussive Plants (Cough Suppresant)

Cough may be nonproductive or productive of sputum. Suppression of the cough or periodic drainage of the sputum is necessary. Expectorants are agents which facilitate coughing in productive cough by thinning the sputum. Some of the plants such as *Eucalyptus* and *Camphor* have expectorant properties. Other plants such *as Physic Nut* and *Boyari* can increase the secretion in the respiratory tract. Plants such as *Daisy* and *Okra* can dilate the bronchial smooth muscles and relieve the tracheal spasms caused by pilocarpine, acetylcholine and histamine.

The antitussives are divided into four major groups; (a) Eliminate cold phlegm with plants that are warm in nature, (b) eliminate heat phlegm with cleansing plants, (c) Antitussive and anti-asthmatic, (d) plants that relieve cough by moistening effect.

5. Chapter 5 The Digestive

The digestive plants can increase the digestion of fat, protein and carbohydrates. Some plants such as *Tamarind* contain lipase and protease. Other plants in this category such as *Bush Rope Bowrialli* and *Sapodilla* can enhance the appetitie by increasing the secretion of gastric acid, digestion and evacuation. Also, some of these plants contain vitamins B and C which assist in regulating the appetite and digestion.

6. Chapter 6 Warming Plants

This group of plants, such as *Fennel,* are used for interior cold syndromes. One condition is caused by pathogenic cold acting on the spleen and stomach, leading to vomiting and diarrhea. The other kind of condition for plants such as *Bay Leaf, Teasam* and *Shiny Bush* is the interior depletion of yang energy, leading to lowered body temperature and cold extremities. The action on the digestive tract are usually stomachic with pungent and spicy essential oils. They can increase the microcirculation and the excretion of gastric acid and protease. Thus they can evacuate gas and relax the intestinal muscles. The action on the cardiovascular system is that of depletion of yang (vital energy) condition such as in the case of shock. Some cardiotonic plants such as *Black Maho* and *Ink Plant* can increase the blood pressure.

7. Chapter 7 The (Energy) Tonics

Chronic patients are usually very weak and depleted. Usually the depletion is caused by asthenia of vital energy, blood, vital essence and vital function. Depletion of these four essence in different organs will reflect different symptoms.

Tonic plants have specific action on the immunity of the body. On nonspecific cellular immunity, they increase the production of T-lymphocytes, prevent the loss of white blood cells caused by cyclophosphamide which is the anti tumor agent. Tonic plants can also increase the phagocytic ability of white blood cells through the reticulo-enthdothelial system and the production of interferon.

On specific humoral immunity they increase the rate of formation of the E-rosette, increase the B-lymphocytes and increase the concentration of the Immunoglobulins of IgG and IgM.

They also increase the adaptability of the body. The tonics can control the activity of the adrenalin, the sudden decrease of blood pressure and excessive gastric bleeding. They have action of the endocrine and the nervous system. The tonics can enhance the action of the adrenal cortex and prevent the degeneration of the thyroid pituitary, adrenal cortex, testis and uterus. This group of plants such as *Sorrel* also have action on Metabolism. The tonics can regulate the metabolism, cholesterol, white blood cells and red blood cells.

The tonic plants can increase the productivity of the body at work. The plants such as *Wild Star Apple*, *Matchood* and *Stinking Toe* can reduce stress and fatigue and improve memory and mentality.

Finally, the tonic plants are divided into the following categories: First, plants such as *Passion Flower* act on the central nervous system (CNS) and sympathetic nervous system. They can increase the cyclic adenosine monophosphate (cAMP) and energy metabolic rate. They can so stimulate cellular bioelectricity. Second, they increase the specific and non-specific immunity of the body by increasing the phagocytosis of the cells. Third, they increase the adaptability and increase the resistance to the invasion of foreign bodies. Fourth, they increase the physical ability and the thinking capability of the brain. Fifth, they regulate the function of the endocrine, increase the function of the sex hormones and the adrenal cortical hormones.

There are a group of plants that can increase the production of peripherial white blood cells and red blood cells. There is a regeneration of the blood cells and the maturation of the reticulocyte. It is believed that the production of vital energy (Qi) can influence the production of blood. The tonics are divided into four groups: vital energy, blood, vital essence and vital function

8. Chapter 8 The Carminatives (Prevents Gas and Bloating in the intestinal Tract)

The stagnation of energy (Qi) flow means the abnormal function of the smooth muscles of the blood vessels, the intestines and the skeletal muscles. Any stagnation of the flow of energy (Qi) in the body/organs/channels will lead to local pain, distention or oppression. The regulatory action on the digestive tract is both excitatory and inhibitory on the smooth muscles of the intestines.

Inhibitory action on the alimentary tract reduce the tension of the intestinal tubules. Plants such *as Cacao* are used for regurgitation, hiccough, diarrhea, abdominal pain and other hyperactive symptoms.

The excitatory action on the alimentary tract can enhance the contraction of the GI-Tubules. Such plants as *Nutmeg* are used for indigestion, abdominal distention, constipation and other hypo-active symptoms. They can also increase the secretion of gastric juice.

Carminatives such as *Anise* have certain kinds of essential oils which can stimulate the local sites, increase the peristalsis of the intestines and the bowel movements, evacuate gas and relieve the distention caused by overeating. Plants such as *Mangrove* helps with the relaxation of the smooth muscles of the bronchi and blood vessels relieving tension of the respiratory skeletal muscles. Accumulation of dampness in the spleen and stomach is related to hypo-function of the digestive tract with symptoms of indigestion, loss of appetite and abdominal distention. *Celery and Prickly Pear* with its aromatic nature contain essential oils which stimulate the movement of the bowels, evacuate the food content and eliminate cellular edema in the gastro intestinal tract.

9. Chapter 9 Blood Stasis - Cholagogue (Stimulates, Cleanses the Liver and Gall Bladder and Increase Bile Flow)

This category of plants can increase the secretion of bile. *Bully Tree* and *Negro-Broom* can regulate the smooth muscles of the liver, bile duct, breast, uterus and the digestive tract. They can also increase the hepatic blood flow to the liver.

Plants for Coagulation and Blood Regulation - Blood stasis is generally caused by bleeding, stagnation of energy flow, low energy, pathogenic heat or cold factors and external trauma. Any blockage in circulation (especially microcirculation) causing inflammation, abnormal growth, fibroid, metabolic or autoimmune disorders can be relieved by eliminating blood stasis.

The plants in this category are divided into two groups (a) inflammatory plants used for angina, atherosclerosis and rheumatoid arthritis and (b) hemostatic plants which can shorten the process of coagulation by increasing the number of platelets and throbin. They can also shorten the bleeding time and construct the local blood vessels. *Black Sage, White Clary, Bloodwood* and *Lionbush* regulate the metabolism of the cardiac muscles, reduce the oxygen consumption, reduce heart beat, prevent ischema condition, dilate the coronary artery and increase the blood flow in the artery and cardiac muscle.

Manicole, Zeb Grass and *Jamoon* can even lower blood pressure by dilating the blood flow to the peripherial blood vessels in the brain and kidney. These plants can also inhibit the agglutination of the platelets, increase the activity of plasmin (fibrinolysin) reduce fibrin stabilizing factors, prevent the formation of thrombus and enhance thrombolysis.They can also Lower blood cholesterol and prevent the formation of altherosclerosis.

10. Chapter 10 Diuretic (Increase the Flow of Urine)

Diuretics are agents which increase the rate of urine flow by their action on the kidneys. There can be increased glomerular filtration or decreased tubular reabsorption. The most effective diuretics influence the excretion of sodium ion rather than the water itself. Diuretics contain increased potassium ion and can increase the excretion of sodium ion or the output of urine. Some plants have antibacterial properties and can also inhibit the growth of bacilli in urinary tract infections.

11. Chapter 11 Anti Inflamitory - Anti Rheumatic Plants

The anti rheumatics include rheumatic arthritis, rheumatoid arthritis, sciatica and all kinds of muscular pain. They are caused by wind, cold and dampness conditions. This group of plants can alleviate pain, increase qi and blood circulation and strengthen the tendons. Another group of plants in this category is the anti inflammatory. They have similar analgesic and antipyretic action as sodium salicylate. *Tulsie* and *Coconut* have some has excitory action on the hypophysis-adrenal gland system. Analgesics such as *Garlic Rope* and *Asashi* can increase the pain threshold in the body. They have sedative action and can relax skeletal muscles. Another group of anti rheumatics is the diuretics such as *Pain-Killer* which can dilate the blood vessels and lower blood pressure.

12. Chapter 12 Sedative Plants

Sedatives are agents used to calm or induce sleeping status. Sleep is a state of rest and repair. Tranquilizers imply mental calmness with depression of mental activity or alertness. Heavy sedatives are the heavy minerals or shells such as *Oyster Shell* and *Cinnabar* that affect the central nervous system (CNS). *Goal-Pimpler* can prolong the sleeping time. Another group of plants in the sedative category is the herbal nourishing sedatives such as *Sour-Sop, Sweet Broom and Blue Vine* which contain protein vitamins and glucosides. They are nourishing to the heart and replenish nouishing fluids in the body. They can improve the integrity, mental spirit and thinking processes of the brain. They can also lower the blood pressure and can be hypnotic and anti convulsive.

13. CHAPTER 13 The Astrigents

Astringent is the category of plants that tend to shrink or constrict fibers, tissues and stops body discharges. The word "astringent" derives from Latin *"adstringere"*, meaning to bind fast. Herbs contracting fibers or tissues and check discharges. Common examples *Pomegranate, Fat Pork, Buri, Worm-Bush, Ant-Bush* and *Bitter Gumma* which contain tannin, organic acids and inorganic salts.

Anti Convulsant Plants

Anticonvulsant, sometimes called antiepileptic (AED) or antiseizure are a diverse group of plants used in the treatment of epileptic seizures. Anticonvulsants are also used in the treatment of bipolar disorder as mood stablizers and in the treatment of neuropathic pain. The goal of anticonvulsants is to suppress the rapid and excessive firing of neurons that start a seizure and offer protection against possible excitotoxic effects that may result in brain damage. Convulsive non epileptic seizures are quite common and will not response to plants that target epileptic reactions. In epilepsy, EEG charts confirm an area of the cortex is typically hyperirritable. Antiepileptic plants help to reduce this area of irritability and thus prevent epileptiform seizures. *Ant's Bush* treats major convulsive seizures (grand mal) or momentary pauses of consciousness (petit mal). These convulsive seizures are related to the imbalance of liver energy, endogenous wind and phlegm with symptoms of spasm, dizziness and convulsions.

Antihelmintics (Expel or Destroy Worms)

The antihelmintic are plants with properties that expel or destroy tapeworms, roundworms, flukeworms and many other parasites in the intestinal tract.

Properties:

This section includes information about two major aspects of the medicinal substances. One is the temperature characteristics. There are five major designations used to describe the temperaments of the plant.

a. Cold
b.Moist/Cool
c. Hot
d. Dry/Warm

The other primary property of the plant is taste. The five tastes are:

1. Acrid/Pungent - The action of the acrid herbs are diaphoretic, nourishing, increasing the circulation of blood and vital energy. The acrid herbs act on the lung meridian.
2. Sweet - The tonic and soothing herbs are generally sweet. They can alleviate pain and spasms. The sweet herbs act on the spleen meridian.
3. Sour - The sour herbs are astringents. They can be used for diarrhea, spermatorrhea and excessive perspiration. The sour herbs act on the liver meridian.
4. Bitter - They have purging and moisture drying action. They are used for asthma, constipation, retention of dampness due to Heat or Cold. They act on the heart meridian.
5. Salt - They are purging and can soften the hard lumps in the body. The salty herbs act on the kidney meridian.

Substances that do not have any of these tastes are said to be bland. Bland substances are diuretics used for edema and dysuria. Substances may also be described as aromatic which describes the ability to penetrate through turbidity and awaken a given function, either the digestive function of the spleen or the cognitive functions of the spirit and orifices.

Another taste attribute to certain plants is astringent. This refers not only to the taste of the substance but also to its ability to prevent the leakage of body fluids. The taste of a medicinal substance partly determines its therapeutic function. Acrid substances disperse and move; sweet substances tonify, harmonize and sometimes moisten; bitter substances drain and dry; salty substances purge and soften; and bland substances leech out dampness and promote urination.

Esoteric Botanica:

In traditional Africa where approximately 80% of the population receive their health care from practitioners of herbal medicine, the healing spirits of the herbs are used to heal physically, mentally and spiritually. Underlying the practice of traditional herbal medicine is the view that disease is the manifestation of malevolent spirits which must be addressed by incantation and rituals in addition to herbal prescription.

Modern day Traditional Chinese Medicine (TCM) has its roots in shamanistic medicine. Aromatic herbs as *Rou Gui*, *Wu zhu Yu* and *Ai Ye* are considered to have magical powers that affect a person's spirit.[93] In the Amazon, the Ayahuasquero divines medical, social and/or spiritual ceremonies for the sick.[94] In Columbia, South America, among the Guahibo Indians, the Curandero treats the 'spiritual side of the (presenting health) condition.[95] The Australian Aboriginal medical system "evolved and depended on spiritual beliefs and the development of herbal medicine."[96]

From the Kallawayan herbalist in the Argentinan Andes, the Obeah healer in Jamaica and Guyana, the Condemble, Santero and Palo spiritualist in Brazil, Mexico and Puerto Rico to the Voodum healer in Haiti, there is one underlying theme. Traditional herbal medicine is the practice of holistic medicine where the spiritual as well as the physical and metal needs are addressed.

---

[93] Bensky, Dan, Andrew Gamble, and Ted Kaptchuk. *Chinese Herbal Medicine: Materia Media.* Washington: Eastland Press, 1993; 4.
[94] Duke, James A., and Rodolfo Vásquez. *Amazonian Ethnobotanical Dictionary*. Boca Raton, FL: CRC, 1994; 7.
[95] Chadwick, Derek J., and Joan Mash. *Bioactive Compounds from Plants: A Wiley-Interscience Publication.* Chichester [etc.: John Wiley & Sons, 1990; 35.
[96] Steiner, Richard P. *Folk Medicine: The Art and the Science*. Washington, D.C.: American Chemical Society, 1986;104.

The spiritual energy of the plants are as follows:[97]

- Amen corresponds to nothingness, the concealed, the original state of peace which is the essential nature of the Supreme Being as well as the essence of Man's being.
- Ausar is the indwelling intelligence guiding all of the functions of the spirit and represents the inner drive felt universally by all to unite.
- Tehuti represents the inner drive to acquire the knowledge needed for success in all undertakings.
- Seker is the divine faculty that is in charge of the life-force which is the formative base of all things in the world.
- Maat corresponds to immutable laws, and the urge to live the truth of the immutable laws of Maat.
- Herukhuti is the divine principle that safeguards one's existence from the injustices of others.
- Heru corresponds to the will or the freedom to follow or reject divine law or emotions.
- Het-Heru corresponds to visual thinking or the imagination.
- Sebek corresponds to thoughts and verbal expression.
- Auset corresponds to devotion, the ability to care for and nurture others, and sacrifice.
- Geb corresponds to the laws governing physical health, i.e.: nutrition, exercise, sleep, breath, wealth, etc.

Governing Organ Systems:

The other means of grouping information is to identify which channels the plant enters. There are five pairs of organ systems and their respective channels:

1. Kidney and Urinary Bladder: Kidney Yin is "the waters of life" and supplies the hormones, blood, and ideas (memories) that support all of life's activities. Kidney Jing corresponds to the hormones, which are the foundation of brain, mental development, emotional and spiritual growth. Kidney yang is the "fire that drives all the vital warmth that makes social activities possible."[98] The kidney yang is the ability "to carry out the power of the will , the power to persevere, ambition's drive, the power to work hard and long, courage , the ability to take risks, sexual vitality (erectile strength and the ability to delay orgasm in men, orgasmic ability in women), good libido, emotional stability and longecity.[99]
2. Liver and Gall Bladder: The ability to relax and to supercharge the imaginative function is governed by the liver/gall bladder energy system. One of its main functions is to provide blood to the ligaments and tendons throughout the body, especially of the upper back, shoulders and neck. Unlike the kidney yang which is the general strength for all of life's activities, the liver yang governs activities directed to a specific end. For this to take place, the blood (liver yin) and motive power (liver yang) must move freely through the body. The free movement of blood and Qi depends on the relaxed state of the body, which in turn depends on the proper nourishment of the tendons and ligaments, which is under the auspices of the liver system. Undertakings require planning which is carried out through the imagination.[100]
3. Heart and Small Intestine: The energy function of the heart system is to provide psychic heat – not heat to drive to drive the functions of the kidney yang, but to provide the warmth for intimacy and social interaction, passion and zest for life and the ability to experience pleasure and joy. Most importantly, it provides the heat that supports man's waking consciousness. The Heart governs the fire/warmth that

[97] See Amen, Ra Un Nefer. *Maat: The 11 Laws of God.* Brooklyn, NY: Khamit Media Trans Visions, 2003.
[98] Amen, Ra Un Nefer. *Qi Gong Success: Prescriptions for Health, Wealth and Happiness.* New York City: Khamit Media Trans Vision, Inc. 2009; 32.
[99] Ibid., 32, 33.
[100] Ibid., 40.

extroverts consciousness. This is the foundation of being observant, sociable (warm), and the source and capacity for enjoyment (Joy is the counterpart of peace in the definition of happiness).[101]

4. Lungs and Large Intestine: Lungs govern our ability to cement bonds (relationships, habits), to set up defensive barriers and structures for self and self-interest protection. It corresponds therefore to the skin, immune system, psychic protection and bonding (aura function), rules, morality, organized information based on experience to safe guard (protect) the success of an undertaking.
5. Spleen and Stomach: The energy of the Spleen/Stomach system directs the functions of digestion, assimilation and incorporation of nutrients into the body, which are mirrored by the reasoning functions of the mind. The Spleen/Stomach governs reasoning (mental catabolism and anabolism), which is the foundation for the formation of convictions—beliefs or truths (according to the premises). Reasoning is the means of centering a person, as it keeps one from acting out of fantasy, if the premise of the reasoning process is based on truth.[102]

These organ channels control the function of their associated organs and their functions extend to the physiological, emotional and mental spheres. The five organ system also serves as a means of organizing information regarding all aspects of man's being – physical, mental, emotional and spiritual. With an understanding of the governing organ systems, one can diagnose problems, set therapeutic treatment and monitor progress for all aspects of life.[103]

Actions and Indications:

The actions and indications refer to the therapeutic functions or actions of the plant and the clinically corresponding symptoms. The concept of a linkage between plants and particular actions or functions refers to a relationship between the tastes and the organs. Sour enters the liver, acridity the lungs, bitterness the heart, salt the kidneys and sweet the spleen.

Cautions and Contraindications:

Traditionally the plants are in general very safe and easy to use. Aside from questions of toxicity, there are a few major types of contraindications or prohibitions in using plants. Contraindications during pregnancy indicates certain plants are absolutely prohibited because they are considered toxic or extremely harsh substances.They are prohibited combinations, prohibitions during pregnancy and dietary prohibitions. Prohibited combinations are certain combinations that should be avoided because they either reduce each other's effectiveness or lead to toxicity or undesirable side effects.

Major Known Ingredients:

This refers to the degree of attention that each plant has received with the limited resources available and should not be construed to mean that a particular plant necessarily has fewer constituents than another upon which research has focused. While in general the most commonly used plants have been studied more than the less commonly used ones, some quite common plants have basically very little recorded research. Sometimes there are specific chemicals that are believed to be a major reason for the plants's action while in other cases the only known ingredients are primarily of general interest.

---

[101] Ibid., 51.
[102] Ibid., 71.
[103] Ibid., 19.

Pharmacological and Clinical Research:

Attemps have been made to understand the actions and properties of these plants through scientific research. Most of the biomedical research into effects and uses of these plants have proceeded along the lines of attempting to isolate their active ingredients and to understand their effects on body tissues.

Toxicity:

This heading details the toxic effects of the substances, usually in doses far in excess of those used clinically. The toxic effects of the substance include symptomatic side effects as well as adverse effects on tissues. One commonly used dose that will kill fifty percent of the experimental animals is referred to as LD_{50}. This test, especially when compared to the recommended values for the therapeutic dose, gives an idea of how toxic the substance is and how careful one must be in using it.

Chapter 1: Diaphoretics

Plants that Increase Perspiration

The medicinal plants discussed in this chapter arc herbal diaphoretics. Diaphoretics are herbs that increase mild perspiration. Sudorifics are herbs that cause severe sweating. When environmental pathogenic influences such as wind, cold and heat attack the immune system a conflict ensues between the person's natural energy system and the pathogen. The immune system realtiates against this attack with symptoms such as chills, muscle aches, headache, stiff neck, general aches, stuffy nose, sinus disorders, sorethroat and fever. This symptom pattern is typically found at the onset of colds, influenza, laryngitis and other acute upper respiratory infections.

Diaphoretic plants are used for relieving the infections in the upper respiratory tract and acute infectious diseases. Most of the diaphoretics are febrifungal/anti-viral. Some plants can induce perspiration and adjust the body temperature. Other plants can adjust the blood flow to the brain and mucosa of the respiratory tract through the process of perspiration while still others can dilate the periphereal capillaries and increase the blood circulation in the skin. The primary function of diaphoretic herbs is to dispel the pathogenic energies of wind, cold and heat. Commonly used western herbs as *sage leaves, elder flowers, lemon balm, wild clover, blessed thistle, yarrow, hyssup bee balm, mint blossoms, burdock root, ragweed and german chamomile* perform similar functions. In Chinese medicine, these are equivalent to such commonly prescribed herbs are *ephedra and cinnamon twig, Jing Jie, xi xin and magnolia flower.* Diaphoretics herbs are penetrating and dispersing by nature and possess a pungent, spicy taste and a dry, warm nature. They are divided into two categories; warming and cooling herbs.

Diaphoretics Plants with Pungent and Warm Nature

Remedies in this category are used for infectious external conditions with acute onset. These conditions are characterized by sensations of chilliness, little or no sweating and fever, aches and pains (especially in the muscles) and a stiff neck. The main function of warm-pungent herbs is to dispel wind and cold when accompanied by chills, fever, absence of sweating and headache. These herbs treat cough, asthma, edema, and pain caused by invasion of wind-damp. Herbs such as *elephant foot, lemon grass, morompo and ginger* have warming properties and induce perspiration

Elephant Foot

Diaphoretics Plants with Pungent and Warm Nature

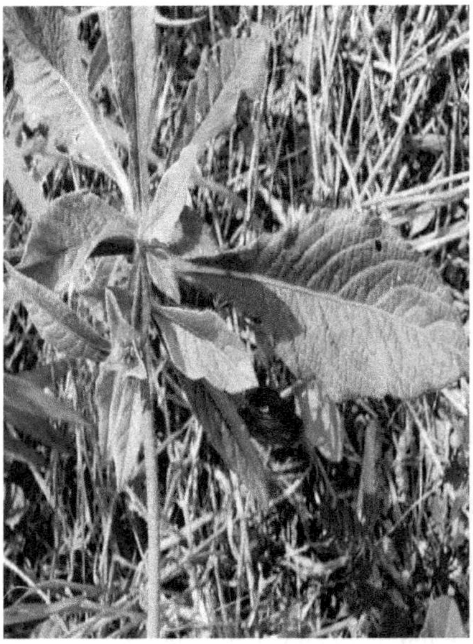

Botanical Name: Elephantopus Mollis.
Family: Asteraceae .
Region Where Grown: Essequibo/West Demerara.
Other Known Names: Ground-itch Bush.
Category: Diaphoretic.
Properties: Acrid, Hot/Moist.
Esoteric Botanica: Maat.
Governing Organs: Liver.
Actions & Indications: Leaf: Used as a tonic or a diaphoretic, or macerated between the hands and the juice then applied externally to relieve itching, especially due to athlete's foot.[104] Its action is on the liver system where there is an accumulation of proteid, and other waste in the blood; liver derangements;. Also invigorates the kidney yang to treat backache, and lumbago, diarrhea and dysentery, and arthritic conditions[105]
Cautions & Contraindications: Use with caution during pregnancy or excessive menstruation..
Major Known Ingredients: Contains the sesquiterpene lactone, deoxyelephantopin, which is an anti-tumor chemical. Extracts of the whole plant significantly inhibit the Walker-256 carcinosarcoma in rats.
Pharmacological & Clinical Research:
Two cytotoxic germacranolides named molephantin and phantomolin and a sesquiterpene lactone named molephantinin were isolated from Elephantopus mollis (E. tomentosus). Molephantinin showed significant inhibitory activity against Walker 256 carcinosarcoma in rats at 2.5 rug/kg, T/C=397%.[106] Elephantopin shows considerable activity against P-388 lymphocyt.ic leukemia (ps) with a *TIC* of 171% at 40 mg/kg and has been selected for further tumor panel evaluation by the National Cancer Institute (NCI). Deoxyelephantopin and molephantinin, isolated from *ElephnntopuB seaber, Elephantopus carolininw/ts,* and *Elephantopus mollis,* have also been shown to be active against. Walker·256 carcinosarcoma in rats with *TIC* values of 226% and 397%, respectively, at the 2.5 mg/kg level.[107]

---

[104] DeFilipps, Robert A., Shirley L. Maina and Juliette Crepin. *Medicinal Plants of the Guianas (Guyana, Surinam, French Guiana)*. Washington D.C.: Dept. of Botany, National Museaum of Natural History, Smithsonian Institute, 2004; 44.
[105] Morton F. Julia. *Atlas of Medical Plants of Middle America: Bahamas to Yucatan.* Springfield, Illinois: Charles C. Thomas Publisher,1981; 1262.
[106] Steiner Richard P., Editor. *Folk Medicine: The Art and The Science.* Washington: American Chemical Society, 1985; 156.
[107] Ibid., 156.

Lemon Grass

Diaphoretics Plants with Pungent and Warm Nature

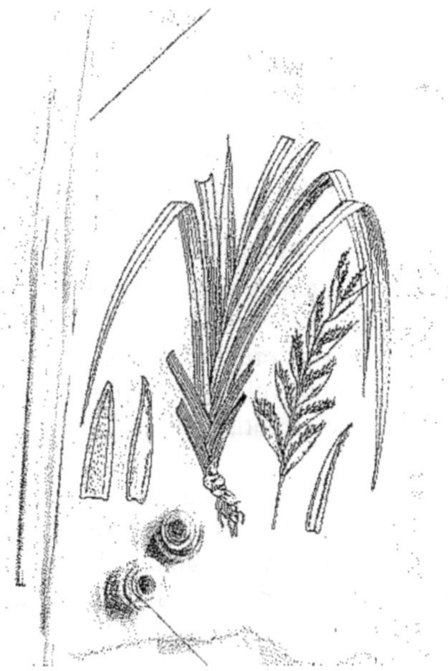

Botanical Name: Cymbopogon Citratus.
Family: Poaceae.
Region Where Grown: Barima-Waini Region.
Other Known Names: Fever grass, Citronella grass, Hierba Luisa.
Category: Diaphoretic.
Properties: Acrid, Cold/Moist.
Esoteric Botanica: Het heru.
Governing Organs: Kidney, Lungs.
Actions & Indications: Whole plant: Used to retard perspiration; ingredient in a herbal bath as a caminative, diaphoretic, depurative and expectorant.[108].
Leaf: Decoction for coughs, colds, fever, sore throat and grippe. Leaves are also used as a digestive aid (AED) to treat stomachaches (SAR)[109] and urinary tract infections. Used for coughs and colds, fevers, malaria and venereal disease and high blood pressure[110]. Dry leaves are boiled and the water drunk as beverage and tonic, an anti-asthmatic, as an anti-pyretic, as an anti-viral and as a treatment for bronchitis, for colds, for coughing, influenza and for tuberculosis. A tea is made, with alcoholic spirits or sweet spirits of nitre, to treat colds; infusion to treat diarrhoea spasms, as a stimulant and antispasmodic; infusion is sudorific and an excellent digestive.[111] Root is used as a contraceptive (VDF) and abortifacient[112] Leaves used to flavor other teas. Lemon grass is also the source of commercial aromatic flavor, fragrance and perfumery[113]
Cautions & Contraindications: Do not use in cases of qi deficiency with profuse sweating, headache due to blood deficiency, or cough due to yin deficiency.
Major Known Ingredients: Lemon grass oil has antispasmodic and antiseptic properties, and is commercially valuable in the perfume industry. From the leaves, its oil is rich in citral, and other terpenes, such as myrcene. Due to its easy polymerization, Myrcene is responsible for the early deterioration of the oil. Pure citral is isolated from the oil and used as a key raw material in the manufacture of Vitamin A.

---

[108] Ross, Ivan A. *Medicinal Plants of the World: Chemical Constituents, Traditional and Modern Medicinal Uses.* Totowa, NJ: Humana, 1999; 120.
[109] Castner, James L., S. Lee. Timme, and James A. Duke. *A Field Guide to Medicinal and Useful Plants of the Upper Amazon*. Gainesville, FL: Feline, 1998; 48.
[110] Ross, Ivan A. *Medicinal Plants of the World: Chemical Constituents, Traditional and Modern Medicinal Uses.* Totowa, NJ: Humana, 1999;119, 120.
[111] Ibid., 120.
[112] Morton F. Julia. *Atlas of Medical Plants of Middle America: Bahamas to Yucatan.* Springfield, Illinois: Charles C. Thomas Publisher, 1981; 1259.
[113] Balandrin, M.F and Klocke, J.A. "Medicinal, Aromatic, and Industrial Materials from Plants, Biotechnology" In Y.P.S. Bajaj (ed.), *Biotechnology in Agriculture and Forestry 4. Medicinal and Aromatic Plant 1.* Berlin: Springer-Verlag, 1988; 14.

Here is a list of other chemical constituents: {+)-limonene, PI, 2 '-O-Rhamnosyl orientin, Lf, 1 A-Cineole, Lf, Alpha citral, PI,Alpha oxobisabolene, PI, Alpha pinene, Lf 1,3%, Benzyl alcohol, PI, Beta myrcene, EO, Beta pinene, Lf EO 1.5%, Beta sitosterol, PI, Beta erpinene, Lf, Beta -(+)-cadinene, PI, Borneol, PI, Camphene, EO 0.90%, Camphor, EO 0.2%, Car-3-ene, EO 0.1 %, Cellulose, PI, Cineal, EO, Citral-B, Lf, Citronella I, EO, Citronellol acetate, Lf 1.3%, Citronellol, EO, Cymbopogenol, Lf, Cymbopogone, Lf, Cymbopogonol, Lf, Cymbopol, Lf, Cynaroside, Lf, D-camphor, PI D-citrone!lic acid, Lf, D-iimonene, EO 5.0%, D-menthone, PI, Dipentene, Lf, Essential oil, PI, Eugenol, Lf
farnesol, Lf EO 2.4%, fenchone, EO 0.3%, furfural, Lf, Geranial, Lf EO 44.9%, Geraniol acetate, Lf EO 9.9% Geraniol, EO, Hept-5-en-2-one,6-methyl, Lf EO 1.10%, Heptan-2-one,3-methyl, Lf EO, Hexacosyl alcohol, Lf Humulene, EO 2,1%, lso-orientin, Lf, L-menthol, Lf, Limonene, Lf EO, Linalool oxide, Lf EO 1.0%, Linalool, Lf, PI, Luteolin, Lf, Luteal i n-7 -O-neohesperidoside, Lf, Menthol, Lf EO 0.6%, Menthane, EO 0.2%), Methyl heplenol, EO, Methyl heptenone, EO, Myrcene, Lf EO, Neral, EO 3.3-33.9%, Nerol acetate, Lf EO 7.50% Nerol, EO, Nerolidol, PI, Ocimene, EO 0.2%, P-Cymene, If, Para-coumaric acid, Lf, Perilla alcohol, EO Phenolic substances, Lf, Phenylethyl alcohol, PI.[114]

Pharmacological & Clinical Research: The essential oil from the leaves is used in aromatherapy, soaps and perfumery. Traditionally, the leaf infusion is widely used to treat colds and fevers. The rhizome has also been used in oral healthcare, as a diuretic, and as an abortifacient. The aerial parts are sold in herbal teas, used commercially in baked foods and confectionary, and also are used in sachets as an insect repellent. The essential oil shows significant antimalarial activity in the four-day suppressive in vitro tests in mice.

Toxicity: Hot water extract of oven dried leaves (2 mg of leaf powder/ISO ml water) administered by gastric intubation to rats at a dose of 20-40 ml/kg daily for eight weeks was inactiveT]2574. The hot water extract taken orally by human adults at a dose of 2-10 gm/day (dry weigbt of plant) was inactive. Serum levels of glucose) urea, crearinine, cholesterol, triglycertdes, lipids, SGOT, SGPT, alkaline phosphatase, total protein, albumin, LDH, CPK, total bilirubin, and indirect bilirubin were unchanged after dosing for two weeks, A slight eleva, don of direct bilirubin and amylase was seen in some patients Til574.[115]

---

114 Ross, Ivan A. *Medicinal Plants of the World: Chemical Constituents, Traditional and Modern Medicinal Uses.* Totowa, NJ: Humana, 1999; 120.

115 Ibid., 120.

Morompo

Diaphoretics Plants with Pungent and Warm Nature

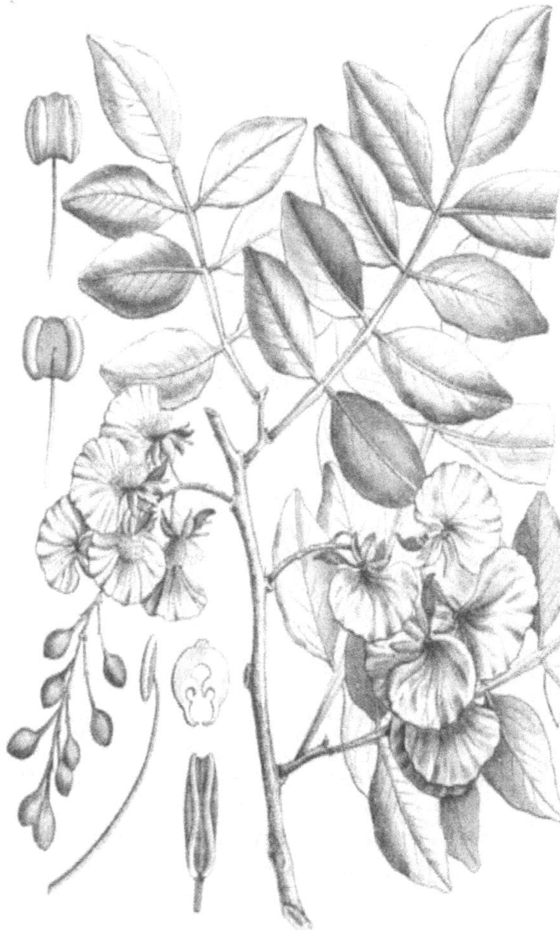

Botanical Name: Swartzia Benthamiana.
Family: Caesalpiniaceae.
Region Where Grown: East Berbice-Corentyne.
Other Names: Okraprabu .
Category: Diaphoretic: Acrid and Warm Nature.
Properties: Sour, Hot/Moist.
Esoteric Botanica: Tehuti.
Governing Organs: Liver, Stomach, Lungs.
Actions & Indications: Sudorific, toothache and tooth decay.
Whole plant: Put the red latex on a piece of cotton which is packed into the cavity of a tooth to relieve toothache.
Stem and Leaf: Crushed leaves and bark are decocted and applied to aching teeth. Also used as a sudorific (cause sweat).[116]
Cautions & Contraindications: If too much is used, or for too long a period of time, it may cause heavy sweating that weakens the body. *Toasting with honey reduces this dispersing property.* Use of the herb may also raise blood pressure or cause restlessness and tremors. Use with caution in cases of deficiency with sweating or wheezing. Do not use for patients with anxiety, heart problems, or insomnia.

---

[116] DeFilipps, Robert A., Shirley L. Maina and Juliette Crepin. *Medicinal Plants of the Guianas (Guyana, Surinam, French Guiana)*. Washington D.C.: Dept. of Botany, National Museaum of Natural History, Smithsonian Institute, 2004; 74.

Ginger

Diaphoretics Plants with Pungent and Warm Nature

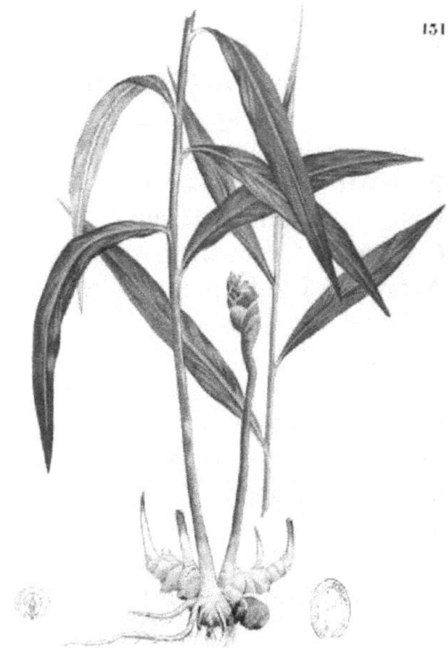

Botanical Name: Zingiber Officinale.
Family: Zingiberaceae.
Region Where Grown: Barima-Waini.
Other Names: Common Ginger .
Category: Diaphoretic.
Properties: Acrid, Hot/Dry.
Esoteric Botanica: Heru.
Governing Organs: Heart, Spleen, Lungs.
Actions & Indications: Ginger is generally used for therapeutic effects on digestion and gastrointestinal function and is widely known as a cooking spice.[117]
Whole plant: Use the boiled plant as a fever wash.
Root: Used to treat hemorrhage and malaria.
Rhizome: Use it in a plaster to relieve headaches; digestive; rubbed on rheumatic areas; sudorific. It is pounded to a paste, which is applied to the abdomen in case of difficult menstruation. This treatment relieves cramps and stimulates the flow of blood. Ginger has numerous physiological effects, including increasing bileantipyretic, vascular pressor, cardiotonic, analgesic, and antiemetic effects. Pressor effects are centrally mediated and produced by shogaol. However, the pressor effects are dose dependent, because low doses of (6)-shogaol and (6)-gingerol had depressor effects. Other effects of ginger are increased bile secretion, antipyretic, and anti~inflammatory effects. (6)-shogaol was found to mediate the antipyretic effect, to a degree comparable with aspirin (Mascolo et al. 1989).[118] Ginger is also used as a carminative, stimulant, diuretic and for its antiemetic properties. The Rhizome is also used for making beverages or for flavoring food.
Cautions & Contraindications: Do not use in cases of Lung heat, or Stomach heat with vomiting.
Major Known Ingredients: Several factors may affect the chemical composition of ginger, including maturity at harvest, agricultural climate, and geographic origin (Mustafa et al. 1993). Ginger has a lipid content of approximately 7%. The oil extract has a high proportion of sesquiterpenes, most nota bly zingiberene, as welT as monot~rpenes and oxygenated compounds. The primary pungent chemical in ginger is an aromatic ketone called gingerol, with homologues varying by carbon atoms in the side chain and designated as (6)-, (8)-, and (10)-gingerol (table 7.5). Gingerols are chemically converted to shogaol, zingerone, and alkanals (hexanal, octanal, and ~ecanal). Shogaol may be further converted to paradol by hydrogenation. It is the commercial preparation that is responsible for some of these reactions, because zingerone and shogaol are found in small amounts in fresh ginger, but in large amounts in stored ginger (Mustafa et al. 1993; Ye et al. 1989). Thus, the composition of fresh and stored ginger may vary, potentially altering its pharmacological effects. The primary terpenoid in ginger is zingiberene. Other terpenes include zingiberol, bisabolene, and galanolactone (figure 7.4). Lesser components of g~nger

117 Spinella, Marcello. *The Psychopharmacology of Herbal Medicine: Plant Drugs That Alter Mind, Brain, and Behavior*. Cambridge, MA: MIT, 2001; 262.
118 Ibid., 262.

include curcuminoids (cassumllnin A and B), and homologues of glOgediol and gingediacetate (Mustafa et al. 1993; Nagano et al. 1997).[119]

Pharmacological & Clinical Research: Few studies have looked at the phannacokinetic properties of ginger constituents. One pharmacokinetic study in rats showed a rapid clearance of (6)-gingerol, with a terminal half-life of 7.23 minutes and a total body clearance of 16.8 rnliminlkg. There was also a high degree of serum binding for (6)-gingerol (92.4%). Further, the disappearance of [6J~gingerol from plasma is mediated by the liver, in part, but not the kidneys. Shogaol has been shown to be metabolized to paradol and dehydroparadol by liver fractions. Four principal mechanisms have been cited to explain the diverse physiological mechanisms of ginger. Broadly, these are (1) eicosanoid inhibition, (2) serotonin antagonism, (3) substance Prelease, and (4) *Ca2+*/ATPase activity.[120]

[119] Ibid., 262.
[120] Ibid., 262.

Diaphoretic Plants with Pungent and Cold Nature

Remedies in this category are used for infectious external conditions with acute onset. They promote sweating and dispel wind cold. The diaphoretic herbs in this category are cool and pungent in property. They are usually used for the treatment of exterior symptom complexes caused by wind and heat. They are not strong enough to promote severe sweating. They are indicated in wind-heat exterior syndrome manifested as high fever, mild chills, thirst, sore throat, scanty or no sweating. Some of these herbs are also effective in promoting the full expression of rashes in measles and are for use on boils and carbuncles on the exterior. The most commonly used herbs in Chinese medicine are *Arctii* (fruit), *Bupleuri* (root), *Clu), samhemi* (flower), *Periostracum cicadae* (flower), *Cimiqfuga* (rhizome), *Dichroae* (root), *Mori* (Jeaf), *Menthae* (herb), *Sojae praparatum* (seed), and *Spirodelae* (herb).

Soldier's Rod can relieve the contraction in the blood vessels of the mucosa caused by the cold, increase the immunity and blood circulation in the body. If there is an exterior cold syndrome, there is reflex contraction in the blood vessels of the mucosa of the upper respiratory tract. The local resistance is reduced, thus the pathogens have the opportunity to invade the body and cause local inflammation.

Soldier Rod

Diaphoretic Plants with Pungent and Cold Nature

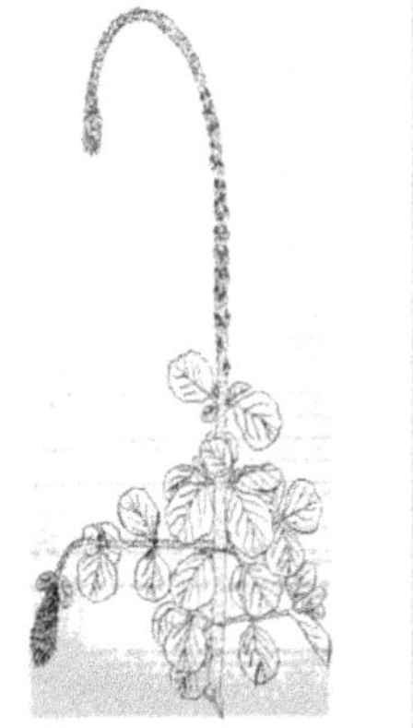

Botanical Name: Achyranthes Indica.
Family: Amaranthaceae.
Region Where Grown: E. Berbice-Corentyne .
Other Names: Cockscomb, Devil's Whip, Cow-Pimpler.
Category: Diaphoretic.
Properties: Bitter, Cold/Moist.
Esoteric Botanica: Het Heru.
Governing Organs:Kidney, Stomach, Liver.
Actions & Indications: Used for colds, coughs, bronchitis, influenza (grippe), sinus congestion, whooping cough, laryngitis, pleurisy, pneumonia, sore throat, pulmonary complaints, hemoptysis, tuberculosis, expectorants and pectorals. Also used as febrifuge, stomachache, colic, syphilis, venereal diseases in general, *(see also* gonorrhea, leucorrhea and hypertension.
Whole plant: Infusion for heart problems. Plant is boiled, and the water drunk as an antipyretic as a treatment for influenza, venereal diseases and as treatment for cold sweat.

Leaf: Decoction for treating high blood pressure,[121] back pain, male potency[122], stomach ache, colic, thrush and colds.
Cautions & Contraindications: Contraindicated in cases of low energy, cough or excess heat ascending to the head. May occasionally cause nausea or vomiting; should this occur, use only a very small dose.
Major Known Ingredients: Extract of plant shows antifertility activity. The seeds have been used as an emetic, the saponin fraction yielded methyl esters of oleanic and maslinic acids.

[121] DeFilipps, Robert A., Shirley L. Maina and Juliette Crepin. *Medicinal Plants of the Guianas (Guyana, Surinam, French Guiana)*. Washington D.C.: Dept. of Botany, National Museaum of Natural History, Smithsonian Institute, 2004; 74.
[122] Leeuwenberg, A. J. M. *Medicinal and Poisonous Plants of the Tropics: Proceedings of Symposium 5-35 of the 14th International Botanical Congress, Berlin, 24 July-1 August 1987*. Wageningen: Pudoc, 1987; 109.

Chapter 2: Purgatives

Plants that Promote Bowel Movement

Herbs in this category either stimulate or lubricate the gastrointestinal tract to facilitate expulsion of stool They are used primarily where the stool has become sluggish, causing abdominal fullness and constipation. These plants stimulate the bowels and induce increasing peristalsis, effectively removing intestinal accumulations and inducing bowel movement. Some Plants contain anthracene glycosides and polyhydroxyanthroquinones from bacterial action in the large bowel. Some substances are irritating and give delayed purging. They may also stimulate nerve plexus in the bowel wall.

Constipation may have various origins. Shallow breathing, a lack, of exercise or fiber in the diet, excessive cheese consumption, insufficient liquid intake, stress, nervous fatigue and emotional upsets, organic disorders (haemorrhoids, colon irritability, inflammation and tumours) are among the major immediate causes of constipation. They may all create certain systemic conditions entailing constipation. Treatment approach is to activate gut motility by bodily exercise and food rich in fibres. If necessary, plant material with swelling or osmotic properties can be used. Stimulant laxatives (with anthranoids) are favoured by patients but should be used with care, since they can lead to chronic constipation. They stimulate the release of histamine and prostaglandins, thus increasing gut motility. The resorption of sodium and chloride ions is reduced thus increasing osmotically the water content in the faeces. In the large intestine, an increased secretion of mucilage takes place. In combination, all these activities lead to a strong laxative effect.

Purgatives - Cathartics/Aperient (Mild Laxative)

Purgative remedies are used to address either immediate or long-term conditions. They lubricate the intestines to move the bowels. These plants in this section are bitter and cold and have strong heat clearing properties and are used for constipation due to accumulation of heat. In western pharmacopaedia there is a wide variety of herbs that range from very mild laxatives, such as yellow dock root, Licorice root and Rhineberry to gentle bulk laxatives (laxatives that swell up when drunk with warm water thereby increasing peristalsis through their sheer bulk in the colon) such as psyllum husks and the bran of grains (e.g., rice or wheat bran), to more active laxatives such as mineral salts (e.g., Glauber's and Epsom salts). Moist laxatives such as *bitter aloes, Senna and buttercup* lubricate the intestines and may cause a certain amount of abdominal griping (cramping). This can be reduced by combining them with *carminatives,* small fruits high in essential oil.

Bitter Aloes

Purgatives: Cathartics/Aperient (Mild laxative)

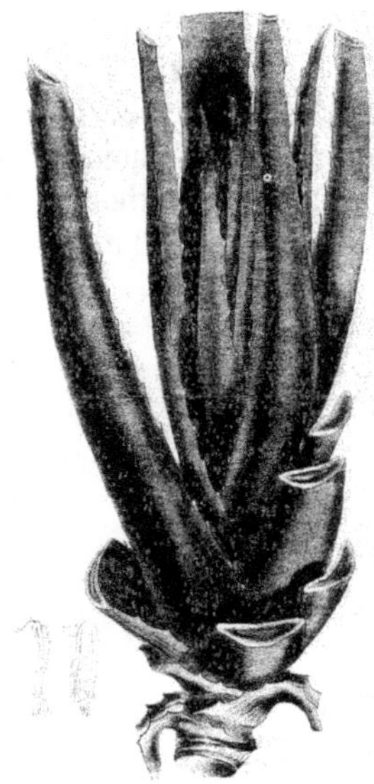

Botanical Name: Aloe Vera.
Family: Aloaceae.
Where Grown: All.
Other Names: Aloes.
Category: Purgatives: Cathartics/Aperient (Mild Laxative).
Properties: Bitter, Cold/Moist.
Esoteric Botanica: Auset.
Governing Organs: Stomach, Liver.
Actions & Indications: Whole plant: Used as a laxative, stomachic and emmenagogue.[123] Used to treat asthma, pneumonia, biliousness and colds. A mild decotion of the leaves is sometimes used as a bitter tonic.
Leaf: Juiced to stop cuts from bleeding.
Juice for a laxative, antimalarial, hairwash, stomach pain remedy, asthma; Infusion of leaf-juice for epilepsy and rheumatism, liver and kidney pain; rubbed on skin to sooth burns from heat or cold[124]; for difficult menstruation.
Leaves also used to treat abcesses and sores as well as for asthma, colds and coughs, malaria, pneumonia; also as a laxative.
The sap from cut or brised leaves is applied to cuts to stop bleeding. Aloe is also used for constipation, dizziness, red eyes and irritability due to heat accumulation. Since it is a mild herb, it may also be used for chronic constipation. Aloe is one of the safest and stimulating purgatives to persons of sedentary habits and phlegmatic constitutions. An ordinary small dose takes up to 18 hours to produce an effect. Its action is exerted mainly on the large intestine, for which reason, also it is useful as a vermifuge.[125]
Cautions & Contraindications: Aloe should not be used by pregnant or breastfeeding women, by children under 12 years of age, or by people with severe intestinal disorders.[126]
Major Known Ingredients: Aloe vera was found to contain aloe-emodin, barbaloin, lupeol, campesterol, cholesterol, sltosterol, chrysophanol, and aloesin. Aloe vera contains aloe-emodin (as does Chinese rhubarb), lupeol, barbaloin, sitosterol, campesterol, aloesin and chrysophanol. Leaf has effective anti-ovulating action on humans. Extracts of aloe are used in commercial skin softening and conditioning creams and cosmetics.
Pharmacological & Clinical Research: Species of Aloe have been used in folk remedies as a cathartic and astringent, and commercially in oitments, cosmetics, lotions and shampoos and for gastrointestinal

---

[123] Keys, John D. *Chinese Herbs: their Botany, Chemistry and Pharmacodynamics*. Rutland, VT: C.E. Tuttle, 1976; 54.
[124] Buchman, Dian Dincin. *Ancient Healing Secrets: Practical Herbal Remedies from around the World that Work Today*. New York: Gramercy Books, 1996; 76.
[125] Grieve, M. *A Modern Herbal; the Medicinal, Culinary, Cosmetic and Economic Properties, Cultivation and Folk-lore of Herbs, Grasses, Fungi, Shrubs, & Trees with All Their Modern Scientific Uses,*. New York: Dover Publications, 1971; 111.
[126] *PDR for Nonprescription Drugs, Dietary Supplements and Herbs*. Montvale, NJ: The Physician's Desk Reference Network, 2010; 424.

disturbances, burns, insect bites and athlete's foot. Polysaccharide obtained from the juice has been used for treating skin and body tissue, wounds including burns, open wounds, ulcers, inset bites and also arthritis. Aloin is commonly used as a laxative and laxative-hypnotic drug combinations consisting of aloe extract are useful in the prophylaxis of drug abuse, e.g. attempted suicide through overdose of sleeping tablets. Extract of Aloe Vera is used in topical compositions as a cosmetic base for decreasing wrinkles and smoothing skin. Antimicrobial activity of the juice has been reported against Pseudomonas aeruginosa and Proteus Vulgaris. Aloe vera extract was bactericidal against several organisms including escherichia coll, streptococcus faecallis and bacillus subtillis and reported antifungal activity.
Toxicity: Erhanol/water (1: 1) extract of dried leaves administered intraperitoneally to mice produced LDsc > l.0 gm/kgA04m. Ethanol/warer (50%) extract of the entire plant administered intraperitoneally to mice produced LDsc 250.0 mg/kg. The maximum tolerated dose was 100.0 mg/kgAO;m[127]

[127] Ross, Ivan A. *Medicinal Plants of the World: Chemical Constituents, Traditional and Modern Medicinal Uses.* Totowa, NJ: Humana, 1999; 77.

Senna

Purgatives: Cathartics/Aperient (Mild laxative

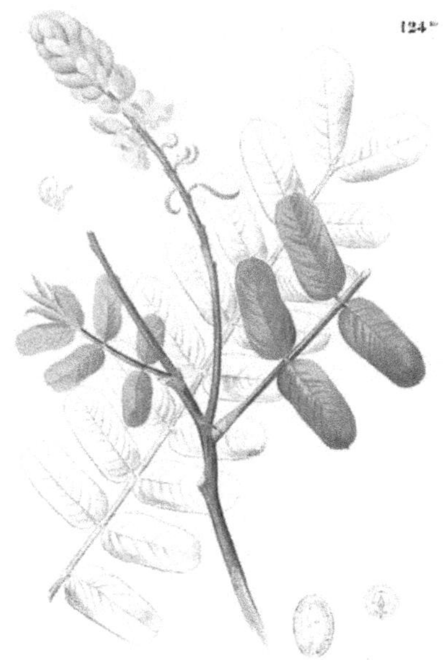

Botanical Name: Senna Alata.
Family: Casesalpinioideae.
Region Where Grown:Demerara-Mahaica.
Other Names: Candle Stick, Christmas Candle, Impetigo Bush, King-of-the-Forest, Money Bush, Tarantan, Ringworm Shrub, River Guava, River Senna.
Esoteric Botanica: Heru.
Category: Purgative (Mild Laxative).
Properties: Sweet, Hot/Dry, Acrid.
Governing Organs: San Jiao, Small Intestine, Spleen, Stomach, Liver, Lungs.
Actions & Indications: Abortifacient, anthelmintic, antimicrobial agent, biliousness, blood cleanser, colds, dermatitis, eczema, hypertension, intestinal worms, purgative.
Root: Infusion for tympanitis. Cooked in water for uterus problems and filaria worm expulsion. Used for diarrhea, bete rouge, as laxative, and for sores and skin fungi. [128]
Flower: Used as laxative and for worms.
Leaf, Flower and Fruit: Mixed in an infusion for stomach problems. Leaf: Infusion for a laxative tea and to cleanse the blood. In a tincture for skin blemishes and ringworm. Finely ground and used alone or mixed with oil to treat various skin conditions, such as tetter, scurf, scaling skin, ulcers, eczema, ringworm, dermatitis; decoction as an externally applied febrifuge.
Seed: Cooked and used as a laxative anthelmintic remedy for intestinal worms. Traditionally, tea made from the leaves is taken as a treatment for constipation and intestinal worms. The leaves are rubbed on the skin to cure eczema and "ringworm".
Cautions & Contraindications: The major symptoms of overdose are griping and severe diarrhoea with consequent losses of fluid and electrolytes. Treatment should be supportive with generous amounts of fluid. Electrolytes, particularly potassium, should be monitored, especially in children and the elderly.[129]
Major Known Ingredients: Leaf contains purgative anthraquinone and shows some antimicrobial activity. Stem contains chrysophanol, emodin, rhein and aloe emodin. Leaf and fruit contain purgative anthracene derivatives of aloe emodin and rhein.[130] The intestinal irritant called emodin acts by stimulating the rhythmic, wave-like muscular contractions (peristalsis) that facilitate the passage of food through the gastrointestinal tract.

---

[128] DeFilipps, Robert A., Shirley L. Maina and Juliette Crepin. *Medicinal Plants of the Guianas (Guyana, Surinam, French Guiana)*. Washington D.C.: Dept. of Botany, National Museaum of Natural History, Smithsonian Institute, 2004; 70.
[129] *WHO monographs on Selected Medicinal Plants Vol 1.* Geneva: World Health Organization Library Cataguing in Publicata data, 1999; 254.
[130] DeFilipps, Robert A., Shirley L. Maina and Juliette Crepin. *Medicinal Plants of the Guianas (Guyana, Surinam, French Guiana)*. Washington D.C.: Dept. of Botany, National Museaum of Natural History, Smithsonian Institute, 2004; 72.

Pharmacological & Clinical Research: Contains not less than 2.5% of hydroxyanthracene glycosides, calculated as sennoside B (*1*, *4*, *5*). Quantitative analysis is performed by spectrophotometry (*1*, *4–8*) and by high-performance liquid chromatography (*20*). Thin-layer chromatography is employed for qualitative analysis for the presence of sennosides A and B (*3–5*). Folium Sennae contains a family of hydroxyanthracene glycosides, the most plentiful of which are sennosides A and B. There are also small amounts of aloeemodin and rhein 8-glucosides, mucilage, flavonoids and naphthalene precursors.[131]
The effects of Folium Sennae are due primarily to the hydroxyanthracene glucosides, especially sennosides A and B. These β-linked glucosides are secretagogues that increase net secretion of fluids and specifically influence colonic motility and enhance colonic transit. They are not absorbed in the upper intestinal tract. They are converted by the bacteria of the large intestine into the active derivatives (rhein-anthrone). The mechanism of action is twofold: (1) effect on the motility of the large intestine (stimulation of peristaltic contractions and inhibition of local contractions), resulting in an accelerated colonic transit, thereby reducing fluid absorption, and (2) an influence on fluid and electrolyte absorption and secretion by the colon (stimulation of mucus and active chloride secretion), increasing fluid secretion. [132]

---

[131] *WHO monographs on Selected Medicinal Plants Vol 1*. Geneva: World Health Organization Library Cataguing in Publicata data, 1999; 244.
[132] Ibid., 245.

Buttercup

Purgatives: Cathartics/Aperient (Mild laxative)

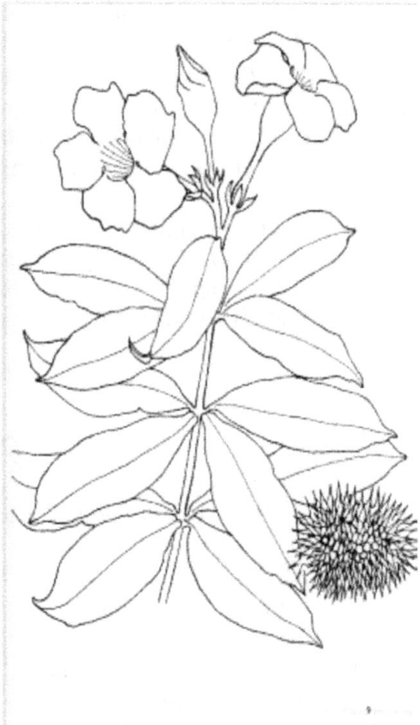

Botanical Name: Allamanda Cathartica.
Family: Apocynaceae.
Region Where Grown: East Berbice-Corentyne.
Other Names: Allamanda, Buttercup, Porcupine-Batty, Wild Senna.
Category: Purgatives: Cathartics/Aperient (Mild Laxative).
Properties: Sweet, Warm.
Esoteric Botanica: Het Heru.
Governing Organs: Kidney, Spleen, Large Intestine.
Actions & Indications: Used as emetic, jaundice, antitussive, anuria, cathartic, dizziness, impotence, laxative and purgative.
Root and Flower: Infusion for jaundice and spleen conditions.
Stem: Bark decoction for a febrifuge.
Leaf and Flower: Decoction for anuria and dizziness.
Flower: Antitussive.
Leaf: Infusion for a cathartic, purgative, emetic and laxative. Used to treat biliousness, malaria and as laxative.
Stem: Latex from bark is purgative.
Cautions & Contraindications: Do not use during pregnancy, menstruation, or with nursing mothers. Do not use with weak patients or those suffering from chronic constipation. Overdose may result in abdominal pain, nausea and vomiting
Major Known Ingredients: An antineoplasmic (antileukemic) iridoid lactone, named allamandine, is present. Flower contains allamandoside, a fungitoxic glycoside. Plant also contains plumericin, isoplumericin, plumieride, flavoplumierin, isoplumierin, beta-sitosterol, allamandin, quercetin.[133]
Pharmacological & Clinical research: Extract of plant is antibiotic against *Staphylococcus.* Root contains isoplumerin, an antifungal sesquiterpenoid.
Toxicity: The toxic iridoids plumericin and isoplumericin have been isolated.

---

[133] DeFilipps, Robert A., Shirley L. Maina and Juliette Crepin. *Medicinal Plants of the Guianas (Guyana, Surinam, French Guiana).* Washington D.C.: Dept. of Botany, National Museaum of Natural History, Smithsonian Institute, 2004; 18.

Purgatives - Emollient (Softening/Moisturizing)

Emollients are simple oil and emulsion which often and lubricate the bowel. They are moist laxatives (mild in nature) that are use to lubricate the intestines. They are suitable for weak and chronic patients. Some plants such as *Plum bark and castor oil c*ontains fatty oil (oleic, linoleic and protein) which lubricates the intestine. They are mild in nature and are most appropriately prescribed for the debilitated, elderly and those who are weakened either from a febrile disease or from childbirth.
In the Chinese parmacopaedia they are Feng Mi, Huo Ma Ren and Yu li Ren.

These laxatives tend to have mildly sweet, cool and moist qualities. They are known as demulcent laxatives because of their high mucilage content. Western herbs such as psyllum, cannabis and flax seeds, prune, peach, apricot and plum kernels all cause bowel contents to slip because of the lubricating effect of their fatty oil. They are particularly suitable for children, pregnant women and the elderly.

Plum Bark

Purgatives: Emollient (Softening/Moisturizing)

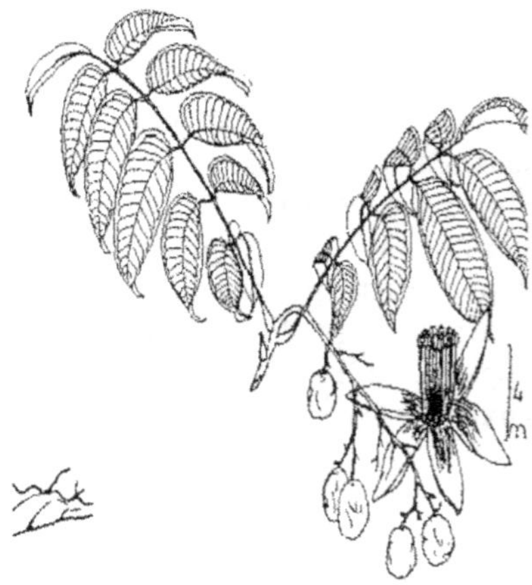

Botanical Name: Spondias Mombin .
Family: Anacardiaceae.
Region Where Grown: Mahaica-Berbice.
Other Names: Hog Plum, Mope, Hubu.
Esoteric Botanica: Tehuti.
Category: Stabilize and Bind .
Properties: Sour, Hot/Moist.
Governing Organs: Liver, Stomach, Large Intestine.
Actions & Indications: Stop diarrhea and dysentery, as eye wash and enema in cases of gonorrhea, hemorroids, and relieve stomach ache, constipation, biliousness, fevers, cystitis, urethritis, and inflammation of eyes, kidneys and throat, cardiac hypertrophy, angina and ulcers of the uterus and vagina.[134]
Root: Infusion for dysentery.
Stem: The bark is decoction as an emetic and treatment for diarrhea, dysentery, gonorrhea and hemorrhoids; Bark used in a gonorrhoea remedy, as an antidiarrhoeic and to remedy stomachache; infusion is sudorific, used to alleviate fatigue.
Stem and Leaf: Decoction for eyewash.
Bark use to treat coughs and colds, hemorrhage and sores.

[134] Morton F. Julia. *Atlas of Medical Plants of Middle America: Bahamas to Yucatan.* Springfield, Illinois: Charles C. Thomas Publisher, 1981; 476-477.

Leaf: A decoction of leaves and nowers is used to relieve stomachache, constlpation, bilious fevers, cystitis, urethritis and inflammation of the eyes and throat.
Decoction for diarrhoea and dysentery; used in an abortifacient preparation.
Fruit: As a mild laxative; stewed and eaten to cure diarrhoea. Leaves used in treatment of diarrhoea, hemorrhage, and sores. [135]
Flower: Infusion for mouth sores.
Cautions & Contraindications: Do not use in cases of internal heat excess and stagnation, or in unresolved exterior disorders.
Major Known Ingredients: The bark contains tannin.
Toxicity: The fruit is said to be bad for the throat.

[135] DeFilipps, Robert A., Shirley L. Maina and Juliette Crepin. *Medicinal Plants of the Guianas (Guyana, Surinam, French Guiana).* Washington D.C.: Dept. of Botany, National Museaum of Natural History, Smithsonian Institute, 2004;10.

Castor Oil Plant

Purgatives: Emollient (Softening/Moisturizing)

Botanical Name: Ricinus Communis.
Family: Euphorbiaceae.
Region Where Grown: Demerara-Mahaica.
Other Names: Palma Christi, Castor Bean, Castor Oil. plant, Ricinus, Recino.
Esoteric Botanica: Sebek.
Category: Purgative.
Properties: Bland, Cool/Dry.
Governing Organs: Large Intestine, Lung.
Actions & Indications: Considered anodyne, antidote, aperient, bactericide, cathartic, cyanogenetic, discutient, emetic, emollient, expectorant, insecticide, lactagogue, larvicidal, laxative, purgative, tonic and vermifuge, castor or castor oil is a dangerous ingredient in folk remedies for abscess, anasarca, arthritis, asthma, boils, burns, cancer, carbuncles, catarrh, chancre, cholera, cold, colic, convulsions, corns, craw~craw, deafness, delirium, dermatitis, dogbite, dropsy, epilepsy, erysipelas, fever, gout, guineaworm, headache, inflammation, moles, myalgia, nerves, osteomyelitis, palsy, parturition, prolapse, puerperium, rash, rheumatism, scald, scrofula, seborrhea, skin, sores, stomachache, strabismus, swellings, toothaches, tuberculosis, lumors, urethritis, uteritis, venereal disease, warts, whitlows and wounds.The oil and seed have been used as folk remedies for warts, cold tumors, indurations of the abdominal organs, whitlows, lacteal tumors, indurations of the mammary gland, corns, moles.[136]

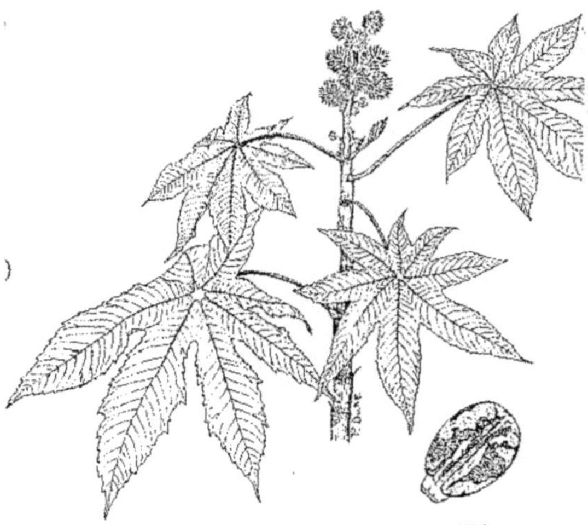

Leaf: Decoction as an external wash to regain health after a high fever. The bruised leaves are applied onto women's breasts in order to slow the secretion of milk. Leaves used in a sunstroke remedy. Leaves are smeared with oil and applied onto painful places on the arm and leg by sufferers of filariasis. Tied onto head to relieve headache, and tied onto ulcers to relieve pain and swelling; infusion for fever. Leaves are boiled, and the water drunk as a treatment for reducing pain or fevers.
Seed: Oil is a purgative, cathartic and used to strengthen the hair; to facilitate expulsion of the placenta in childbirth; liniment for painful muscles and spots of filariasis.[137] Cotton saturated with warm castor oil is effectively applied to the anus for piles. Oil is used for grippe and colic. The seed is eaten as a purgative; crushed and placed on the stomach of women in labor; laxative; oil used to relieve pain of constipation and as an ingredient in a curative herbal bath. The oil is also used for hair loss.[138]

[136] Duke, James A. *CRC Handbook of Medicinal Herbs*. Boca Raton, FL: CRC, 1985; 408.
[137] Ibid., 149.
[138] Buchman, Dian Dincin. *Ancient Healing Secrets: Practical Herbal Remedies from around the World That Work Today*. New York: Gramercy Books, 1996; 83.

Cautions & Contraindications: Do not use in cases of deficiency cold in the spleen or stomach. Use with great caution during pregnancy or with nursing mothers

Major Known Ingredients: The seeds of *R. communis* are the source of 50--55 % of Castor oil. The oil consists mainly of ricinolein, which is the triglyceride of' the unsaturated ricinoleic acid; the neutral fat is not active, but becomes so upon saponification in the intestine, where it yields glycerin and ricinoleic acid; liquid; soluble in alcohol, acetone, ether, chloroform); the cathartic effect is due mainly to motor stimulation of the small intestine. The seeds also contain 2 substances which do not pass to the oil, the highly toxic albumin ricin (white powder; soluble in 10 % sodium chloride solution) and a toxic alkaloid ricinine (ricidine; $C_8H_SN_20_2$; brilliant needles or prisms; m.p. 201-5°; sparingly soluble in water, alcohol, chloroform, ether)[139].

Pharmacological & Clinical Research: Seed contains the toxalbumin ricine and the alkaloid ricinine; vitamin E is plentiful. Leaf shows antimicrobial activity. Contains a tumor cell agglutinator, and has been proposed as a cancer treatment. Ricinoleic acid, which *is* formed from triglycerides under the influence of lipase in the small intestine, enhances the formation of prostaglandin E2, endogenous NO and the release of serotonin and histamine. These properties reduce the net resorption of fluids and electrolytes, and stimulate peristalsis.[140]

Toxicity: The plant contains the toxic protein ricin which is most comcentrated in the seeds and a potent allergen. The seeds are also rich in purgative oil that owes its action to a triglyceride of ricinoleic acid.[141]

---

[139] Keys, John D. *Chinese Herbs, Their Botany, Chemistry, and Pharmacodynamics*. Rutland, VT: C.E. Tuttle, 1976; 105.

[140] Van, Wyk Ben-Erik., and Michael Wink. *Medicinal Plants of the World: An Illustrated Scientific Guide to Important Medicinal Plants and Their Uses*. Portland: Timber, 2004; 274.

[141] Morton F. Julia. *Atlas of Medical Plants of Middle America: Bahamas to Yucatan*. Springfield, Illinois: Charles C. Thomas Publisher, 1981; 464, 465.

Cathartics (Drastic Purgatives)

Drastic purgatives increase peristalsis action of the intestines and the reabsorption of the intestine. They are very strong diuretics that induce pronounced diarrhea. Very specific water accumulation problem presenting with distended abdomen or stagnation of fluids in the thoracic cavity . The harsh expellants drive out excess water and induce pronounced diarrhea. In western terms this pattern generally corresponds to pleurisy or ascites The *Sandbox Tree* is suited for more robust individuals. Because of their violent effect they are only used in very severe cases for short periods of time. They have their equivalent in the Chinese pharmacopaedia in such herbs as ba dou, da ji and gan sui. These herbs are also contraindicated in pregnancy.

Sandbox Tree

Purgatives Drastic Purgatives

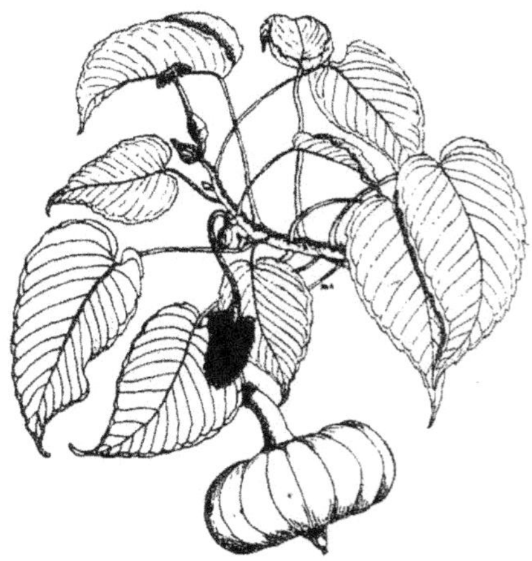

Botanical Name: Hura Crepitans .
Family: Euphorbiaceae.
Region Where Grown:Demerara-Mahaica.
Other Names: Poison Tree, Sandbox, Monkey's Dinner Bell.
Category: Purgative (Drastic).
Properties: Sweet, Cold/Moist.
Esoteric Botanica: Auset.
Governing Organs: Stomach, Spleen, Liver.
Actions & Indications: Reported to be anodyne, antidotal, aperient, canicidal, carcinogenic, dentifuge, emetic, insecticidal, piscicidal, poison, purgative, and vermifuge, sandbox tree is a folk remedy for elephantiasis, leprosy, rheumatism, skin ailments and sores.[142]
Stem: Decoction of bark used as a purgative and emetic; sap in bark reputedly is a remedy for leprosy. Warmly unblocks and vigorously purges – for severe cold accumulation in the interior leading to constipation and abdominal fullness, distention, and pain.
Leaf: Infusion as a body-rub for leprosy. The leaves, crushed in water, are poulticed on rheumatism. The sap is given as a vermifuge at the rate of 30 cg in a cup of water. Promotes the healing of abscesses and

[142] Duke, James A., and Rodolfo Vásquez. *Amazonian Ethnobotanical Dictionary*. Boca Raton, FL: CRC, 1994; 235.

ulcers – used topically for abscesses that have suppurated but not yet ulcerated to accelerate the ulcerating process; milky sap is caustic and irritant.
Seed: Viscous oil is a very strong (drastic) purgative and emetic.
Cautions & Contraindications: Use with caution in weak and debilitated patients. Do not use during pregnancy. Do not take hot liquids while taking this herb.
Major Known Ingredients: The phytohaemagglutinin crepitin has been isolated. Seed contains a glucosamine lectin having mitogenic and haemagglutinating properties. Latex contains hurine (similar to cardol), inositol, huratoxin (C"1H.'KOH)' a proteinase caHed hurain, 24-methylencycloartenol, cycloartenol, and butyrospermol. Leaves contain kaempferol, p~coumaric acid, and ferulic acid. Seeds contain oil and a toxalbumin, crepitin, similar to ricin. Extracts are mitogenic and useful in lymphocytic stimulation. Hura seeds contain several very active proteases and the agglutinating ability of these acting with red blood cells is enhanced by pretreatment with trypsin. Huratoxin is a cocarcinogenic daphnane ester. [143]
Toxicity: Latex contains the toxic diterpene hura-toxin. Ingestion of raw seeds may cause violent vomiting and diarrhea. They contain a purgative oil and the toxic protein hurin or crepitin which has been found to be a potent lymphatic mitogen.[144]

---

[143] Ibid., 235.
[144] Morton, Julia F. *Atlas of Medical Plants of Middle America: Bahamas to Yucatan*. Springfield: Charles C. Thomas, 1981; 446-447.

Diuretics (Increase the flow of urine – get rid of excess water)

Diuretics: There is an increase in the glomerular filtration or decrease in the tabular absorption. The increased output of urine can alleviate the edema condition in the glomerular nephritis or congestive heart failure. Some plants such as *Inflammation Bush* contain pharbitin which is decomposed in the intestine on contact with bile and intestinal fluid. It stimulates the intestinal mucosa, increases the secretion and thus causes peristalsis. It has a diuretic effect and is usually used for patients with edema and constipation. Bacterial infections may occur internally, either from blood or lymphmic tissues, or from outside, via the urethra. These infections are favomed by urinary obstructions and can lead to inflammation.

Diuretic herbs are often applied in combination with antibacterial drugs to reduce symptoms of increased urine production. In severe cases, treatment with antibiotics becomes necessary. Inflammation of the urinary tract (including urolithiasis and nephrolithiasis) Inflammation of the kidneys and urinary tract can be caused by bacterial infections, urinary gravel and stones (formed from urate, oxalate, cystin, xanthine or creatine). Diuretic drugs containing terpenoids, coumarins, furanocounlarins, flavonoids, saponins, cardiac glycosides, or their metabolic products, lead to increased urine formation and have an anti-inflammatory effect in the urinary tract. More diluted urine prevents stone formation.

Minnie Root

Purgatives Diuretics (Increase the flow of urine and get rid of excess water)

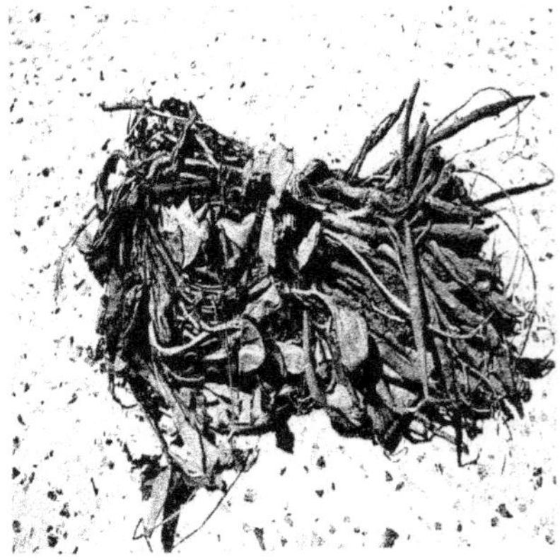

Botanical Name: Ruellia Tuberosa.
Family: Acanthaceae.
Region Where Grown: Cuyuni-Mazaruni.
Other Names: Bluebell, Menow Weed, Duffy Gun, Manny Roots.
Category: Stabilize and Bind.
Properties: Sour, Hot/Moist.
Esoteric Botanica: Maat.
Governing Organs: Liver, Urinary bladder, Kidney.
Actions & Indications: Used to bathe sores and wounds, and is taken to relieve chest ailments, pulmonary catarrh, asthma, influenza and ordinary colds, febrifuge and sudorific; relieve toothache, painful swellings, emetic and purgative.[145]
Whole plant: To treat bladder diseases and frequent micturition;[146] It is also used to bathe sores and wound and is taken to relieve chest ailments, pulmonary catarrh, asthma, influenza and ordinary colds.

---

[145] Morton, Julia F. *Atlas of Medical Plants of Middle America: Bahamas to Yucatan*. Springfield: Charles C. Thomas, 1981; 846.

[146] DeFilipps, Robert A., Shirley L. Maina, and Juliette Crepin. *Medicinal Plants of the Guianas (Guyana, Surinam, French Guiana)*. Washington, D.C.: Dept. of Botany, National Museum of Natural History, Smithsonian Institution, 2004; 2.

Root: The root is primarily decoted as a diuretic in uriary problems, especially in cases of gonorrhea and syphilis, as well as an emetic and purgative. Infusion for kidney diseases - stabilizes the kidneys and retains the essence – for leakage of fluids due to weak essence with such symptoms as excessive urination, incontinence, spermatorrhea, clear and copious vaginal discharge and excessive sweating; in a syrup for whooping cough; infusion or decoction for a diabetes remedy; tubers in a tea used for cleansing the blood. It was formerly used in treating leprosy.[147]
Leaf: Decoted in a tea used for alleviating retention of urine and to remedy weakness. Mainly used as a febrifuge and sudorific.
Cautions & Contraindications: Do not use in cases of painful and difficult urination or with damp-heat, or other acute syndromes with pathogens present.
Major Known Ingredients: Leaf contains apigenin and luteolin. Seed oil yields myristic, capric and lauric acids

[147] Morton, Julia F. *Atlas of Medical Plants of Middle America: Bahamas to Yucatan.* Springfield: Charles C. Thomas, 1981; 845.

Ziba Grass

Purgatives Diuretics (Increase the flow of urine and get rid of excess water)

Botanical Name: Cynodon Dactylon.
Family: Poaceae.
Region Where Grown: Barima/Waimi.
Other Names: Bahama Grass, Bermuda Grass, Devil Grass.
Category: Drain Dampness – leech out water.
Properties: Sour, Hot/Moist.
Esoteric Botanica: Tehuti.
Governing Organs: Liver, Urinary Bladder, Stomach, Lung.
Actions & Indications: Decoction of whole plant used to treat anuria ("stoppage of water"), stomachache, abdominal distention, or ascites due to dampness accumulation and in baths to prevent itching. [148] Expels dampness and stops itching – used both internally and topically for damp skin disorders and other dermatological problems where itching is a major symptom, such as eczema and scabies. Also for damp-heat in the external genitals.
Cautions & Contraindications: Use with caution in cases of yin deficiency
Major Known Ingredients: Extracts have a high phagocytic index; shoot apex may produce cyanogenetic glycosides[149]

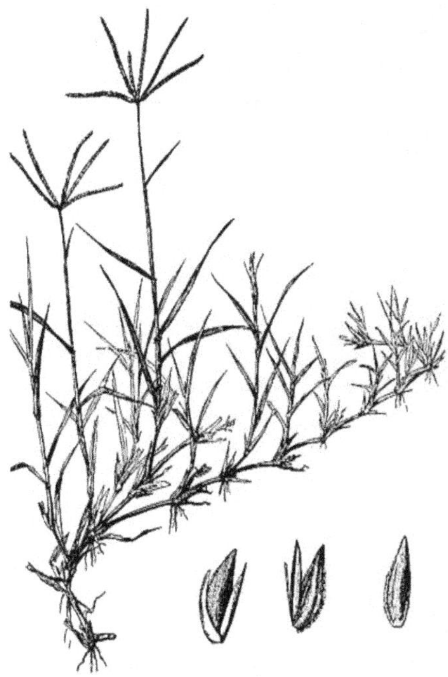

[148] DeFilipps, Robert A., Shirley L. Maina, and Juliette Crepin. *Medicinal Plants of the Guianas (Guyana, Surinam, French Guiana)*. Washington, D.C.: Dept. of Botany, National Museum of Natural History, Smithsonian Institution, 2004; 231.
[149] Ibid., 231.

Man Grass

Purgatives Diuretics (Increase the flow of urine and get rid of excess water)

Botanical Name: Eleusine Indica.
Family: Poaceae.
Where Grown: Demerara-Mahaica.
Other Names: Goose Grass, Goosefoot Grass.
Esoteric Botanica: Tehuti.
Category: Tonify Qi.
Properties:Hot/Moist, Acrid.
Governing Organs: Liver, Large Intestine, Urinary Bladder, Lungs.

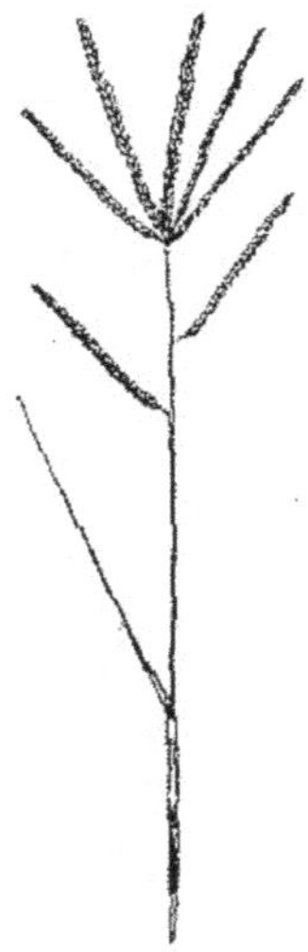

Actions & Indications: Whole plant: Infusion as aperitive and refresher; antidiarrhoeic and used for dysentery and convulsions. Strengthens the spleen and tonifies the stomach – for lethargy, lack of appetite, chest and abdominal distention, diarrhea or even prolapse in severe cases. Decoction is diuretic, enema and bladder disorders; relieve pain caused by straining the abdominal muscles and is applied to open wounds to stop bleeding. Decoction for children's convulsions and jaundice.
Leaf: Macerated in a decoction applied to skin rashes. Used as contraceptive, for hemorrhage and for loss of hair.
Root: The root infusion is used for diarrhea; leaf decoction for dysentery, swellings and oliguria.[150]
Seed: The seed used for dysentery, diarrhea and contusions.
Cautions & Contraindications: Do not use in cases of yin deficiency with heat signs, heat excess or in the absence of significant qi deficiency. Use with caution for patients with untreated hypertension.
Major Known Ingredients: Contains cyanogenetic heterosides.[151]
Pharmacological & Clinical Research:
Toxicity: The seeds contain a significant amount of HCN. Under certain conditions the grass may aaccumulate toxic levels of nitrate.[152]

---

[150] Duke, James A. *CRC Handbook of Medicinal Herbs*. Boca Raton, FL: CRC, 1985; 70.
[151] DeFilipps, Robert A., Shirley L. Maina, and Juliette Crepin. *Medicinal Plants of the Guianas (Guyana, Surinam, French Guiana)*. Washington, D.C.: Dept. of Botany, National Museum of Natural History, Smithsonian Institution, 2004; 231.
[152] Morton, Julia F. *Atlas of Medical Plants of Middle America: Bahamas to Yucatan*. Springfield: Charles C. Thomas, 1981; 30.

Inflammation Bush

Purgatives Diuretics (Increase the flow of urine and get rid of excess water)

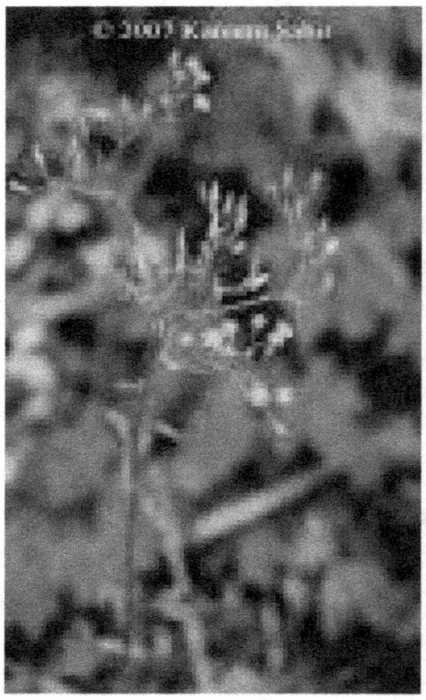

Botanical Name: Cyanthillium Cinereum.
Family: Asteraceae.
Region Where Grown: Cuyuni/Mazaruni.
Other Names: Blue Fleabane, Strongman bush, Tropical fleabane.
Esoteric Botanica: Auset.
Category: Dains Dampness.
Properties: Bitter, Cold/Moist.
Governing Organs: Liver, Spleen, Stomach.
Actions & Indications: Used as a blood cleanser, diuretic, kidney. ailments, menstruation, including menstral flow pains, placenta expulsion, sprains and swellings.
Stem and Leaf: Decoction for diuretic, kidney disorders, swellings, inflammation, lower abdominal pains and menstrual pains, Breaks up blood stasis – used as an auxiliary herb for amenorrhea due to blood stasis; also to expel the placenta and as an abortifacient.[153] For abdominal distention or ascites due to accumulation of dampness. Alleviates pain – damp-heat collecting in the channels with such symptoms as fever and red, swollen, hot and painful joints and muscular strains.
It is considered a more potent abortifacient and better treatment for menstrual pains.
Cautions & Contraindications: Do not use during pregnancy or in cases with spleen or kidney yang or qi deficiency.
Major Known Ingredients: Plant contains triterpenes and sterols; oil contains vernolic acid. Various extracts of the plant are antiviral, anticancer and diuretic.

[153] DeFilipps, Robert A., Shirley L. Maina, and Juliette Crepin. *Medicinal Plants of the Guianas (Guyana, Surinam, French Guiana)*. Washington, D.C.: Dept. of Botany, National Museum of Natural History, Smithsonian Institution, 2004; 43.

Stinging Nettle

Purgatives Diuretics (Increase the flow of urine and get rid of excess water)

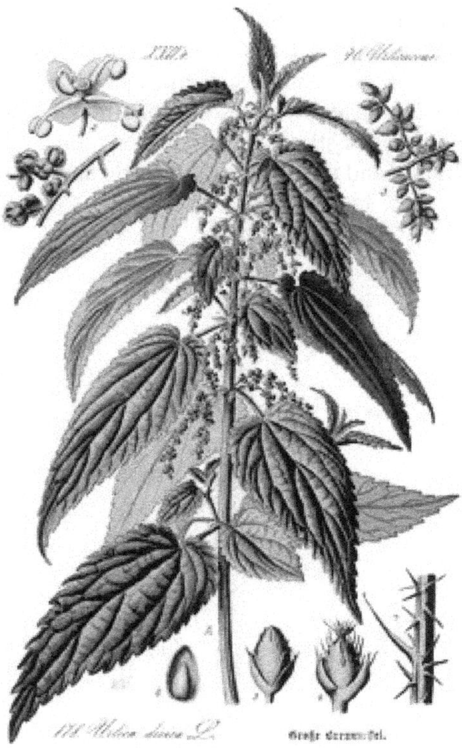

Botanical Name: Laportea Aestuans.
Family: Urticaceae.
Region Where Grown: Potaro-Siparuni.
Other Names: None.
Category: Drains Dampness.
Properties: Sweet, Cool/Dry, Astringent .
Esoteric Botanica: Sebek.
Governing Organs: Urinary Bladder, Lung, Kidney, Liver, Lung.
Actions & Indications: The entire plant, collected just before flowering, has had a lengthy reputation in folk medicine as a specific for antiasthmatic, cleansing tonic and purifier. It has also been given as an expectorant, antispasmodic, diuretic, astringent and tonic. Applying nettle to scalp, especially in the form of the fresh juice, stimulates hair growth. Chronic rheumatism have been treated by placing nettle leaves directly on the afflicted area.[154]
Stem and Leaf: Boiled for a preparation to remedy urine retention and as a diuretic and laxative. Nettle is also anti-asthmatic: the juice of the leaves mixed with honey or sugar will relieve bronchial and asthmatic trouble.[155] The seeds have also been used in consumption. The seeds and flowers sometimes given in wine as a remedy for ague. An infusion of the bark and stems is taken in cases of syphilis.
Root: The root has beneficial effect upon enlarge prostate glands.
Cautions & Contraindications: Do not use during pregnancy. Use with caution in cases of exhausted yang qi, or spermatorrhea due to Kidney deficiency or exhaustion from overwork. Warning: Stinging Nettle should not be used by people who suffer from fluid retention due to impaired cardiac or kidney function.
Major Known Ingredients: Both the flowers and root of the Stinging Nettle plant contain beneficial compounds used in various conditions. The flower is used intemally and externally for rheurnatism. It is also used internationally for urinary tract infections and kidney and bladder stones. The root is used for irritable bladder and to help relieve symptoms of benign prostatic hyperplasia (obstructed urinary flow),

---

[154] Foster Steven and Varro E. Tyler. *Tyler's Honest Herbal: A Sensible Guide to the Use Herbs and Related Remedies*. London: Haworth Herbal: 1984; 269.
[155] Grieve, M. *A Modern Herbal; the Medicinal, Culinary, Cosmetic and Economic Properties, Cultivation and Folk-lore of Herbs, Grasses, Fungi, Shrubs, & Trees with All Their Modern Scientific Uses,*. New York: Dover Publications, 1971; 111.

although it does not reduce prostate enlargement.[156] Nettle leaf contains minerals, (especially silicic acid; up to 5%), amines (histamine, acetylcholine, serotonin), flavonol glycosides, phenolic acids, scopoletin, β-sitosterol and tannins.[157] Roots contain polysaccharides, a lectin (UDA), several phenolics (including lignans, coumarins) and sterols, including P-sitosterol, *7α,* and 7β - hydroxysitosterol and their glycosides, The stinging hairs an like miniature syringes and inject histamine and acetylcholine, causing extreme irritation.[158]

Pharmacological & Clinical Research: The stinging hairs cause burning and infl ammation on contact with the skin but not, as severely as those of *U. baccilera.*[159] Leaves show a mild diuretic, analgesic, and anti-inflammatory action (the dose of non-steroidal anti-inflammatory drugs i.n the treatment of arthritis can be reduced, if Urtica is taken concomitantly - phenolic compounds are responsible for this activity. Nettle roots interact with testosterone-binding proteins, 5α-reductase and aromatase. Nettle lectins appear to be an immune stimulant. Controlled clinical studies support efficacy for the treatment of benign prostate hypertrophy and the traditional diuretic and anti-inflammatory uses in treating arthritis.[160]

---

[156] *PDR for Nonprescription Drugs, Dietary Supplements, and Herbs.* Montvale, NJ: PDR Network, 2010; 427.
[157] Van, Wyk Ben-Erik., and Michael Wink. *Medicinal Plants of the World: An Illustrated Scientific Guide to Important Medicinal Plants and Their Uses*. Portland: Timber, 2004; 332.
[158] Ibid., 332
[159] Morton, Julia F. *Atlas of Medical Plants of Middle America: Bahamas to Yucatan.* Springfield: Charles C. Thomas, 1981; 155.
[160] Van, Wyk Ben-Erik., and Michael Wink. *Medicinal Plants of the World: An Illustrated Scientific Guide to Important Medicinal Plants and Their Uses*. Portland: Timber, 2004; 332

Chapter 3: Antipyretics/Febrigugals

Plants that Lower Body Temperature or Alleviate Fever

The antipyretics can reduce the temperature of the body either by decreasing oxygenation or by inhibiting the heat center in the brain. The plants in this category are usually cold or cool in nature. They are used to alleviate the heat symptoms such as heat in the face, blood shot eyes, bleeding, constipation, amberurine, delirium, mania, abscess and inflammation. The antipyreticPlants can lower the body temperature while the anti-hypertensive herbs can lower the blood pressure.

Antipyretics or Febrifugals - Plants that can Eliminate Heat and Fire

These plants can inhibit the central nervous system, sympathetic nervous system, decrease the basal metabolic rate and heat production. They are diuretic and can lower the blood pressure and decrease blood volume, insomnia, tension and restlessness. They are used for high fever, inflammation, hypertension, delirium. The “fire” is related to lung, liver, heart and stomach fire. It is usually related to high fever and the excitory activity of the central nervous system.

Anxiety and fear have the subjective feeling of dangerous threat (even mortal terror), and suffer from psychological and vegetative symptoms, such as nervousness, concentration problems, head aches, paleness, perspiration, trembles, heartbeat, raised blood pressure and diarrhoea. Anxiety, accompanied by tension and restlessness can continue for weeks. Anxiety is treated with anxiolytics or tranquillisers. The aim is to separate the influence of psychic conditions on the vegetative system. Activation of the GABA receptor with benzodiazepins (at the "benzodiazepin" receptor), leads to attenuation of the limbic system, to muscle relaxation, sedation and spasmolytic effects.

Patients with insomnia suffer from a bad sleep quality, difficulties falling asleep and sleeping without interruptions. Patients worryy much about their insomnia, fear negative consequences and go through mood swings. They show an increased irritability, general tiredness, often also tension and restlessness. Insomnia, tension and restlessness can be treated with GABA receptor agonists and other sedatives. A number of plant extracts affect the GABA receptor. Plants with essential oils can be regarded as mild spasmolytic drugs that also alleviate nervousness and tension.

A distinction is made between primary wounds caused by cuts, stabs, abrasions and scratches and secondary wounds caused by bites, fissures, burns or contusions (bruises with damaged veins below intact skin). Primary wounds heal within six to eight days without loss of tissue after a scab or scurf has been formed. Secondary wounds are slower to heal since new tissue (granuL:ltion tissue) has to be formed and the process is often accompanied by infections and haematomas. Wounds are treated with medicines or medicinal plants that have haemostyptic, disinfectant, wound cleaning, analgesic, anti-inflammatory and astringent properties. Some of these may also promote the formation of granulation tissue and new epithelia. Responsible compounds include flavonoids, tannins, essential oils, sesquiterpenes, saponins, allantoin, benzoylesters, alkylamides, polysaccharides (e.g. mucilage), fatty oils and enzymes (e.g. papain, bromelain).

Psoriasis is a complex disorder (influenced by inherited and psychosomatic factors) and characterised by an enhanced proliferation of epidermal cells (keratocytes) that leads to the extensive production of scales. This disorder is often accompanied by inflammation of the skin. Psoriasis *is* mainly treated symptomatically. Inflammation can be controlled by anti-inflammatory medicines and the proliferation of epidermal cells by chemotherapy. Phytotherapy plays a role in the treatment of psoriasis. Plants with cytotoxic alkaloids, such as berberine, with dianthranols or with phototoxic furanocoumarins (e.g. abundant in members of the Apiaceae) are employed. Furanocoumarins, such as 8-methoxypsoralen, are lipophilic and easily penetrate the skin. Inside the cells furanocoumarins intercalate DNA. If the skin is then exposed to UV light (360 nm) these compounds are activated and can form covalent bonds with thymine bases in the DNA. The alkylation stops DNA replication and induces cell death. Longterm utilisation of this treatment (known as phototherapy), which uses mainly isolated compounds, such as 8-methoxypsoralen, can cause skin cancer. Salicylic acid has also been used to treat psoriasis because of its keratolytic properties; vitamin A derivatives, such as retinoids can influence inflammation and cell proliferation.

Vitiligo is characterised *by* the occurrence of white patches on the skin that can be rmmd or irregular in shape. The origin of vitiligo is uncertain but has been linked to disorders of the nervous system or an inhibition of pigment formation by genetic or immunological factors. Furanocoumarins, such as psoralen, in combination with UV light (UV-A) induce repigmentation of skin parts with vitiligo. Carotenoids, such as P-carotene or canthaxanthin, are deposited in the epidermis and can slightly compensate for the pigment deficiency.

Eczemas are dermal inflammations that affect either the epidermis or cutaneous-vascular tissues. Certain types affect the skin epidermis, e.g. contact dermatitis, allergies and contact eczema, diaper dermatitis and atopic dermatitis (neurodermatitis). The second type of dermatitis includes exanthema caused by chemicals and medicines, plant allergies. urticaria, Quincke's oedema, and photoallergies.. Chronic eczema can be caused by disturbances of the metabolism and a sensible treatment is to improve the basic underlying problems and to induce physiological changes. Treatment with medicinal plants includes the topical application of fatty ointments to protect the skin from unspecific irritations, anti-inflammatory compounds (that block the cascade leading to prostaglandins and leucotrienes: e.g. acid and corticomimetics) and compounds that suppress itching.

Fit-Weed

Antipyretics or Febrifugals: Plants that can Eliminate Heat and Fire

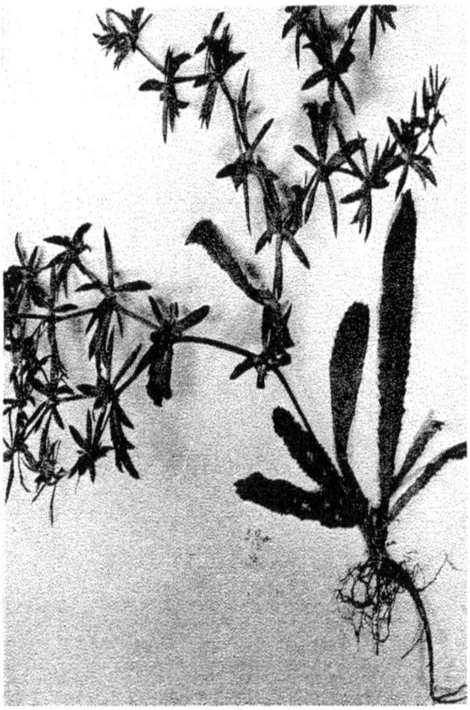

Botanical Name: Eryngium Foetidum.
Family: Apiaceae.
Region Where Grown: Barima-Waini.
Other Names:Cilantro, Coulante, Culantro, Fit Bush, Coriander, Spirit Weed, Nanna-a-run, Stinking weed.
Category: Antipyretics or Febrifugals: Plants that can eliminate heat and fire.
Properties: Acrid, Aromatic, Cook/Dry.
Esoteric Botanica: Sebek.
Governing Organs: Lung, Gall Bladder, Stomach.
Actions & Indications: Whole plant: Plant is boiled and the water drunk as an anti-malarial. Plant is boiled and the water used for an herbal bath or as a medication for chicken pox or for measles. Clears heat and relieves toxicity – for various manifestation of fire toxin in the upper or superficial aspects of the body. It is commonly used for sore teeth, swollen or painful gums, ulcerated lips or gums, canker sores, painful and swollen throat, sores or blotches from warm-febrile diseases.[161] Used for treatment of hemorrhage.
Leaf: Infusion for chills, grippe, febrifuge, head colds, children's purgative; decoction of crushed leaves for children's leprosy and children's convulsions or "fits".[162] and for a febrifuge bath; Leaves are boiled and the water drunk as an anti-pyretic or as a medication for colds. Leaves are used for flavoring food. They are used for coughs and colds, epilepsy and for headaches.
Root: Infusion for a febrifuge, sudorific, hydropsy, stomach pain and abortifacient. It is used traditionally in an infusion taken for fevers, flu, diabetes and constipation, as a diuretic and as an anti-convulsant treatment. In cooking, the leaves are used for their unique pungent aroma as an important seasoning for foods, such as meat dishes, sauces, chutneys and preservatives.
Cautions & Contraindications: Do not use in cases of heat due to yin deficiency, and for patterns where the upper is excessive and the lower is deficient. Also contraindicated in cases of fully erupted measles and in patients with breathing difficulty.
Major Known Ingredients: Leaf shows antimicrobial activity. The aerial parts are rich in calcium, iron and riboflavin, with approximately 0.1- 0.95% essential oil and a peculiar saponin. The aerial part of the plant is high in calcium, iron and carotene and has a good amount of riboflavin.[163]

---

[161] DeFilipps, Robert A., Shirley L. Maina, and Juliette Crepin. *Medicinal Plants of the Guianas (Guyana, Surinam, French Guiana)*. Washington, D.C.: Dept. of Botany, National Museum of Natural History, Smithsonian Institution, 2004; 47
[162] Leeuwenberg, A. J. M. *Medicinal and Poisonous Plants of the Tropics: Proceedings of Symposium 5-35 of the 14th International Botanical Congress, Berlin, 24 July-1 August 1987*. Wageningen: Pudoc, 1987; 56.
[163] Morton, Julia F. *Atlas of Medical Plants of Middle America: Bahamas to Yucatan*. Springfield: Charles C. Thomas, 1981; 647

Pharmacological & Clinical research: The plant has been studied for its anti-inflammatory and other pharmacological properties.

Yarula

Antipyretics or Febrifugals: Plants that can Eliminate Heat and Fire

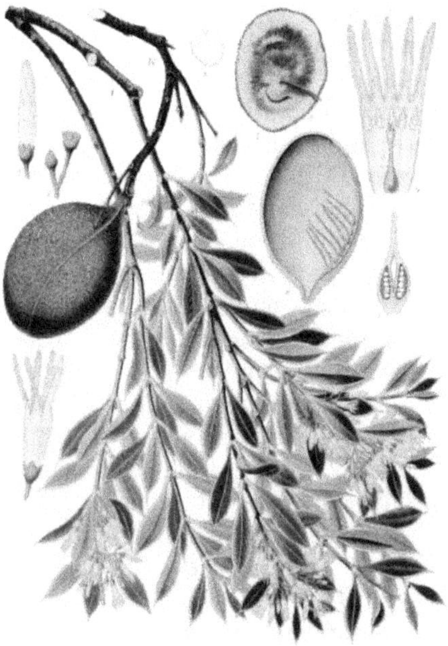

Botanical Name: Aspidosperma Excelsum Bentham.
Family: Apocynaceae.
Region Where Grown: Potaro-Siparuni.
Other Names: Paddlewood, Yaruru, Musara.
Category: Antipyretics or Febrifugals.
Properties: Acrid, Bitter, Cold/Dry.
Esoteric Botanica: Seker.
Governing Organs: Speen, Liver, Stomach, Lung.
Actions & Indications: Bark is boiled and the water drunk as an anti-malarial. Juice from the bark is applied as a medicament for eye infections. Bark is boiled with water and used for washing the skin as medicament for chicken pox.[164] Use to treat malaria. White latex is absorbed on cotton wool and inserted into cavities as an analgesic for toothaches and pain. White latex is mixed with water and inhaled as a medicament for migraine headaches.
Stem: Inner bark is used to treat toothache, and roasted for a warm application to sore eyes red eyes and headache, fever, cough and a sore, red, swollen throat. Clears heat and relieves toxicity – for red swellings, carbuncles, erythemas, mumps and acute febrile maculopapular rashes. Vents rashes – for the early stages of measles when there is incomplete expression of the rash. Moistens intestines – for wind-heat constipation.
Cautions & Contraindications: Do not use for patterns of qi deficiency and diarrhea or open sores and carbuncles.
Major Known Ingredients: Alkaloids of stem-bark show antimicrobial activity

[164] DeFilipps, Robert A., Shirley L. Maina, and Juliette Crepin. *Medicinal Plants of the Guianas (Guyana, Surinam, French Guiana)*. Washington, D.C.: Dept. of Botany, National Museum of Natural History, Smithsonian Institution, 2004; 19

Pop Bush

Antipyretics or Febrifugals: Plants that can Eliminate Heat and Fire

Botanical Name: Physalis Pubescens .
Family: Solanaceae.
Region Where Grown: Demerara-Mahaica.
Other Names: None.
Category: Antipyretics or Febrifugals: Plants that can eliminate heat and fire.
Properties: Bitter, Hot/Dry.
Esoteric Botanica: Heru.
Governing Organs: Heart, Small Intestine, Urinary Bladder, Spleen
Actions & Indications: Aperitive, cholagogue, condiment, diuretic, Whole plant: Infusion used as a narcotic.[165]
Root: Bitter, aperitive, tonic, febrifuge. Used for ground itch,[166] as a diuretic in edema and colic of the kidneys and worms. for Kidney deficiency and waning essence with lower back pain, light headedness, prematurely gray hair, impotence, spermatorrhea and weakness of he lower extremities. Tonifies the spleen and augments the qi – for weakness, shortness of breath, lassitude, reduced appetite and loose stools due to spleen and stomach deficiency.
Leaf: Infusion for a cholagogue. Boiled in a preparation for urine retention. Used to treat swelling. Fruit: Infusion as a diuretic, laxative; vermifuge; and edible condiment when macerated in vinegar. Also used for a successful, but secret, dropsy cure.

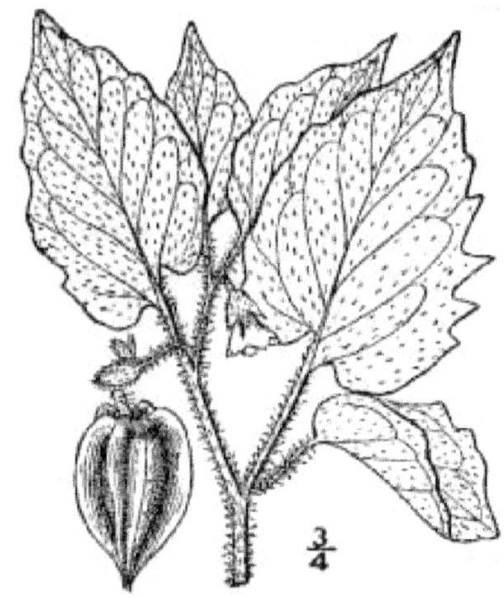

Cautions & Contraindications: Do not use in cases of excess, especially when there is fullness due to dampness, stagnation or accumulation. The fruit contains alkaloid fisaline and is high in niacin. The root contains the alkaloid hygrine.[167]
Major Known Ingredients: Genus *Physalis* contains with anolide lactonic steroids. Physaline is a substance recommended as a quinine substitute for intermittent fevers.[168]

---

[165]DeFilipps, Robert A., Shirley L. Maina, and Juliette Crepin. *Medicinal Plants of the Guianas (Guyana, Surinam, French Guiana)*. Washington, D.C.: Dept. of Botany, National Museum of Natural History, Smithsonian Institution, 2004; 271.
[166] Morton, Julia F. *Atlas of Medical Plants of Middle America: Bahamas to Yucatan*. Springfield: Charles C. Thomas, 1981; 798.

[168] DeFilipps, Robert A., Shirley L. Maina, and Juliette Crepin. *Medicinal Plants of the Guianas (Guyana, Surinam, French Guiana)*. Washington, D.C.: Dept. of Botany, National Museum of Natural History, Smithsonian Institution, 2004; 271.

Spanish Needle

Antipyretics or Febrifugals: Plants that can Eliminate Heat and Fire

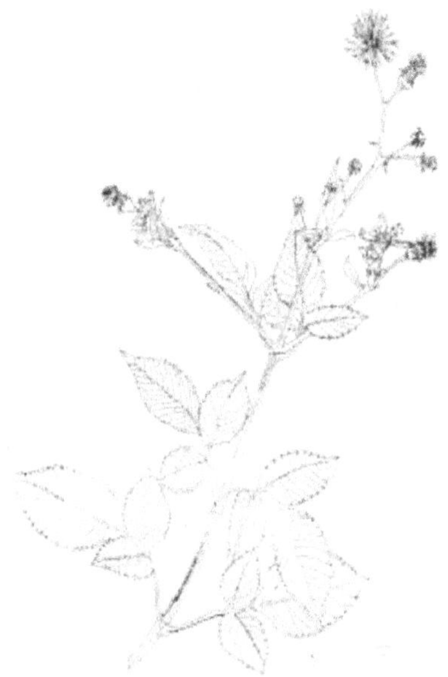

Botanical Name: Bidens Cynapiifolia
Family: Asteraceae
Region Where Grown:Potaro/Siparuni.
Other Names: None.
Category: Antipyretics or Febrifugals: Plants that can eliminate heat and fire.
Properties: Bitter, Acrid, Hot/Dry.
Esoteric Botanica: Tehuti.
Governing Organs: Liver, Gall Bladder.
Actions & Indications: This plant treats an array of medical problems including mouth sores, sore throat, dysentery, chills, toothache and headache; diabetes, jaundicc, hepatitis and it is also used for external cuts and sores.[169]
Whole plant: Rubbed with salt and applied to headache; infusion is antidiarrhoeic; hypotensive; for fevers, eyewash, diabetes and "fluttering heart"[170] or fibrillation. Plant is boiled and the water drunk as an analgesic, antimalarial or antipyretic. Used for diabetes, thrush and ground itch.
Sap: Used for irritated eyes.
Leaf: Juice is antiseptic, for cicatrizing wounds. Juice from macerated leaves is used as an eye drop for treating infections of red, painful or swollen eyes, or headache and dizziness. Also used for eye pain that increases in the evening.
Cautions & Contraindications: Contraindicated for pregnant women. Also used with caution in cases of spleen or stomach deficiency.[171]
Major Known Ingredients: Leaf has antimicrobial activity on Gram-positive bacteria and yeast.[172]

---

[169] Castner, James L., S. Lee. Timme, and James A. Duke. *A Field Guide to Medicinal and Useful Plants of the Upper Amazon*. Gainesville, FL: Feline, 1998; 25.
[170] DeFilipps, Robert A., Shirley L. Maina, and Juliette Crepin. *Medicinal Plants of the Guianas (Guyana, Surinam, French Guiana)*. Washington, D.C.: Dept. of Botany, National Museum of Natural History, Smithsonian Institution, 2004; 42.
[171] Ibid., 42.
[172] Ibid., 42.

Once-a-Mile

Antipyretics or Febrifugals: Plants that can Eliminate Heat and Fire

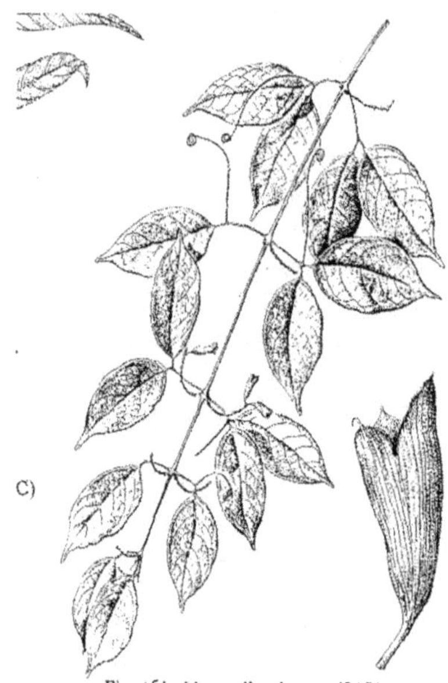

Botanical Name: Martinella Obovata.
Family: Bignoniaceae.
Region Where Grown: Pomeroon-Supenaam.
Other Names: Eye Vine, Akoacorollii, Uquilla, Kamoro
Category: Antipyretics or Febrifugals: Plants that can eliminate heat and fire.
Properties: Sweet, Cold/Moist.
Esoteric Botanica: Auset.
Governing Organs: Stomach, Liver, Lung.
Actions & Indications: Different parts of the plants used for various ailments including conjunctivitis or other eye irritations, chronic wounds, vermifuge and antipyretic.[173]
Root: Juice from the freshly cut tuberous roots is used as an eyedrop to treat infections and relieve sore or irritated eyes.[174] Used for sores and sore eyes, conjunctivitis,[175] for itchy, red and painful eyes and sensitivity to light due to externally-contracted wind-heat. Clears the liver and benefits the eyes – for patterns of liver yang rising with such symptoms as headache, red and painful eyes, excessive tearing, or sensitivity to light.
Leaf: Boiled leaves for treating colds. Clears the eyes and remove superficial visual obstruction – for wind-heat eye problems such as red, painful and swollen eyes or blurry vision. Also treat such common symptoms as red, sore, dry or painful eyes, or spots in front of the eyes.
Cautions & Contraindications: Do not use in cases of exterior deficiency.

C)

[173] Duke, James A., and Rodolfo Vásquez. *Amazonian Ethnobotanical Dictionary*. Boca Raton, FL: CRC, 1994; 112.
[174] DeFilipps, Robert A., Shirley L. Maina, and Juliette Crepin. *Medicinal Plants of the Guianas (Guyana, Surinam, French Guiana)*. Washington, D.C.: Dept. of Botany, National Museum of Natural History, Smithsonian Institution, 2004; 52.
[175] Lewis W.E., M. Elvin-Lewis and M.C. Gnerre. "Introduction to the Ethnobotanical Pharmacopoeia of the Amazonian." *Medicinal and Poisonous Plants of the Tropics.* Ed., A. J. M. Leeuwenberg. Wageningen: Pudoc, 1987; 100.

Wild Coffee

Antipyretics or Febrifugals: Plants that can Eliminate Heat and Fire

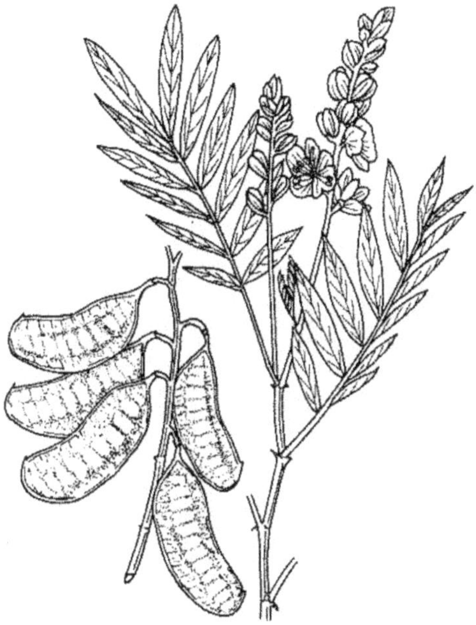

Botanical Name: Senna Occidentalis.
Family: Caesalpiniaceae.
Region Where Grown: All Regions.
Other Names: Cafie Balli, Mayamal, Wild Coffee. Tumuka.
Category: Antipyretics or Febrifugals: Plants that can eliminate heat and fire.
Properties: Sour, Hot/Moist.
Esoteric Botanica: Tehuti.
Governing Organs: Liver, Stomach, Kidney, Small Intestines.
Actions & Indications: Purgative, bilious fever, cholagogue, diabetes, eczema, emetic, febrifuge, kidney stones, leishmaniasis and rheumatism.
Whole plant: Decoction for hypertension, diabetes, biliousness and fever[176]; grippe, thrush; boiled and gargled for throat trouble; pounded and mixed with wood-ash and rubbed on areas of leishmaniasis and eczema. Used for coughs, colds and for "lining cold" (puerperal fever).
Root: Tincture rubbed onto rheumatic areas; decoction for a purgative and emetic; infusion for cholagogue and skin diseases. Infusion for bilious fever, ordinary fever, stomachache and to ease menstruation. Tea made from roots and dried flowers is used for colds, upset stomach and diarrhea.
Leaf: Remedy for renal calculi. Leaves are made into a tea for treating afterbirth problems. Used for treating fevers, coughs and colds, headaches, hemorrhage and thrush. Flower: In a preparation to reduce stomach acid in children.
Seed: Dried, pulverised and roasted as a coffee substitute and for use as a febrifuge.[177] Infusion is drunk to calm one's nerves. Used for treating kidney problems, hemorrhage, worms and cleaning womb and tubes.
Cautions & Contraindications: Contraindicated during pregnancy, menstruation and in nursing mothers. Also, contraindicated for weak patients and those suffering from chronic constipation. Overdose may result in abdominal pain, nausea, and vomiting. [178]
Major Known Ingredients: Extracts of leaf and seed show antibiotic activity. Leaf contains flavonoid glycosides, anthraquinone and bianthraquinone. Seed contains N-methyl morpholine, campesterol and beta-sitosterol glucosides.[179]

---

[176] DeFilipps, Robert A., Shirley L. Maina, and Juliette Crepin. *Medicinal Plants of the Guianas (Guyana, Surinam, French Guiana)*. Washington, D.C.: Dept. of Botany, National Museum of Natural History, Smithsonian Institution, 2004; 72.
[177] Ibid., 73.
[178] Bensky, Dan, Andrew Gamble, and Ted J. Kaptchuk. *Chinese Herbal Medicine: Materia Medica.* Seattle, WA: Eastland, 1993; 118.

Pharmacological & Clinical Research: Folium Sennae contains many anthraquinone glycoside derivatives. Therefore, it has a strong laxative action that may be accompanied by abdominal pain. In addition, the hepatic metabolite of sennoside A and B stimulates the pelvic ganglion, which causes contraction of the colon and diarrhea . In a clinical series of 100 cases, granules of Folium Sennae dissolved in warm water were very effective in treating post partum constipation.[180]

---

[179] DeFilipps, Robert A., Shirley L. Maina, and Juliette Crepin. *Medicinal Plants of the Guianas (Guyana, Surinam, French Guiana)*. Washington, D.C.: Dept. of Botany, National Museum of Natural History, Smithsonian Institution, 2004; 73.

[180] Bensky, Dan, Andrew Gamble, and Ted J. Kaptchuk. *Chinese Herbal Medicine: Materia Medica*. Seattle, WA: Eastland, 1993; 119.

Carrion Crow Bush

Antipyretics or Febrifugals: Plants that can Eliminate Heat and Fire

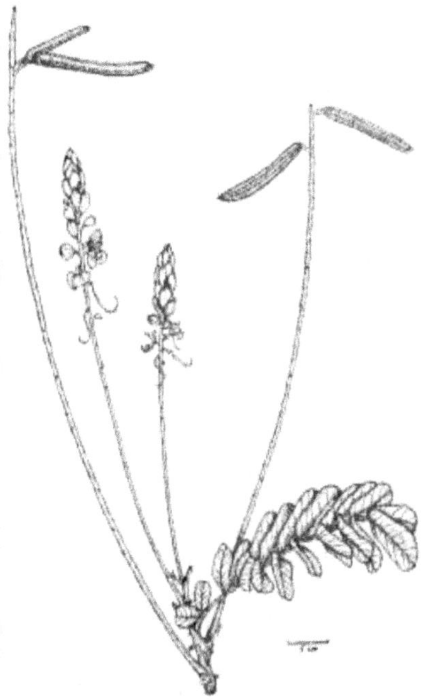

Botanical Name: Senna Reticulata.
Family:Caesalpiniaceae.
Region Where Grown: All Regions.
Other Names: None.
Category: Antipyretics or Febrifugals: Plants that Clear Heat. and Relieve Toxicity .
Properties: Acrid, Bitter, Cold/Dry.
Esoteric Botanica: Sebek.
Governing Organs: Lungs, Large Intestine.
Actions & Indications: Purgative, eczema, emetic, ringworm and skin eruption. Senna is used to treat venereal and skin problems, ringworm and as an insect repellent and against fungal infections.[181]
Whole plant: Decoction for hypertension, diabetes, biliousness and fever; grippe and thrush. [182]
Leaf and Flower: Clears heat, relieves fire toxicity, expels wind and dries dampness – for wind-heat or damp-heat sores, carbuncles and rashes. These are marked by much pus or leaking of yellow fluid, moist skin and pruritus. Crushed in water for treating eczema and other skin eruptions, the crushed leaves being used as a sponge.
Leaf: For the cure of ringworm. Clears damp-heat from the skin – for recurrent ulcers or other hot skin lesions. Used for treating fevers and pneumonia and as a laxative. for the early stages of warm-febrile diseases with such symptoms as simultaneous chill and fever with chill predominating; little or no sweating, cough, slight sensitivity to wind, sore throat, headache, and a rapid and floating pulse.
Flower: As an emetic and as a laxative.
Seed: The boiled seeds are used for the treatment of Bright's disease. Exhaustion or deficiency of Lung and kidney yin with heat (night sweats, steaming bone disorder, irritability, afternoon or low-grade fevers, malar flush, five center fever, insomnia, irritability and bleeding gums. Also for such kidney vacuity heat signs as spermatorrhea, nocturnal emissions and abnormally elevated sexual drive. Generates fluids and clears heat – for oral ulcers & inflammation due to yin deficiency as well as wasting and thirsting disorder (diabetes).
Cautions & Contraindications: Do not use in cases of diarrhea due to spleen deficiency.

---

[181] Castner, James L., S. Lee. Timme, and James A. Duke. *A Field Guide to Medicinal and Useful Plants of the Upper Amazon*. Gainesville, FL: Feline, 1998; 114.
[182] DeFilipps, Robert A., Shirley L. Maina, and Juliette Crepin. *Medicinal Plants of the Guianas (Guyana, Surinam, French Guiana)*. Washington, D.C.: Dept. of Botany, National Museum of Natural History, Smithsonian Institution, 2004; 72.

Pap-Bush

Antipyretics or Febrifugals: Plants that can Eliminate Heat and Fire

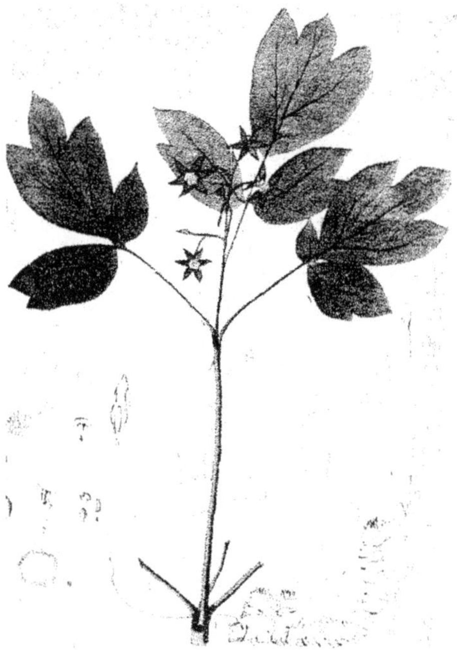

Botanical Name: Physalis Angulata.
Family: Solanaceae.
Region Where Grown: U. Takutu-U. Essequibo.
Other Names: Monkey-Gun, Papoose .
Category: Antipyretics or Febrifugals: Plants that can eliminate heat and fire.
Properties: Bitter, Hot/Dry.
Esoteric Botanica: Herukhuti.
Governing Organs: Heart, Stomach, Kidney.
Actions & Indications: Antiabortive and carminative. Leaves and fruits used as narcotics the decoction as an inflamatory and disinfectant for skin diseases (Leaf juice used for worms, earache, liver, malaria and rheumatism). Leaf infusion is drunk as a diuretic and for asthma. [183] Root infusion used for hepatitis. The sap is usded for earache.[184]
Whole plant: Decoction used to treat upset stomach and Bright's disease[185]; Infusion is a remedy for indigestion, nephritis and fever.[186] Whole plant is antidote for poison and good for cold and to relieve boils in the rectum.[187] Used in treatment of skin diseases. Clears heat and dries dampness – for damp-heat dysenteric disorder, hot painful urinary dysfunction and eczema. Clears damp-heat from the skin – for recurrent ulcers or other hot skin lesions.
Decocted fruit cures swelling, fever and is diuretic.
Cautions & Contraindications: Do not use in cases of spleen deficiency with or without diarrhea.

---

[183] Duke, James A., and Rodolfo Vásquez. *Amazonian Ethnobotanical Dictionary*. Boca Raton, FL: CRC, 1994; 136.
[184] Ibid., 136.
[185] DeFilipps, Robert A., Shirley L. Maina, and Juliette Crepin. *Medicinal Plants of the Guianas (Guyana, Surinam, French Guiana)*. Washington, D.C.: Dept. of Botany, National Museum of Natural History, Smithsonian Institution, 2004; 220.
[186] Morton, Julia F. *Atlas of Medical Plants of Middle America: Bahamas to Yucatan*. Springfield: Charles C. Thomas, 1981; 797.
[187] Astschull, S. Von R. *Drugs and Foods from Little-known Plants Notes in Harvard University Herbaria* Cambridge: Harvard University, 1973; 269.

Stinkwood

Antipyretics or Febrifugals: Plants that can Eliminate Heat and Fire

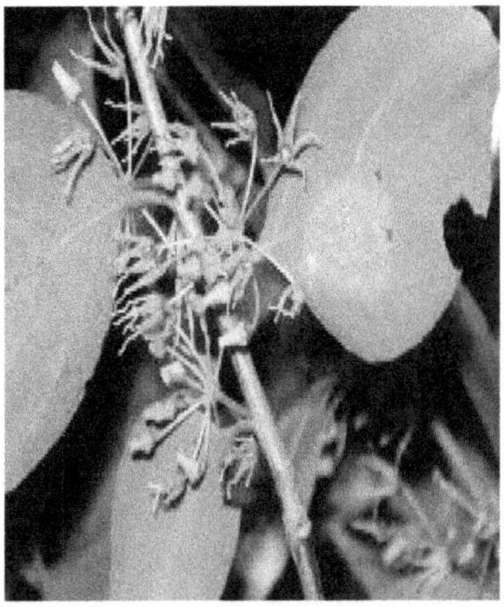

Botanical Name: Goupia Glabra.
Family: Celastraceae.
Region Where Grown: E. Berbice-Corentyne.
Other Names: Goupi.
Category: Antipyretics or Febrifugals: Plants that can eliminate heat and fire.
Properties: Astringent, Acrid, Cold/Dry.
Esoteric Botanica: Sebek.
Governing Organs: Lung, Liver, Large Intestine.
Actions & Indications: Fever, astringent, dental analgesic, headache, syphilis, toothache, tooth decay and as a vermifuge.
Bark is used for soothing a toothache.[188] Clears heat and eliminates irritability – for heat patterns with irritability and thirst. Also used for mouth sores and swollen, painful gums due to heat in the heart or stomach channels. It is used for toothache and to treat chickenpox and eczema. Clears heat and relieves fire toxicity – primarily for dysenteric disorders, especially those due to damp-heat in the stomach or intestines.
Stem: Juice from fresh inner bark is applied to cotton wool and inserted in an aching tooth cavity as an excellent dental analgesic.
Bark decoction drunk for malaria. Cold water infusion of bark is drunk for a vermifuge.
Sap of inner bark drunk as vermifuge.
Leaf: Decoction used as a wash to treat headache and fever. Leaves are used in an astringent decoction to treat syphilis and chicken pox. It is also used for eye disorders such as cataracts.[189]
Cautions & Contraindications: Do not use in cases of chronic dysenteric disorders with injured spleen and stomach qi.

---

[188] DeFilipps, Robert A., Shirley L. Maina, and Juliette Crepin. *Medicinal Plants of the Guianas (Guyana, Surinam, French Guiana)*. Washington, D.C.: Dept. of Botany, National Museum of Natural History, Smithsonian Institution, 2004; 81
[189] Duke, James A., and Rodolfo Vásquez. *Amazonian Ethnobotanical Dictionary*. Boca Raton, FL: CRC, 1994; 82

Antipyretics or Febrifugals - Plants that can Eliminate Heat by Cooling the Blood

These plants are antipyretic, cardiotonic and cholagogue. They can inhibit the sympathetic nervous system, decrease the basal metabolic rate, heat production and lower the blood pressure.

Iguana Wood

Antipyretics or Febrifugals: Plants that can eliminate heat by cooling the blood

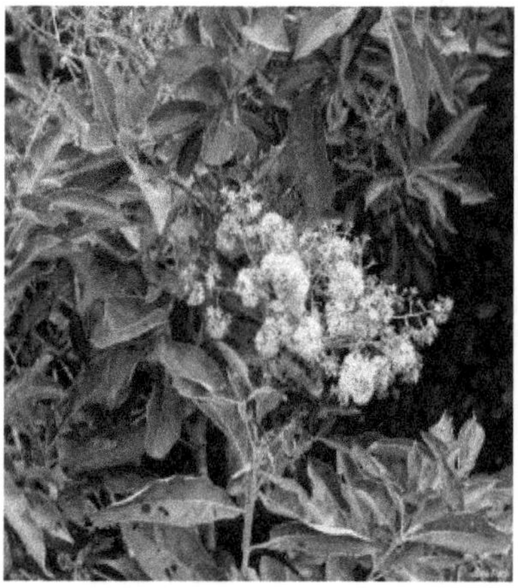

Botanical Name: Cordia Tetrandra.
Family: Boraginaceae.
Region Where Grown: E. Berbice-Corentyne.
Other Names: Clammy Cherry, Table Tree, Torch Tree, Turkey Berry, Yuwanaro.
Category: Antipyretics or Febrifugals: Plants that Eliminate Heat by Draining Fire.
Properties: Bitter, Hot/Dry.
Esoteric Botanica: Herukhuti.
Governing Organs:Stomach, Liver.
Actions & Indications: Leaf: Decoction of dried, finely crushed leaves in water is used for high blood pressure.[190] Clears the Liver and brightens the eyes – for ascending liver fire with red, painful, swollen eyes or headache and dizziness. Also used for eye pain that increases in the evening due to liver deficiency, especially when the eyes are neither red nor swollen. Clears heat and dissipates nodules – for any neck lumps or nodules as in scrofula, lipoma, swollen glands or goiter due to phlegm-fire. Also used for similar nodules in the inguinal canal and other parts of the body. Treats hypertension – recently used for this purpose, especially when accompanied by liver fire or ascendant yang patterns. Drains damp-heat from the liver and gallbladder channels – for damp-heat in the upper portion of the gallbladder channel with such symptoms as red, swollen sore throat and eyes, swollen and painful ears or sudden deafness. Also for damp-heat in the liver or gallbladder channels (especially the lower parts) with such symptoms as jaundice, pain, swelling or dampness in the genital area or foul-smelling vaginal discharge and itching. Drains and pacifies excessive liver fire – for liver fire blazing upward with headache or red eyes. Also for liver wind-heat with fever, spasm, convulsions or flank pain.
Cautions & Contraindications: Use with caution in cases of cold in the middle burner, or with a restless fetus due to cold in the blood. Do not use in cases of spleen or stomach deficiency with diarrhea.

---

[190] DeFilipps, Robert A., Shirley L. Maina, and Juliette Crepin. *Medicinal Plants of the Guianas (Guyana, Surinam, French Guiana)*. Washington, D.C.: Dept. of Botany, National Museum of Natural History, Smithsonian Institution, 2004; 58.

Powis Eye

Antipyretics or Febrifugals: Plants that can eliminate heat by cooling the blood

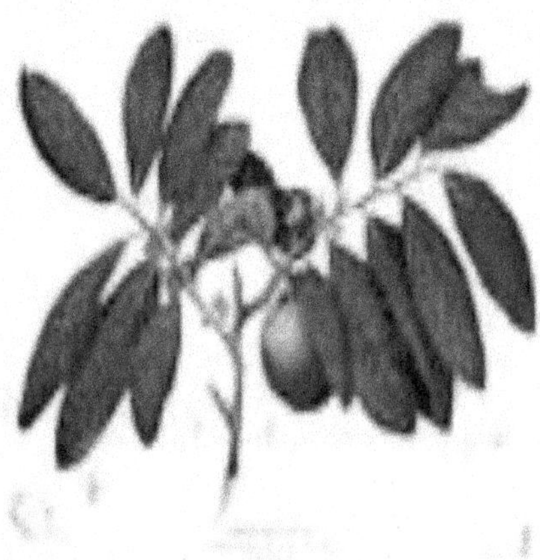

Botanical Name: Diospyros Guianensis.
Family: Ebenaceae.
Region Where Grown: U. Takutu-U. Essequibo.
Other Names: Pedakuruk, Barabara.
Category: Antipyretics or Febrifugals: Plants that can eliminate heat .
Properties: Bitter, Hot/Dry.
Esoteric Botanica: Herukhuti.
Governing Organs: Heart, Large Intestine, Lung
Actions & Indications: Stem: Bark decoction as a wash for fevers.
Leaf: Leaves are crushed in a little oil and the juice is applied to certain eczematous dermatoses.[191] Vents rashes – used in the early stages of rashes (e.g. measles) to induce the rash to come to the surface to speed recovery. Clears heat and relieves toxicity – for red swellings, carbuncles, erythemas, mumps and acute febrile maculopapular rashes. Also used as a febrifuge.
Cautions & Contraindications: Do not use in cases of exterior deficiency or yin deficiency with heat signs. Not recommended for nursing mothers as the herb may lead to insufficient lactation.
Major Known Ingredients: Stem-bark contains a naphthaquinone which alleviates certain dermal lesions and the terpenes lupeol, betulinol and betulinic acid.[192]

[191] DeFilipps, Robert A., Shirley L. Maina, and Juliette Crepin. *Medicinal Plants of the Guianas (Guyana, Surinam, French Guiana)*. Washington, D.C.: Dept. of Botany, National Museum of Natural History, Smithsonian Institution, 2004; 113.
[192] Ibid., 113.

Dove Weed

Antipyretics or Febrifugals: Plants that can eliminate heat by cooling the blood

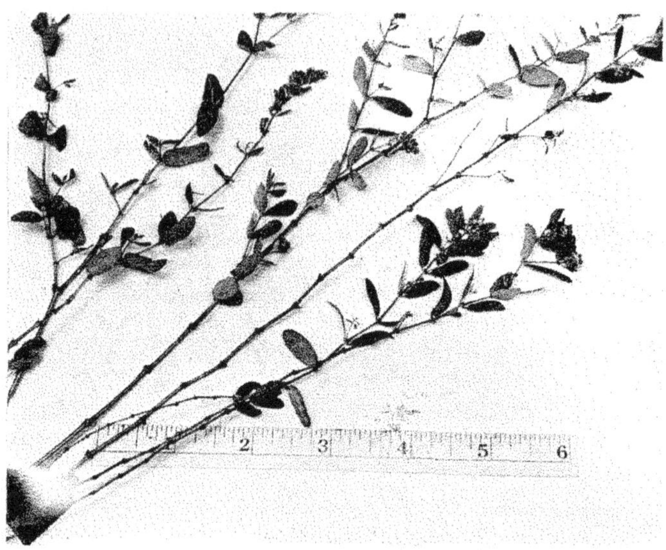

Botanical Name: Chamaesyce Hirta.
Family: Euphorbiaceae.
Region Where Grown: Demerara-Mahaica.
Other Names: Milkweed.
Category: Antipyretics or Febrifugals: Plants that can eliminate heat by cooling the blood
Properties: Sweet, Hot/Dry
Esoteric Botanica: Herukhuti
Governing Organs: Stomach, Spleen
Actions & Indications: Whole plant: Anti-inflammatory as applied to insect bites and snakebite; infusion is cholagogue, febrifuge and used to remedy intestinal afflictions, colds and flatulence;[193] An infusion of the entire plant is used as a febrifuge, diuretic, antispasmodic and antiasthmatic.[194]
Leaf: Infusion used as a cholagogue and to treat diarrhea. Crushed, smoked in a cigarette to relieve asthma. Bruised or chopped leaves employed in a restorative cataplasm to treat adenitis and abscesses. Leaf is also decoted to stop dysentery, also as a diuretic in bladder and kidney diseases and to dissolve kidney stones.[195] It is also used as a remedy for influenza, fever, measles, hypertension and urinary burning.
Cautions & Contraindications: Do not in cases of spleen or stomach cold from deficiency with loose stools, or in exterior conditions.
Major Known Ingredients: Contains shickimic acid, which is an antispasmodic principle, as well as taxerol, friedeline, beta sitosterol and ellagic acid. [196] The plant also contains leucocyanidol, quercitol, camphol, quercitrin and quercitrol derivative containing rhamnose and a chlorophenolic acid.
Pharmacological & Clinical Research: This plant is used in European medicine for cardiac asthma.

---

193 DeFilipps, Robert A., Shirley L. Maina, and Juliette Crepin. *Medicinal Plants of the Guianas (Guyana, Surinam, French Guiana)*. Washington, D.C.: Dept. of Botany, National Museum of Natural History, Smithsonian Institution, 2004; 115.
194 Morton F. Julia, *Atlas of Medical Plants of Middle America: Bahamas to Yucatan*. Springfield, Illinois: Charles C Thomas Publisher, 1981; 425.
195 Leeuwenberg, A. J. M. *Medicinal and Poisonous Plants of the Tropics: Proceedings of Symposium 5-35 of the 14th International Botanical Congress, Berlin, 24 July-1 August 1987*. Wageningen: Pudoc, 1987;99.
196 DeFilipps, Robert A., Shirley L. Maina, and Juliette Crepin. *Medicinal Plants of the Guianas (Guyana, Surinam, French Guiana)*. Washington, D.C.: Dept. of Botany, National Museum of Natural History, Smithsonian Institution, 2004; 115

Toxicity: In experimental animals, the plant produces bronchial dilatation but depresses respiration and heart action. In large doses, it irritates the stomach and causes nausea and vomiting. Handling the plant may cause dermatitis.[197]

---

[197] DeFilipps, Robert A., Shirley L. Maina, and Juliette Crepin. *Medicinal Plants of the Guianas (Guyana, Surinam, French Guiana)*. Washington, D.C.: Dept. of Botany, National Museum of Natural History, Smithsonian Institution, 2004; 426

Breadfruit

Antipyretics or Febrifugals: Plants that can eliminate heat by cooling the blood

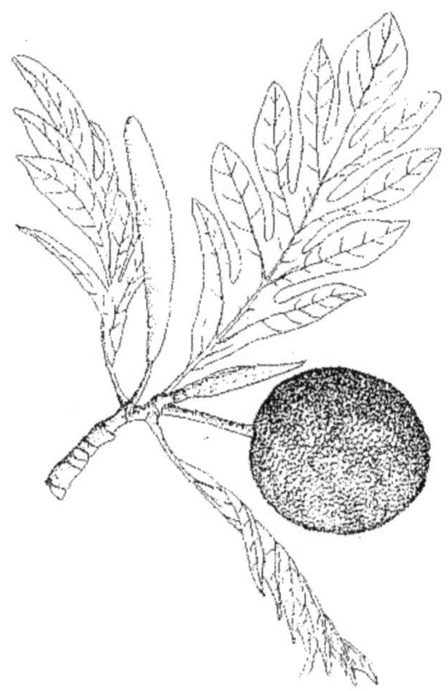

Botanical Name: Artocarpus Altilis.
Family: Moraceae .
Region Where Grown: All Regions.
Other Names: None.
Category: Antipyretics or Febrifugals: Plants that can Eliminate Heat by Cooling the Blood.
Properties: Acrid, Cold/Dry.
Esoteric Botanica: Sebek.
Governing Organs:Lung, Liver, Urinary Bladder.
Actions & Indications: Effective against hypertension. Used for boils, burns, diabetes, gout, oliguria, rheumatism, sores and tumors. Stem: Exudate used to treat abcesses, bruises and sprains. for warm-febrile diseases accompanied by extreme heat or heat signs and for very high fevers at the nutritive or blood level with reckless movement of blood. Fire toxins may be either severe fevers or pustulate damp-heat sores (boils, carbuncles, or appendicitis). Leaf: Used in a decoction which is drunk to reduce hypertension[198] and diabetes.[199] Leaf used to treat urinary tract ailments. Clears heat and promotes urination – for such disorders as damp-heat in the Small Intestine, painful urinary dysfunction, and hot edema.
Cautions & Contraindications: Use with great caution during pregnancy. Should only be used for excessive disorders. Do not use for rashes in cases of qi deficiency or where there is no high fever.
Major Known Ingredients: Fruit contains artocarpine and the enzyme papayotine. Leaf contains the phenols quercetin and camphorol, and gamma-aminobutyric acid, which lowers the blood pressure. Stem-bark and fruit contain cyclopropane sterols.
Pharmacological & Clinical Research:
Toxicity: Leaves contain quercetin and camphorol.[200]

---

[198] Leeuwenberg, A. J. M. *Medicinal and Poisonous Plants of the Tropics: Proceedings of Symposium 5-35 of the 14th International Botanical Congress, Berlin, 24 July-1 August 1987*. Wageningen: Pudoc, 1987; 99
[199] DeFilipps, Robert A., Shirley L. Maina, and Juliette Crepin. *Medicinal Plants of the Guianas (Guyana, Surinam, French Guiana)*. Washington, D.C.: Dept. of Botany, National Museum of Natural History, Smithsonian Institution, 2004; 197.
[200] Morton F. Julia, *Atlas of Medical Plants of Middle America: Bahamas to Yucatan*. Springfield, Illinois: Charles C Thomas Publisher, 1981; 426.

Antipyretics or Febrifugals - Plants that can Eliminate Heat and Toxin

These plants have strong antibiotic effect. Some inhibit the growth of virus, fubgus, bacteria and even cancer cells. Some inhibit the immunity function of the body. They can destroy toxins produced by pryogens. They can enhance the function of the adrenals.

Duka

Antipyretics or Febrifugals: Plants that can Eliminate Heat and Toxin

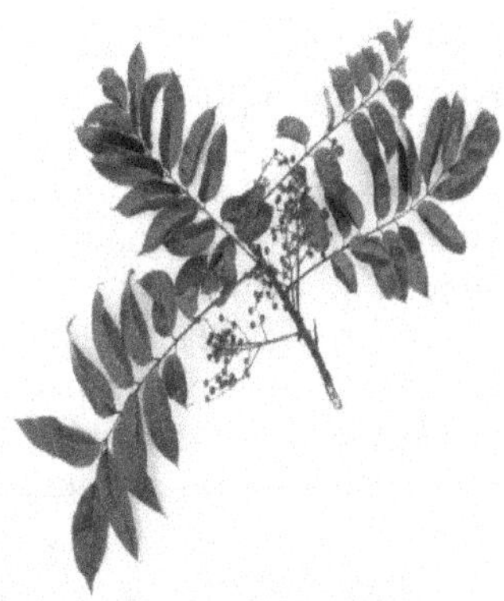

Botanical Name: Tapiriria Guianensis.
Family: Anacardiaceae.
Region Where Grown: U. Takutu-U. Essequibo.
Other Names: Makarin, Warimia, Atapereri.
Category: Antipyretics or Febrifugals: Plants that can Eliminate Heat and Toxins.
Properties: Sour, Hot/Moist.
Esoteric Botanica: Tehuti.
Governing Organs: Liver, Gall Bladder.
Actions & Indications: Treats dysuria, fever and thrush.
Bark: Finely ground bark is ingested for children's thrush; bark decoction used as a fever bath; bark infusion for washing ulcers; treats warm-febrile diseases accompanied by extreme heat or heat signs and for very high fevers at the nutritive or blood level with reckless movement of blood. Fire toxins may be either severe fevers or pustulate damp-heat sores (boils, carbuncles or appendicitis). Inner bark used to dress cuts and sores and to treat snakebite. Relieves toxicity – for toxic sores, swollen and painful throat and snakebite. Bark used in treatment of sores and for wounds/cuts. Also used as a purgative.
Flowers: Tea from flower is used by elderly persons experiencing painful urination.
Cautions & Contraindications: Do not in cases of spleen or stomach cold from deficiency with loose stools or in exterior conditions.
Pharmacological & Clinical Research: Stem yields an abundant oleoresin fluid which is recommended for syphilitic ulcers.

Buri

Antipyretics or Febrifugals: Plants that Eliminate Heat and Dampness

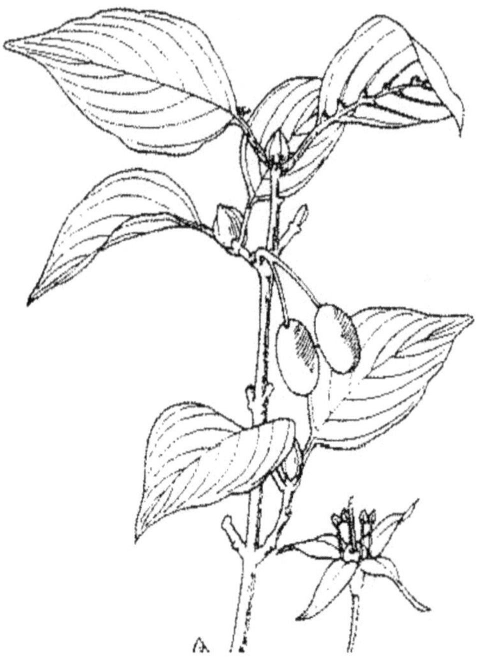

Botanical Name: Tabernaemontana Undulata.
Family: Apocynaceae.
Region Where Grown: U. Takutu-U. Essequibo.
Other Names: Dogwood.
Category: Antipyretics or Febrifugals: Plants that can Eliminate Heat and Toxins.
Properties: Bitter, Hot/Dry.
Esoteric Botanica: Heru.
Governing Organs: Heart, Liver, Large Intestine, Lung
Actions & Indications: Febrifuge, astringent and diaphoretic.
Whole plant: Latex used for removing "mosquito worms" from body, and placed on cotton plug for toothache.[201]
Root: Used to treat headaches .
Stem: Grated bark used in a plaster for headache, and as a resolvent for small abscesses; latex extracted from the trunk is placed on absorbent cotton as a tampon for painful dental cavities.
Leaf: Macerated for an eyewash to remedy conjunctivitis. Petiole-latex applied to penis for gonorrhoea. Also used to soothe bites and for skin irritations and snakebite wounds.
Cautions & Contraindications: Do not use in cases of spleen or stomach cold from deficiency with loose stools or in exterior conditions.
Major Known Ingredients: Alkaloids in stem-bark include conopharyngine, jollyanine, voacangine, isovoacangine, ibophyllidine, coronaridine and heyneanine. Leaf contains the alkaloids angustine, pleiocarpamine, tubotaiwine, hydroxycoronaridine and hydroxyheyneanine. [202]

---

[201] DeFilipps, Robert A., Shirley L. Maina, and Juliette Crepin. *Medicinal Plants of the Guianas (Guyana, Surinam, French Guiana)*. Washington, D.C.: Dept. of Botany, National Museum of Natural History, Smithsonian Institution, 2004; 25.
[202] Ibid., p. 26

Bitter Tally

Antipyretics or Febrifugals: Plants that Eliminate Heat and Dampness

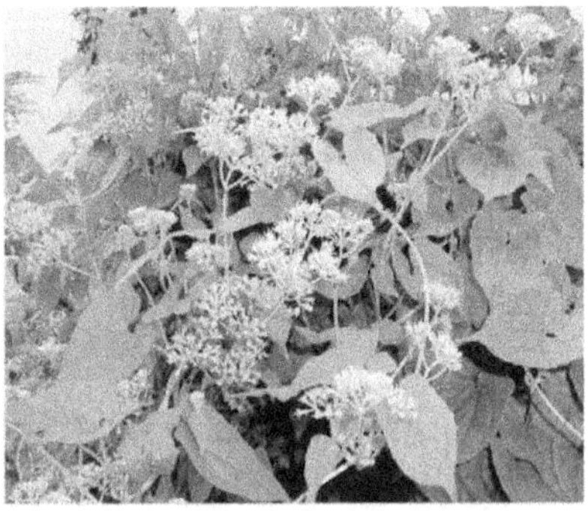

Botanical Name: Mikania Micrantha.
Family: Asteraceae.
Region Where Grown:Upper Demerara/Berbice.
Other Names: None.
Category: Antipyretics or Febrifugals: Plants that can Eliminate Heat and Toxins.
Properties:Sweet, Cold/Dry.
Esoteric Botanica: Seker.
Governing Organs: Stomach, Spleen, Liver.
Actions & Indications: Used as an antimalarial, antisyphilitic, and for treating skin ulcers and indigestion. [203]
Whole plant: Tea for stomachache and to clean out the uterus (dilation and curettage). Boiled with other plants for tonic to reduce malarial fever.
Stem and Leaf: Decoction for a children's clyster. Used to treat malaria and eczema.
Leaf: Juice for external ulcers and itch. Infusion for snakebite and syphilis; bowels; cholagogue. Leaf in liquid mixture for children's anal thrush, and placed in hot water bath for women after confinement for pregnancy. Decoction for a febrifuge bath; in a diuretic tea. Infusion used for washing rashes, skin eruptions and smallpox. Leaves are boiled, and the water drunk as an anti-menorrhagic. Leaves are boiled, and the water used for washing the skin as a treatment for chicken pox or for measles. Juice from macerated leaves is applied to persistent sores and "bush-yaws". Macerated leaves are vigorously rubbed on skin as a treatment for wounds, bruises, tumors and syphilitic sores.[204]
Cautions & Contraindications: Do not use for measles. Use with caution in cases of Spleen or Stomach deficiency, as the herb had a mild laxative effect.
Major Known Ingredients: The leaves contain guacin and tannins. The ground leaves and stems contain the sesquiterpene lactones mikanolide and dihydromikanolide.[205]

---

[203] DeFilipps, Robert A., Shirley L. Maina, and Juliette Crepin. *Medicinal Plants of the Guianas (Guyana, Surinam, French Guiana)*. Washington, D.C.: Dept. of Botany, National Museum of Natural History, Smithsonian Institution, 2004; 46.
[204] Morton F. Julia, *Atlas of Medical Plants of Middle America: Bahamas to Yucatan.* Springfield, Illinois: Charles C Thomas Publisher, 1981; 948.
[205] Ibid., p. 948.

Phootee

Antipyretics or Febrifugals: Plants that Eliminate Heat and Dampness

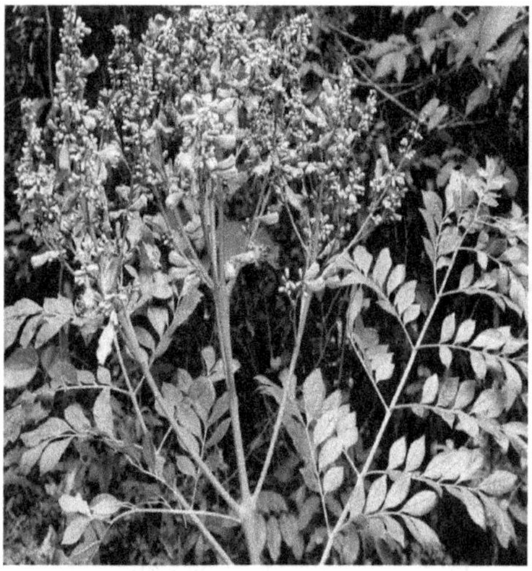

Botanical Name: Jacaranda Copaia.
Family: Bignoniaceae.
Region Where Grown: Potaro-Siparuni
Other Names: Aku, Pasai, Futui, Copaia, Pasa.
Category: Antipyretics or Febrifugals: Plants that can Eliminate Heat and Toxins.
Properties: Acrid, Cool/Dry.
Esoteric Botanica: Sebek.
Governing Organs: Lungs, Spleen, Large Intestine.
Actions & Indications: Fever, dysentery, insect repellant, leishmaniasis, purgative, ringworm, skin diseases, syphilis,
Stem: Leafy branches burned in the dry season to repel insects;
Bark: Used in an antisyphilitic powder as a purgative and for dysentery.[206]
Leaf: In a plaster with soap to treat leishmaniasis (bos-yaws).
Leaf decoction for bronchitis, fever and rheumatism.[207]
Decoction for fevers; in a pomade for skin diseases such as ringworm.
Juice from the young leaves is warmed and applied to persistent sores. Used for fevers, sores, syphilis, toothache and leishmaniasis.
Leaf and Wood: Leaves and wood are used for smoking as an insect repellant. Used for treating skin sores and ulcers. Considered cathartic and emetic.
Crushed leaves are used for treating sores, wounds, and infected cuts.[208]
Cautions & Contraindications: Do not use in cases of spleen or stomach cold from deficiency with loose stools or in exterior conditions.

---

[206] DeFilipps, Robert A., Shirley L. Maina, and Juliette Crepin. *Medicinal Plants of the Guianas (Guyana, Surinam, French Guiana)*. Washington, D.C.: Dept. of Botany, National Museum of Natural History, Smithsonian Institution, 2004; 51.
[207] Duke, James A., and Rodolfo Vásquez. *Amazonian Ethnobotanical Dictionary*. Boca Raton, FL: CRC, 1994; 98.
[208] Leeuwenberg, A. J. M. *Medicinal and Poisonous Plants of the Tropics: Proceedings of Symposium 5-35 of the 14th International Botanical Congress, Berlin, 24 July-1 August 1987*. Wageningen: Pudoc, 1987; 100.

White Cedar

Antipyretics or Febrifugals: Plants that Eliminate Heat and Dampness

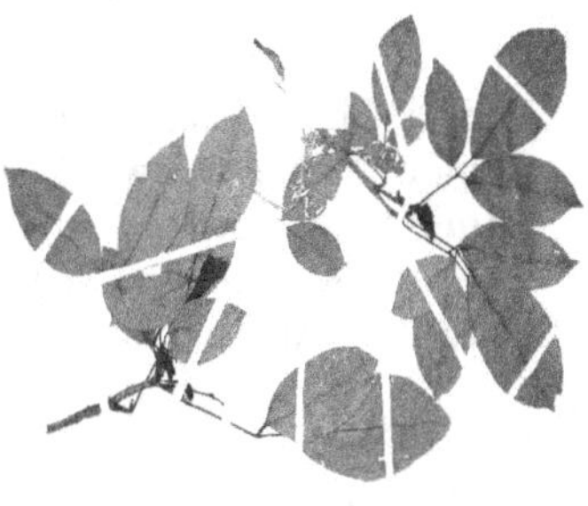

Botanical Name: Tabebuia Insignis.
Family: Bignonia.
Region Where Grown: U. Takutu-U. Essequibo.
Other Names: Warakuri, Greenheart, Ironwood.
Category: Antipyretics or Febrifugals: Plants that can Eliminate Heat and Toxins.
Properties: Sweet, Cold/Moist.
Esoteric Botanica: Auset;
Governing Organs: Stomach, Lung.
Actions & Indications: Bark: Used for malaria. Infusion of bark employed for treating skin diseases and syphilis.[209] Clears heat, cools the blood and relieves fire toxicity while venting rashes – for encouraging rashes to surface, or if the course of a disease like chickenpox or measles is not going well, for encouraging the complete expression of the rash. Often used for fire toxin with very dark purple rashes. Clears damp-heat from the skin – applied topically for damp-heat skin lesion or vaginal itching. Also used for burns. Used for treating skin diseases. Clears heat and toxin and dissipates nodules – for hard, hot sores such as boils and carbuncles. Expels externally-contracted wind-heat - for the early stages of warm-febrile diseases with such symptoms as simultaneous chills and fever with chill predominating with little or no sweating.
Cautions & Contraindications: Do not use in cases of diarrhea due to spleen and stomach cold from deficiency. Also use with caution with yin-deficiency (non-healing) sores.

[209] DeFilipps, Robert A., Shirley L. Maina, and Juliette Crepin. *Medicinal Plants of the Guianas (Guyana, Surinam, French Guiana)*. Washington, D.C.: Dept. of Botany, National Museum of Natural History, Smithsonian Institution, 2004; 54.

Counta

Antipyretics or Febrifugals: Plants that Eliminate Heat and Dampness

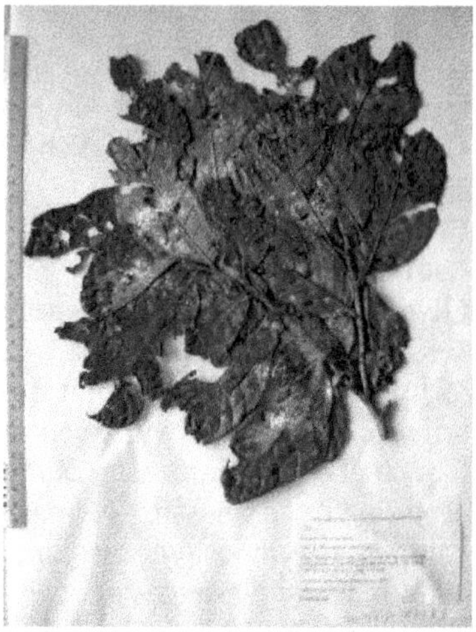

Botanical Name: Licania Heteromorpha.
Family:Chrysobalanaceae.
Region Where Grown: Barima-Waini.
Other Names: Man Wattle, Counta, Tensen. Kairiballi.
Kariballi, Kautaballi. Carib: Yapopare. Wapishana: Tiwowatan.
Category: Antipyretics or Febrifugals: Plants that can Eliminate Heat and Toxins.
Properties: Bitter, Hot/Dry.
Esoteric Botanica: Herukhuti
Governing Organs: Heart, Stomach, Large Intestine, Spleen
Actions & Indications: Whole plant: Sap is applied externally to sores and skin blemishes such as "lotta" - a fungal infection. Cools the blood and reduces blotches – for blotches or other skin eruptions due to heat in the blood. Often used in cases with intense fever, irritability and changes in consciousness
Stem: Infusion of bark used to treat gonorrhoea and diarrhoea; drains heat, relieves fire toxicity, cools the blood and benefits the throat – for warm-febrile diseases, warm epidemic disorders, mumps and painful swollen throat conditions.
Powdered outer bark is sprinkled on wounds to keep them clean and dry.
Cautions & Contraindications: Do not use in cases where the patient is weak, or in the absence of fire toxin.

Coraila

Antipyretics or Febrifugals: Plants that Eliminate Heat and Dampness

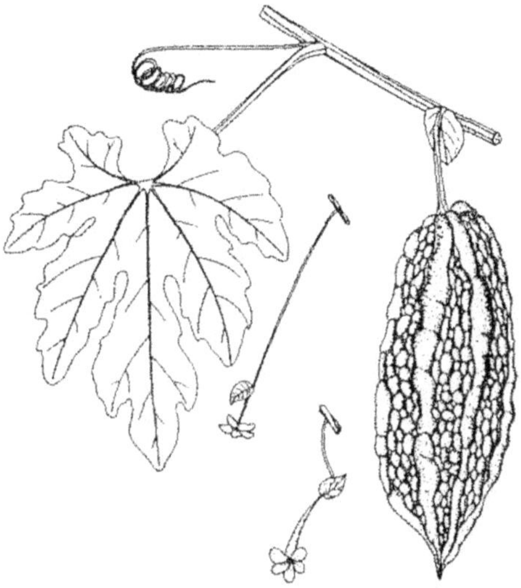

Botanical Name: Momordica Charantia.
Family: Cucurbitaceae.
Region Where Grown: Demerara-Mahaica.
Other Names: Baan-Caryla, Carailli, Caryla, Wild Caryla. Carilla Bush. Bitter Melon, Bitter gourd, Clasam pear, Balsam Pear, Balsam Apple, Cerasee, Karela, Sorrow Seed
Category: Antipyretics or Febrifugals: Plants that can Eliminate Heat and Toxins.
Properties: Cool/Dry, Acrid.
Esoteric Botanica: Sebek
Governing Organs: Lung, Large Intestine
Actions & Indications: Plant decoction used for colic, and worms. The plant is considered vermicidal stomachic, emmenagogue and very effective in the expulsion of *Trichocephaios.* Decoction used as febrifuge and emetic.
Whole plant is boiled and the water used as a tonic and anti-diarrheal. The vine is boiled and the decotion taken before and after childbirth as a cleanser. Plant is boiled and a pinch of table salt is added to the water, which is drunk to treat biliousness.
Stem, Leaf and Fruit: Decoction for diabetes, cancer, external ulcers and sores, bitter tonic.[210] Drains heat and relieves fire toxicity – for any heat disorder, especially Liver heat with red, swollen and painful eyes. Reduces abscesses and dissipates nodules – for abscesses and sores, particularly if they are firm and hard; especially useful for breast and intestinal abscesses.
Stem and Leaf: Dried leaves and stems are boiled and the water drunk as an antidiabetic, as an anti-hypertensive or as a treatment for biliousness.
Leaf: In an antiseptic bath for children; infusion is febrifuge; juice in a vermifuge infusion, also drunk for malaria and hepatitis, fevers and biliousness.[211] The leaf is also cooked as a children's anthelmintic and for scabies or itch. Infusion for stomach cramps. Leaves used in a tea for cleansing the blood. Leaves are boiled and the water drunk as an anti-hypertensive, as an antidiabetic or to purify the blood. Leaves are boiled and the water used as an antidiuretic and to also treat malaria.
Flower: Flowers and young leaves are boiled and the water drunk as a medication for hepatitis.
Cautions & Contraindications: This is a relatively safe herb. Overdose can cause mild diarrhea.

---

[210] DeFilipps, Robert A., Shirley L. Maina, and Juliette Crepin. *Medicinal Plants of the Guianas (Guyana, Surinam, French Guiana).* Washington, D.C.: Dept. of Botany, National Museum of Natural History, Smithsonian Institution, 2004; 103.

[211] Leeuwenberg, A. J. M. *Medicinal and Poisonous Plants of the Tropics: Proceedings of Symposium 5-35 of the 14th International Botanical Congress, Berlin, 24 July-1 August 1987.* Wageningen: Pudoc, 1987; 99.

Major Known Ingredients: Contains antileukemic, estrogenic and hypoglycemic chemicals. Seed contains abortifacient proteins, as well as the glucosidic steroid charantine which has an insulin-like hypoglycemic activity, and the oncostatic drug momordin.[212]
Pharmacological & Clinical Research: Momordica Charantia has been confirmed to possess antiviral properties (against polio, herpes simplex 1, and HIV). The active constituent appears to be a 28.6 kD protein named MRK29 that inhibits HIV-l reverse transcriptase.[213]

---

[212] Morton F. Julia, *Atlas of Medical Plants of Middle America: Bahamas to Yucatan.* Springfield, Illinois: Charles C Thomas Publisher, 1981; 893.
[213] Yaniv, Zohara, and Uriel Bachrach. *Handbook of Medicinal Plants*. New York: Food Products; Haworth Medical, 2005; 338.

Sandpaper Tree

Antipyretics or Febrifugals: Plants that Eliminate Heat and Dampness

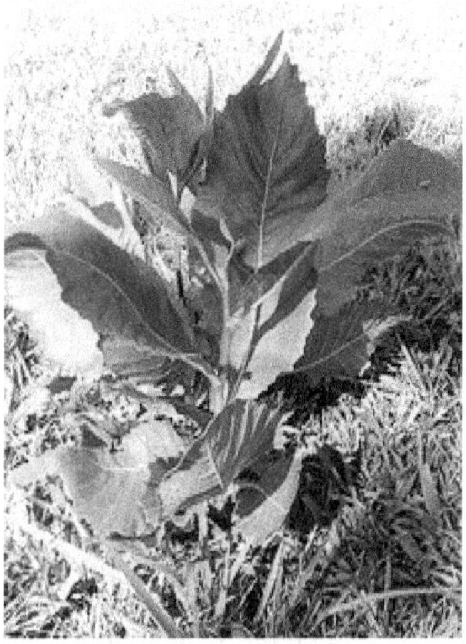

Botanical Name: Curatella Americana .
Family: Dilleniaceae.
Region Where Grown: Potaro-Siparuni.
Other Names: Mimili, Sandpaper tree, Uratkiye, Iminyar.
Category: Antipyretics or Febrifugals: Plants that can Eliminate Heat and Toxins
Properties: Astringent, Sour, Hot/Moist.
Esoteric Botanica: Tehuti.
Governing Organs: Liver, Gall Bladder, Heart.
Actions & Indications: Stem: Macerated bark is boiled and the water drunk to prevent ulcers or to treat jaundice. [214] Drains heat, relieves fire toxicity, cools the blood and benefits the throat – for warm-febrile diseases, warm epidemic disorders, mumps, and painful swollen throat conditions.
Bark is boiled with water and used for treating hepatitis. Bark employed as a sedative. Clears heat, strongly relieves fire toxicity and reduces abscesses – for intestinal abscess, toxic sores, ulcerations, and swellings
Leaf: Infusion of the leaves is used as an astringent. It is considered an effective treatment for sysphilis.[215]
Cautions & Contraindications: Do not use in cases where the patient is weak or in the absence of fire toxin. Use with caution during pregnancy.

[214] DeFilipps, Robert A., Shirley L. Maina, and Juliette Crepin. *Medicinal Plants of the Guianas (Guyana, Surinam, French Guiana)*. Washington, D.C.: Dept. of Botany, National Museum of Natural History, Smithsonian Institution, 2004; 109.
[215]Morton F. Julia, *Atlas of Medical Plants of Middle America: Bahamas to Yucatan.* Springfield, Illinois: Charles C Thomas Publisher, 1981; 560.

Pirapisi

Antipyretics or Febrifugals: Plants that Eliminate Heat and Dampness

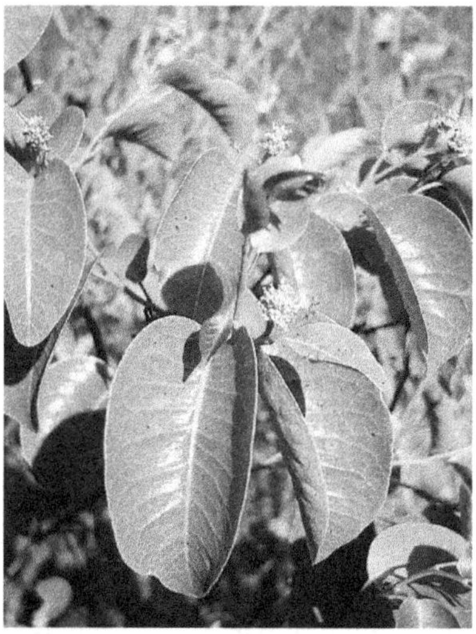

Botanical Name: Maprounea Guianensis.
Family: Euphorbiaceae.
Region Where Grown: Cuyuni-Mazaruni.
Other Names: Footie, Awati.
Category: Antipyretics or Febrifugals: Plants that can Eliminate Heat and Toxins.
Properties: Acrid, Cool/Dry.
Esoteric Botanica: Sebek.
Governing Organs: Lung, Liver.
Actions & Indications: Plant is ised as an antibacterial and antifungal agent, for athlete's foot, douche after childbirth, eczema, measles, venereal disease and ringworms.
Stem: Bark is used in a decoction to remedy venereal chancres, and pustules which form on the legs; [216]Clears heat, relieves fire toxicity, expels wind and dries dampness – for wind-heat or damp-heat sores, carbuncles and rashes. These are marked by much pus or leaking of yellow fluid, moist skin and pruritus.
Bark and leaves in a decoction or drinkable maceration to relieve diarrhoea.
Bark grated and pressed onto navel of infants to accelerate cicatrization of umbilicus.
Leaf: Decoction for bathing patient with measles and as a douche for mothers after childbirth.
Leaves cooked with salt are applied as a treatment for fungal diseases such as athlete's foot and ringworm, and for remedying eczema and skin rashes. Used for itches and sores. Cools the blood and reduces blotches – for blotches or other skin eruptions due to heat in the blood.
Cautions & Contraindications: Do not use in cases of spleen or stomach cold from deficiency. Use with caution during pregnancy.
Major Known Ingredients: Contains compounds which show antibacterial and antifungal properties.

[216] DeFilipps, Robert A., Shirley L. Maina, and Juliette Crepin. *Medicinal Plants of the Guianas (Guyana, Surinam, French Guiana)*. Washington, D.C.: Dept. of Botany, National Museum of Natural History, Smithsonian Institution, 2004; 121.

Soapwood

Antipyretics or Febrifugals: Plants that Eliminate Heat and Dampness

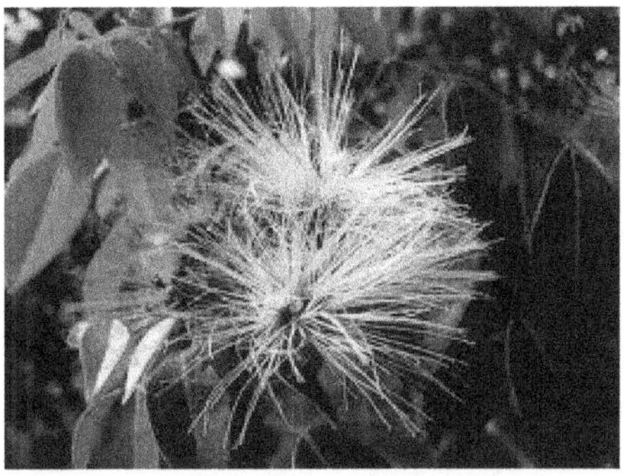

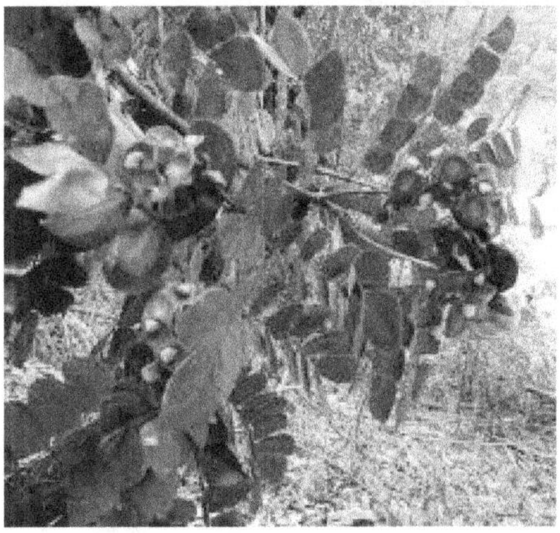

Botanical Name: Abarema Jupunba.
Family: Mimosaceae.
Region Where Grown: Essequibo Isl-W. Demerara.
Other Names: Bread-and-Cheese, Soapwood.
Category: Antipyretics or Febrifugals: Plants that can Eliminate Heat and Toxins.
Properties: Bitter, Cold/Moist.
Esoteric Botanica: Het Heru.
Governing Organs: Kidney, Urinary Bladder, Stomach.
Actions & Indications: General uses include fertility, hair growth stimulant and for parasitic worms.
Whole plant: Reputedly a parasiticide.
Root: Infusion of scraped roots is used to treat dandruff and to stimulate hair growth.[217]
Bark: Macerated bark is used as a shampoo and a soap. Inner bark is used for treating itchy scalp. Soap with anti-parasitic properties is extracted from the bark.
Bark and Leaf: Macerated leaves and inner bark are used as a detergent or as a treatment for itchy and scaling scalp. Clears heat and dries dampness – primarily for dysenteric disorder, vaginal discharge, jaundice, and sores. Disperses wind, kills parasites and stops itching – for damp toxin skin lesions or infestation with chronic itching and bleeding.
Seed: Swallowed by young women just before engaging in sexual intercourse as a fertility drug.
Cautions & Contraindications: Use with caution during pregnancy.

[217] DeFilipps, Robert A., Shirley L. Maina, and Juliette Crepin. *Medicinal Plants of the Guianas (Guyana, Surinam, French Guiana)*. Washington, D.C.: Dept. of Botany, National Museum of Natural History, Smithsonian Institution, 2004 ; 190.

Antipyretics or Febrifugals - Plants that Eliminate Heat and Dampness

The plants that belong to this category can inhibit the growth of bacteria and are used for dysentery. Heat and moisture are the required factors for the growth of yeast, bacteria, amoebiae and trichomonas. Also many of the herbs in this category are used in the treatment of various cancer.

The liver is the main organ of metabolism (e.g. lipid metabolism, protein biosynthesis; glycogen storage) and detoxification in our body. Viral, bacrerial and parasitic infections or toxins (toxins from mushrooms, lower fungi, plants or chemical industry) that destroy liver cells, can be life threatening. Liver cirrhosis as a result of long-term alcohol abuse can be considered in this context. Some compounds damage the endothelia of blood vessels in the liver, such as pyrrolizidine alkaloids, arsenic and other toxins. On the other hand, the liver has a high regeneration capability, so that new cells can easily replace the destroyed tissue. Medicinal plants e can alleviate severe liver damage. Basicaliy, secondary metabolites, such as lignans help to stabilise and seal membranes of liver cells, so that toxins cannot enter. Silymarin is a radical scavenger, stimulates RNA transcription and protein biosynthesis and supports the regeneration of damaged liver tissue.

Sarsaparilla

Antipyretics or Febrifugals: Plants that Eliminate Heat and Dampness

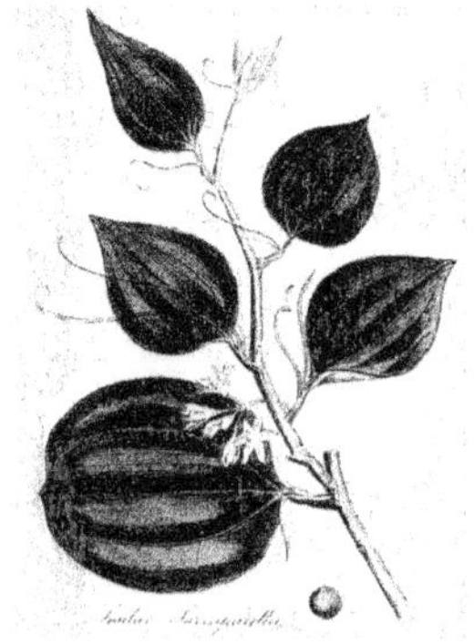

Botanical Name: Philodendron Fragrantissimum.
Family:Araceae.
Region Where Grown: Barima-Waini.
Other Names: Bucuruna.
Category: Antipyretics or Febrifugals: Plants that can Eliminate Heat and Dampness.
Properties: Acrid, Cool/Dry.
Esoteric Botanica: Sebek.
Governing Organs:Lung, Large Intestine, Kidney,Urinary Bladder.
Actions & Indications: Commonly use as a aphrodisiac, demulcent, diuretic and edema.
Root: Ingredient in liquid aphrodisiac and tea.
Stem and Leaf: Decoction for febrifuge, demulcent, diuretic. Used as aphrodisiac. Leaf: For reducing the pain and inflammation of chronic diseases as rheumatism [218] and scrofula.[219] Leaves are heated and rubbed on edematous areas.

---

[218] DeFilipps, Robert A., Shirley L. Maina, and Juliette Crepin. *Medicinal Plants of the Guianas (Guyana, Surinam, French Guiana)*. Washington, D.C.: Dept. of Botany, National Museum of Natural History, Smithsonian Institution, 2004; 30.

[219] Weiner, Michael A., Janet Weiner, and Norman R. Farnsworth. *Weiner's Herbal: The Guide to Herb Medicine*. New York: Stein and Day, 1980; 169.

The extracts of the roots have been used to treat various conditions including skin infections. Root extracts also are widely used in the food industry to flavour soft drinks, ice-cream, confectionery and bakery products.
Major Known Ingredients: The very limited phytochemical studies done so far, have suggested the presence of saponins (glycosides) in the plant. Sarsaparilla contains a mixture of saponins derived mainly from sarsapogenin and smilagenin. The saponins have a strong diuretic action as well as some diaphoretic, expectorant and laxative properties. In addition, the plant material is a moderately useful flavoring agent.[220]
Pharmacological & Clinical Research: In recent times, sarsaparilla has been widely promoted as one of the ingredients in various herbal combination products intended to serve athletes and bodybuilders as legal replacements for illegal steroidal drugs.[221]

---

[220] Steven Foster, Tyler Varro E. *Tyler's honest Herbal: A Sensible Guide to the Use of Herbs and Related Remedies*. Binghamton, NY: The Haworth Herbal Press, 2000; 335.
[221] Ibid., pp. 335-336

Wild Marron

Antipyretics or Febrifugals: Plants that Eliminate Heat and Dampness

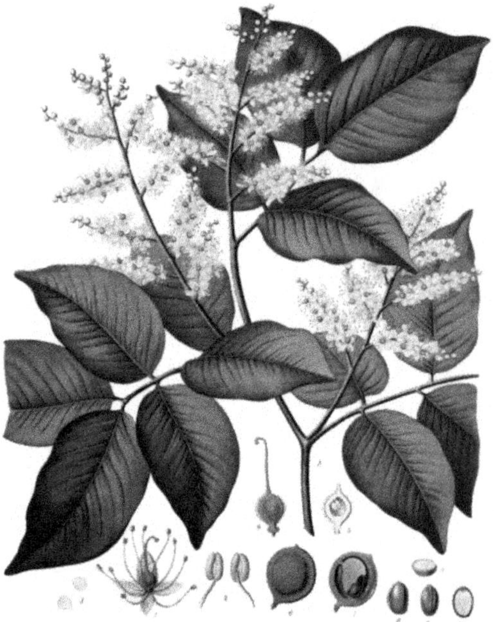

Botanical Name: Pityrogramma Calomelanos.
Family: Adiantaceae.
Region Where Grown: E. Berbice-Corentyne
Other Names: Aisegay, printing fern, Silver Fern, Silverback Fern, Marran, Wild Maran.
Category: Tonics: Vital Function.
Properties: Sour, Hot/Moist.
Esoteric Botanica: Maat.
Governing Organs: Liver, Kidney, Lung, Gall Bladder, Stomach.
Actions & Indications: Whole Plant: Infusion is used for sexual debility and to "strengthen men's backs", i.e., to increase male sexual stamina and to treat female hemorrhaging.[222] Decotion is drunk or applied locally to treat venereal disease, amenorrhea and hypertension[223]. Also used for asthma, cough, cold, pneumonia, tuberculosis and whooping cough. Plant infusion used as depurative, mild astringent and pectoral, especially recommended in infusions for pulmonary affections.[224] Root: Infusion for a bechic to treat pulmonary conditions. Leaf: Crushed leaves used to promote healing of ulcers and cuts. Boiled in water for a bronchitis remedy. Macerated leaves (or leaf-juice) may be placed on wounds to stop bleeding. Infusion drunk to remedy stomach pains. Decoction is drunk to relieve colds. Fresh leaves are macerated and placed on cuts and wounds to stop bleeding.
Major Known Ingredients: Contains the sesquiterpene lactones pterosin (reportedly antibiotic) and calomelanolactone.[225]
Pharmacological & Clinical Research: The resin from undetermined species of *Copaifera* is used to anoint wounds, due to its ability to coagulate blood.

---

222 DeFilipps, Robert A., Shirley L. Maina, and Juliette Crepin. *Medicinal Plants of the Guianas (Guyana, Surinam, French Guiana)*. Washington, D.C.: Dept. of Botany, National Museum of Natural History, Smithsonian Institution, 2004; 3.
223 Morton F. Julia, *Atlas of Medical Plants of Middle America: Bahamas to Yucatan*. Springfield, Illinois: Charles C Thomas Publisher, 1981; 14.
224 Duke, James A., and Rodolfo Vásquez. *Amazonian Ethnobotanical Dictionary*. Boca Raton, FL: CRC, 1994; 138.
225 DeFilipps, Robert A., Shirley L. Maina, and Juliette Crepin. *Medicinal Plants of the Guianas (Guyana, Surinam, French Guiana)*. Washington, D.C.: Dept. of Botany, National Museum of Natural History, Smithsonian Institution, 2004; 4.

Parrot-Beak

Antipyretics or Febrifugals: Plants that Eliminate Heat and Dampness

Botanical Name: Centropogon Cornutus.
Family: Campanulaceae.
Region Where Grown: Cuyuni-Mazaruni.
Other Names: Saint John.
Category: Antipyretics or Febrifugals: Plants that can eliminate heat and Dampness.
Properties: Sour, Hot/Moist.
Esoteric Botanica: Tehuti.
Governing Organs: Liver, Kidney, Urinary Bladder.
Actions & Indications: Whole plant: Boiled and the liquid is drunk to remedy venereal disease.[226] Drains damp-heat, especially from the lower burner – for such problems as thick yellow vaginal discharge, urinary tract infections, STDs, foul-smelling diarrhea, or dysenteric disorder. Exudate: Used for irritated eyes. Drains damp-heat from the liver and channel with such symptoms as red, swollen sore eyes, swollen and painful ears or sudden deafness. Also for damp-heat in the liver channel (especially the lower parts) with such symptoms as jaundice, pain, swelling or dampness in the genital area or foul-smelling vaginal discharge and itching. Drains and pacifies excessive liver fire – for liver fire blazing upward with headache or red eyes. Also for liver wind-heat with fever, spasm, convulsions, or flank pain.

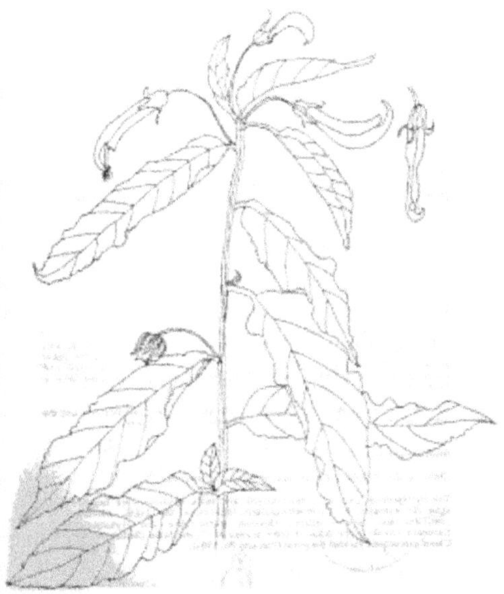

Leaf: Used for a tonic and abortive decoction. Also used for bed wetting and to treat urinary tract problems. Drains kidney fire – for ascending kidney fire with signs of yin deficiency such as steaming bone disorder, night sweats, insomnia, anxiety, irritability, dry skin, malar flush, five center fever, dry mouth with thirst, thin pulse, mirror tongue and all symptoms of menopause. Also for damp-heat jaundice.
Cautions & Contraindications: Do not use in cases of Spleen deficiency with or without diarrhea
Major Known Ingredients: Contains chelidonic acid.

---

[226] DeFilipps, Robert A., Shirley L. Maina, and Juliette Crepin. *Medicinal Plants of the Guianas (Guyana, Surinam, French Guiana)*. Washington, D.C.: Dept. of Botany, National Museum of Natural History, Smithsonian Institution, 2004; 75.

Water Sawari

Antipyretics or Febrifugals: Plants that Eliminate Heat and Dampness

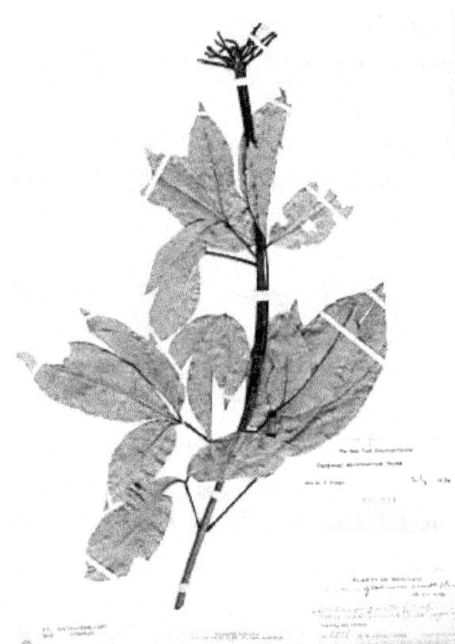

Botanical Name: Caryocar Microcarpum.
Family: Caryocaraceae.
Region Where Grown: E. Berbice-Corentyne.
Other Names: Bats Sawari, Kula, Imbo, Hora, Alokomali, Butternut, Imba.
Category: Antipyretics or Febrifugals: Plants that can Eliminate Heat and Dampness.
Properties: Salty, Cold/Moist.
Esoteric Botanica: Het Heru.
Governing Organs: Kidney, large Intestine.
Actions & Indications: Whole plant: Used for a febrifuge. Clears heat and drains fire, especially from the upper burner – for heat patterns with high fever, irritability, thirst, cough and expectoration of thick yellow sputum, or for hot sores and swellings. For patterns of wind-heat with fever and headache.
Bark used for mycoses and filarial.[227] Bark also used to treat back pain. Tonifies the kidneys and fortifies the yang – for deficient kidney yang patterns with such symptoms as fatigue, impotence, cold extremities, lightheadedness, tinnitus, soreness and weakness in the lower back and knees, and frequent, copious, clear urination. Augments the kidney and tonifies the yang – for impotence and sore and weak lower back and lower extremities from kidney yang deficiency.
Fruit: Nuts are used as a fish poison. Fruit: Edible, tasty
Cautions & Contraindications: Use cautiously in exterior conditions.
Major Known Ingredients: Stem and leaf contain triterpene saponins, free triterpenes and tannins. Fruit contains ichthyotoxic and ant-repellent chemicals.[228]

---

227 Duke, James A., and Rodolfo Vásquez. *Amazonian Ethnobotanical Dictionary*. Boca Raton, FL: CRC, 1994; 44.
228 DeFilipps, Robert A., Shirley L. Maina, and Juliette Crepin. *Medicinal Plants of the Guianas (Guyana, Surinam, French Guiana)*. Washington, D.C.: Dept. of Botany, National Museum of Natural History, Smithsonian Institution, 2004; 78.

Leaf-of-life

Antipyretics or Febrifugals: Plants that Eliminate Heat and Dampness

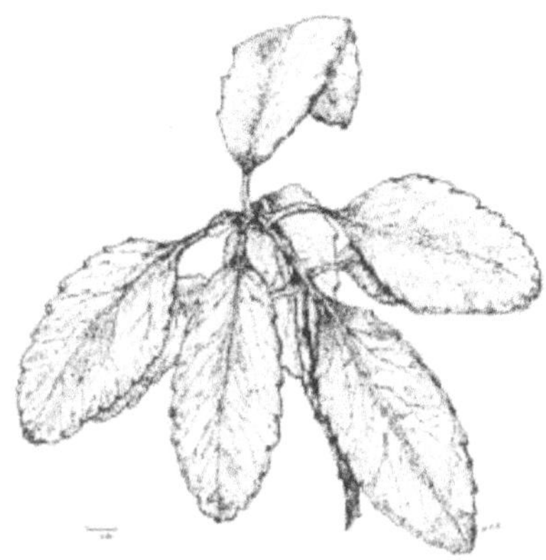

Botanical Name: Kalanchoe Pinnata.
Family: Crassulaceae.
Region Where Grown: U. Takutu-U. Essequibo
Other Names: Balsam, Sagiwanor, Tree of Life, Wonderblad.
Category: Antipyretics or Febrifugals: Plants that can eliminate heat and Dampness.
Properties: Salty, Cold/Dry.
Esoteric Botanica: Seker.
Governing Organs:Spleen, Large Intestine, Liver, Lungs, Kidney.
Actions & Indications: Whole plant: Infusion for a febrifuge, headache, earache, heartburn, eye irritations, bronchitis, and to promote the healing of sores.[229]
Leaf: Leaf-juice (or flower) put into eyes to treat conjunctivitis.[230] Clears the vision and expels wind-heat – for itchy, red and painful eyes and sensitivity to light due to externally-contracted wind-heat Clears heat and drains fire, especially from the upper burner – for heat patterns with high fever, irritability, thirst, cough and expectoration of thick yellow sputum or for hot sores and swellings (applied topically or taken internally). Also drunk with salt for colds, coughs, grippe, loose bowels and teething babies; for sores, ulcers and swelling Crushed stems and leaves are emollient and hemostatic. They are applied on skin diseases.[231] Leaves are also soaked in water and left outside overnight; the next morning this water is drunk to relieve heartburn.[232] Leaves are also diuretic and are seen as a cure for urethritis (tract inflammation). They also clear the liver and benefits the eyes – for patterns of liver yang rising with such symptoms as headache, red & painful eyes, excessive tearing or sensitivity to light. Poultice of roasted leaves or juice from macerated leaves is used for treating ringworm. May be use for fire toxin anywhere in the body, especially in the throat or Lungs. Also macerated leaves are soaked in water, and used as shampoo.
Leaves used for sore eyes, coughs and colds, sores and wounds. Warmed leaves applied to hernia pain.

---

229 Duke, James A., and Rodolfo Vásquez. *Amazonian Ethnobotanical Dictionary*. Boca Raton, FL: CRC, 1994; 69.

230 DeFilipps, Robert A., Shirley L. Maina, and Juliette Crepin. *Medicinal Plants of the Guianas (Guyana, Surinam, French Guiana)*. Washington, D.C.: Dept. of Botany, National Museum of Natural History, Smithsonian Institution, 2004; 99.

231 Morton F. Julia, *Atlas of Medical Plants of Middle America: Bahamas to Yucatan.* Springfield, Illinois: Charles C Thomas Publisher, 1981; 258.

232 Duke, James A., and Rodolfo Vásquez. *Amazonian Ethnobotanical Dictionary*. Boca Raton, FL: CRC, 1994; 101.

Major Known Ingredients: Plant contains fumaric acid, and saponins having cicatrizant properties.[233] The plant also has high level of calcium and chloride; malic, citric lactic and succinct acid.
Pharmacological & Clinical Research: Three glycosides have been isolated; glycoside A, glycoside B (quercetin 3-diarabinoside) and glycoside C (kaemferol 3-glucoside). The phenols, p-coumaric, ferulic, syringic and caffeic acids. In addition p- hydroxybenzoic acid was detected. The juice of heated leaves has exhibited antibacterial activity against Staphylococcus aureus, Bacillus subtilis, Escherichia coli and Pseudomonas aeruginosa.[234]

[233] DeFilipps, Robert A., Shirley L. Maina, and Juliette Crepin. *Medicinal Plants of the Guianas (Guyana, Surinam, French Guiana)*. Washington, D.C.: Dept. of Botany, National Museum of Natural History, Smithsonian Institution, 2004; 100.
[234] Morton F. Julia, *Atlas of Medical Plants of Middle America: Bahamas to Yucatan*. Springfield, Illinois: Charles C Thomas Publisher, 1981; 259.

Pain-Cure

Antipyretics or Febrifugals: Plants that Eliminate Heat and Dampness

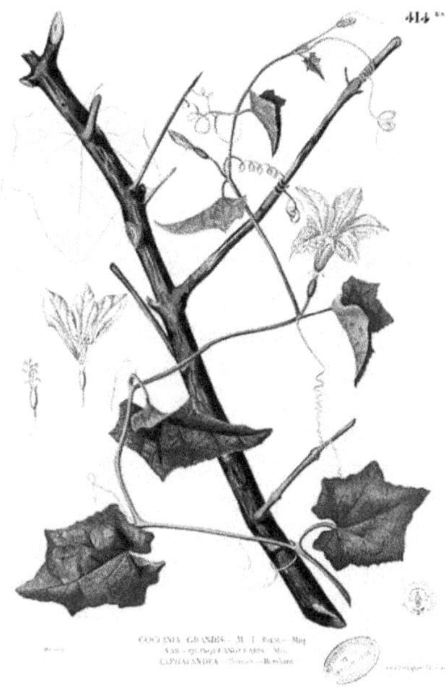

Botanical Name: Coccinia Grandis.
Family: Curbitaceae.
Region Where Grown: Demerara-Mahaica.
Other Names: None
Category: Antipyretics or Febrifugals: Plants that can eliminate heat and Dampness.
Properties: Sweet, Cold/Dry.
Esoteric Botanica: Seker.
Governing Organs: Spleen, Stomach, Lungs, Liver.
Actions & Indications: Whole plant: Crushed and externally applied to affected areas to relieve pain of headache and rheumatism.[235] The plant dispels wind-dampness – for stiffness and migratory pain in the joints. Disperses wind-cold and strengthens the sinews and bones – for paralysis, weak knees and legs, spasms, stiffness and pain in the lower back, and cold pain in the bones. Dries dampness, transforms phlegm, expels wind, stops spasm – for wind-phlegm affecting the head resulting in wind-stroke, facial paralysis, hemiplegia, or migraine headaches. Expels wind-cold-dampness and alleviates pain – for dizziness, severe lateral headaches, numbness, facial pain, facial weakness or any head pain with signs of damp-cold or wind-dampness.
The plant is also decocted for chest colds. Strongly releases the exterior and disperses cold – for Tai Yang repletion patterns (fever & chills with chills predominating, scratchy throat, body aches, headaches and absence of sweating).
Leaf: Used for scrotal hernias.Transforms blood stasis and dissipates clumps – for postpartum abdominal pain and clumps due to blood stasis. Also for hernial disorders, abdominal masses, cysts and fibroids.
Cautions & Contraindications: Do not use in cases of spleen or stomach deficiency with diarrhea.

235 DeFilipps, Robert A., Shirley L. Maina, and Juliette Crepin. *Medicinal Plants of the Guianas (Guyana, Surinam, French Guiana)*. Washington, D.C.: Dept. of Botany, National Museum of Natural History, Smithsonian Institution, 2004; 100.

Cow Itch

Antipyretics or Febrifugals: Plants that Eliminate Heat and Dampness

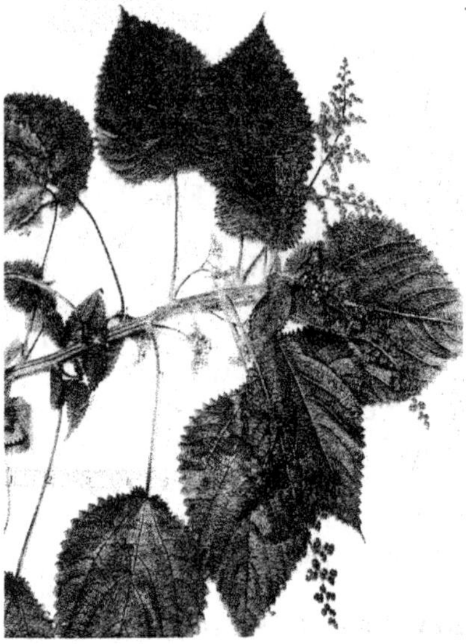

Botanical Name: Mucuna Urens.
Family: Fabaceae.
Region Where Grown: Potaro-Siparuni.
Other Names: Horse eye, Ox-eye.
Category: Antipyretics or Febrifugals: Plants that can eliminate heat and Dampness.
Properties: Bitter, Hot/Dry.
Esoteric Botanica: Herukhuti.
Governing Organs: Heart, Small Intestine, Liver.
Actions & Indications: Who Plant use to treat gonorrhea and migraine.[236] The plant is decoted (including the root) and is taken as a diuretic, especially in venereal diseases; it is also drunk to expel the placenta after childbirth.[237]
Stem and Seed: Cataplasm of the bark and ground seeds is recommended for inguinal hernia and intestinal worms. Transforms blood stasis and dissipates clumps – for postpartum abdominal pain, clumps due to blood stasis, hernial disorders, abdominal masses, cysts and fibroids. Promotes the movement of qi and alleviates pain – for stagnant qi that manifest with such symptoms as chest pain, abdominal pain, menstrual pain, hernial disorders and especially epigastric pain.
Fruit: Hairs on the fruit cause severe itching on the skin.
Seed: Used for itch and for treating intestinal worms. Kills parasites – while best for treating tapeworms, it is also useful in killing a wide variety of intestinal parasites,[238] including Fasciolopis (intestinal flukes), pinworms and roundworms, as well as blood flukes. The ability of this herb to drain downward helps in expelling the bodies of the parasites. Clears heat and relieves fire toxicity – primarily for dysenteric disorders, especially those due to damp-heat in the stomach or intestines.
Cautions & Contraindications: Use with caution in cases of collapse of the middle qi. Do not use during pregnancy.
Pharmacological & Clinical Research: The indole bases have been shown to have an unspecified spasmolytic action on spasms induced in smooth muscles by acetylcholine, histamine or oxytocin. Two of them, 5-methoxy-N-N-dimethyltryptamine and 5-oxyindole-3-alkylamine, produce a block of a mbocurarine type and indole-3-alkylamine causes blockade of the striated muscle of the frog abdomen. In the anaesthetized dog, 5-oxindole-3-alkylamine and 5-methoxy-N, N-dimethyltryptamine cause severe depression of respiration and the blood pressure with spasm of the bronchi, which can lead to death. In the rat, to the contrary, they induce hyperactivity. In view of the presence of L-DOPA and serotonin in the

236 Duke, James A., and Rodolfo Vásquez. *Amazonian Ethnobotanical Dictionary*. Boca Raton, FL: CRC, 1994; 120.
237 Morton F. Julia, *Atlas of Medical Plants of Middle America: Bahamas to Yucatan.* Springfield, Illinois: Charles C Thomas Publisher, 1981; 152.
238 DeFilipps, Robert A., Shirley L. Maina, and Juliette Crepin. *Medicinal Plants of the Guianas (Guyana, Surinam, French Guiana)*. Washington, D.C.: Dept. of Botany, National Museum of Natural History, Smithsonian Institution, 2004; 135.

plant, its possible use in Parkinson's disease has been suggested. The plam also has a hypoglycaemic and cholesterol lowering effect.
Toxicity: Contact with the plant causes instant stinging and rash.[239]

Neem

Antipyretics or Febrifugals: Plants that Eliminate Heat and Dampness

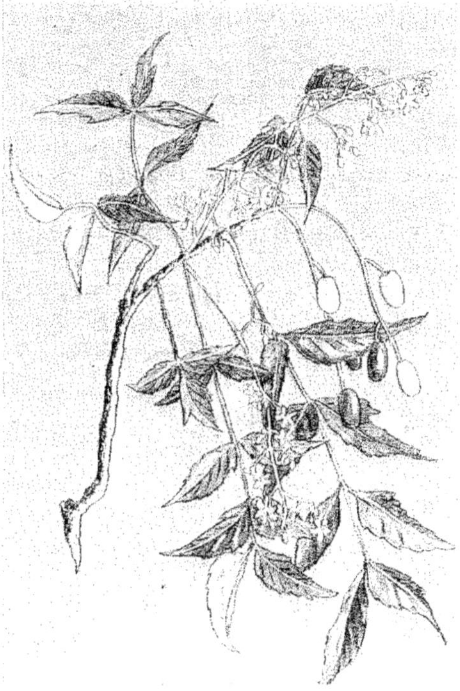

Botanical Name: Azadirachta Indica.
Family: Meliaceae.
Region Where Grown: U. Takutu-U. Essequibo.
Other Names: None.
Category: Antipyretics or Febrifugals: Plants that can eliminate heat and Dampness.
Properties: Sour, Hot/Moist.
Esoteric Botanica: Tehuti.
Governing Organs: Liver, Large Intestine, Lung.
Actions & Indications: Stem: Bark decoction for antifungal properties in treating malarial fever.[240]
Treats malarial disorder – for chronic malarial disorder with signs of qi and blood deficiency
Stem, Leaf and Flower: Decoction used as an abortifacient.
Leaf: Infusion to combat fever and intestinal worms; Kills parasites – while best for treating tape worms. It is also useful in killing a wide variety of intestinal parasites, including Fasciolopis (intestinal flukes), pinworms and roundworms, as well as blood flukes. Expels intestinal parasites and reduces stagnation – for roundworm or tapeworm infestation and food stagnation. Decoction as a bitter tonic for wasting and thirsting disorder diabetes and jaundices. Drains heat, relieves fire toxicity, cools the blood, and benefits the throat – for warm-febrile diseases, warm epidemic disorders, mumps and painful swollen throat conditions. Also for damp-heat jaundice. Relieves toxicity, kills parasites, dries dampness and alleviates itching – used as an external wash for scabies, ringworm and rashes due to dampness or damp-heat. Also for swollen and painful throat or eyes as well as jaundice.
Leaves used in a bath for measles; Clears heat and relieves toxicity – for red swellings, carbuncles, erythemas, mumps and acute febrile maculopapular rashes. Vents rashes – for the early stages of measles when there is incomplete expression of the rash. Leaves are also spread on a patient's bed to relieve itching.
Seed: Seed-oil is used against scabies and other skin diseases.

---

[239] Oliver-Bever, Bep. *Medicinal Plants in Tropical West Africa*. Cambridge: Cambridge UP, 1986; 102.
[240] DeFilipps, Robert A., Shirley L. Maina, and Juliette Crepin. *Medicinal Plants of the Guianas (Guyana, Surinam, French Guiana)*. Washington, D.C.: Dept. of Botany, National Museum of Natural History, Smithsonian Institution, 2004; 182.

Cautions & Contraindications: Do not use in cases of deficiency without heat signs or excessive heat patterns. This herb retains and preserves pathogenic influences and should therefore not be used in the early stages of a warm-febrile disease.
Major Known Ingredients: Among the active constituents in Neem is avaginal contraceptive and an insect and pest repellant. Its antibacterial properties have been most explored against Staphylococcus mutans and lactobacilli for use in tooth preservative preparations. Mahmoodin, a tetranor triterpenoid, has been isolated from neem and demonstrated to be antibacterial.[241]
Pharmacological & Clinical Research: Evidence in support of the antimalarial effect of the Neem plant reported a fall in parasite count in chloroquine-sensitive strains of Plasmodium berghci-infected mice when the mice were treated with a decoction of the leaves. Another study reported the growth-inhibitory effect of this leaf extract on P. falciparum culture and the antimalarial effect of the boiled leaf was found to be approximately half of the therapeutic dose of chloroquine sulphate on dry weight basis. Investigations have also been carried out on Neem with a view to finding some scientific evidence for its other uses in traditional medicine.[242] Neem is a powerful insect antifeedant that disrupts metamorphosis in moth larvae at extremely low concenrmtions. The main focus of research on Neem has been on the insecticidal properties but in recent years investigations have expanded to the medicinal utilizations. Several studies have shown antifungal and antibacterial activity in extracts of Neem leaves and seeds, likely to be due to the limonoids. A volatile fraction of Neem seed oil (coded as NIM-76) was shown to have potent in vitro spermicidal activity. The activity has been linked to various free fatty acids and their methylesrers. A large number of studies have been published on the medical properties of Neem and Neem extracts, covering a wide range of indications and ailments.[243]
Toxicity: Ethanol (70%) extract of the fresh bark and leaf, when administered by gastric intubation to mice, resulted in LD_{50} 13.0 gm/kg. Ethanol/warer (1:1) extract of the dried seed, administered intraperitoneally to mice of both sexes, resulted in LD_{50} 681.0 mg/kg. Ethanol/water (l: 1) extract of the stembark, administered intraperitoneally to mice) resulted in $LD_{50} > 1.0$ gm/kg AlmOJ. Ethanol/water (1:1) extract of the stemwood, administered intraperitoneal1y to mice, resulted in $LD_{50} > 1000$ mg/kg. Ethanol/water (1: 1) extract of the dried root, fruit pulp, root wood) and leaf, when administered intraperitoneally to mice, resulted in LD_{50} 681.0 mg/kg.[244]

---

241 Yaniv, Zohara, and Uriel Bachrach. *Handbook of Medicinal Plants*. New York: Food Products; Haworth Medical, 2005; 343.
242 Sofowora, Abayomi. *Medicinal Plants and Traditional Medicine in Africa*. Chichester, West Sussex: Wiley, 1982; 177.
243 Van, Wyk Ben-Erik., and Michael Wink. *Medicinal Plants of the World: An Illustrated Scientific Guide to Important Medicinal Plants and Their Uses*. Portland: Timber, 2004; 64.
244 Ross, Ivan A. *Medicinal Plants of the World: Chemical Constituents, Traditional, and Modern Medicinal Uses*. Vol. 2. Totowa, NJ: Humana, 1999; 100.

Wild Guava

Antipyretics or Febrifugals: Plants that Eliminate Heat and Dampness

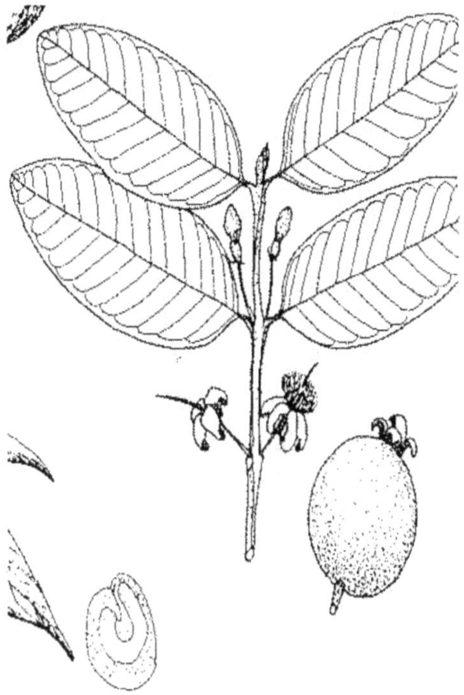

Botanical Name: Calycolpus Goetheanus.
Family: Myrtaceae.
Region Where Grown: Essequibo Isl-W. Demerara.
Other Names: kakirio, Pika.
Category: Antipyretics or Febrifugals: Plants that can eliminate heat and Dampness.
Properties: Sweet, Warm, Acrid.
Esoteric Botanica: Het Heru.
Governing Organs: Stomach, Spleen, Liver, Lung.
Actions & Indications: Bark: Juice from macerated bark is used for treating cuts and wounds. Juice from macerated inner bark is used for treating discolored rashes ("lotta"is a skin infection) and for treating ringworm. Decotion from bark is drunk as an anti-diarrheal. Decotion of bark or young fruit is used to treat dysentery, diarrhea and colic.[245] Guava can be used for poor circulation, cataracts, vertigo, to help kidneys eliminate waste, to support the heart, reduce the risk of cancer, obesity, lower cholesterol, asthma, diabetes, constipation, arthritis, expels placenta, prolonged menstruation, to fight free radicals, protects the prostrate and to control hypertension and cholesterol. It is also an antiseptic, cough suppressant, an astringent, aids with sore throats, conjunctivitis, bacterial infections, blood cleansing, gastroenteritis, respiratory problems, shock, ulcers, toothache, vaginal discharge, yeast and other imbalances.
Cautions & Contraindications: Use with caution over prolonged periods. Do not use alone for heat from yin deficiency.
Major Known Ingredients: Properties are calcium, iron, ash, protein, carbohydrates, potassium, magnesium, Vitamin A, a very high concentration of Vitamin C, omega-3 and omega-6, polyunsaturated fatty acids and dietary fibre.
Pharmacological & Clinical Research: Guava contains more than 30 chemicals and each chemical can have a healing effect on the body. Guava leaf contains Quercetin which is thought to contribute to its anti-diarrhoea effect. In addition, the lectin chemicals in guava were shown to bind to E-coli, thus preventing its adhesion to the intestinal wall and thus preventing infection which can cause diarrhoea.

[245] DeFilipps, Robert A., Shirley L. Maina, and Juliette Crepin. *Medicinal Plants of the Guianas (Guyana, Surinam, French Guiana)*. Washington, D.C.: Dept. of Botany, National Museum of Natural History, Smithsonian Institution, 2004; 205.

Periwinkle

Antipyretics or Febrifugals: Plants that Eliminate Heat and Dampness

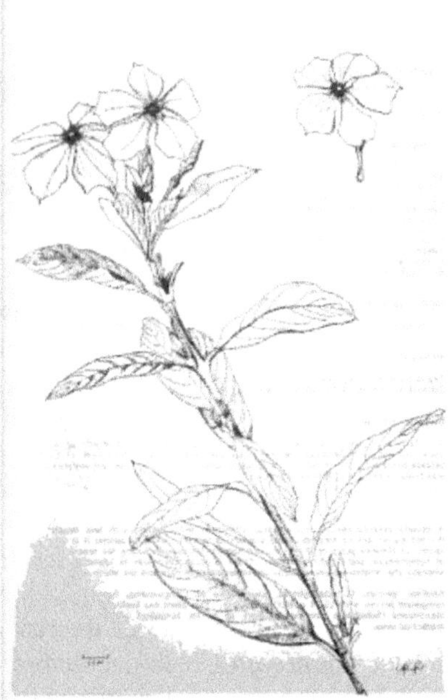

Botanical Name: Catharanthus Roseus.
Family:Apocynaceae.
Region Where Grown: E. Berbice-Corentyne.
Other Names: Never-done, Old maid.
Category: Antipyretics or Febrifugals: Plants that can eliminate heat and Dampness.
Properties: Bitter, Acrid , Cold/Moist.
Esoteric Botanica: Auset.
Governing Organs: Stomach, Spleen, Urinary Bladder, Kidney.
Actions & Indications: Plant treats, edema, hypertension, menstruation (including menstrual cramps), flow and pain.
Stem and Leaf: Leafy branches in remedy to cure inhibited menstruation.
Leaf: Leaves are used for diabetes and as a purgative in chronic constipation, dyspepsia and indigestion.[246] Infusion or decoction used for hypertension.
Flower: Infusion for mild diabetes. Treats wasting and thirsting disorder – i.e. diabetes, cleansing the blood, and for a cholagogue and aperitif (appetite stimulant). Used to treat urinary tract ailments. Tonifies the kidneys and fortifies the yang – for impotence, urinary incontinence and nocturnal emission from deficient kidney yang. Decoction of roots is astringent, diaphoretic, emmenagogue, stomachic and tonic and is said to cause abortion.[247]
Cautions & Contraindications: Use with caution in cases of yin deficiency.
Major Known Ingredients: A few alkaloids have been isolated from the plant: ajmalicine, akuammicine, akuammine, alstonine, ammocaline, carosidine, carosine, catharanthine, catharicine, catharine, catharosine, cavincidine, cavincine, cleavaminc, deacety Ivincalcucoblastine, deaeety Ivindoltne, dihydrositsirikine, isoeurodine, isositsirikine, leurocristine, leurosidine (vinrosidine), leurosidine, leurosine, leuwsivine, lochnericine, lochnerine, lochnerinine, lochnerivine, lochrovidine, lochrovine, maandrosine, mitraphylline, neoleurocristine, neoleurosidine, pericalline, permividinc, perimivine, perivine, perosine, pieurosine, reserpine, rovidine, rovidine sulfate, serpentine, sitsirikine, teoil containing aldehydes, sesquiterpenes, and sulfur compounds, furfural, ochnerol and lochnerallol, two glycosides (adenosine, roseoside), deoxyloganin, loganin, tannin, carotene, sterols and a flavone derivative. Some of the alkaloids have both antitumor and tumorigenic attributes.[248] The dimeric alkaloids vincristine (leucocristine) and vinblastine (vincaleukoblastine) are used to treat children's leukemia and Hodgkin's disease. More than 70 other alkaloids have been isolated.[249]

---

[246] Yaniv, Zohara, and Uriel Bachrach. *Handbook of Medicinal Plants*. New York: Food Products ; Haworth Medical, 2005; 106.
[247] Ibid., p,106.
[248]Ibid., pp, 106 – 107.
[249] Ciba Foundation Symposium Bioactive Compounds from Plants. England: John Wiley and Sons, 1990; 14.

Pharmacological & Clinical Research: Periwinkle was used as an oral insulin substitute in the Philippines during World War II when insulin became unobtainable[250]. In the early 1960s it was discovered that the leaves of the Neem plant significantly prolong the life of mice in which leukemia had heen clinically induced. This finding eventually led to the discovery of the potent anticancer drugs, vincaleukohlastine (vinblastine, VLB) and leurocristine (vincristine, VCR), both of which are used in the treatment of human cancer. Vincristine is one of the most important anticancer drugs in the treatment of childhood leukemias. Vinblastine is of lesser importance, but is effective in treating certain types of Hodgkin's disease. Since vincristine does have neurotoxic side effects and vinblastine can cause a marked decrease in the number of white blood cells, these must be considered as very potent drugs.[251] As the most important plant source of anticancer drugs, leaves are consumed in the U.S. at an estimated 1000 MT, with another 1000 for England, Italy, Netherlands, and West Germany.[252]

Toxicity: Two vincaleukoblastine or vinblastine and leukocristine or vincristine have been employed in cancer chemotherapy. There are several glycosides, including ademosine and roseoside, in the leaves and the alkaloids reserpine, alstonine, ajmalicine and vinceine in the roots.[253]

---

[250] Ciba Foundation Symposium Bioactive Compounds from Plants. England: John Wiley and Sons, 1990; 14.

[251] Weiner, Michael A., Janet Weiner, and Norman R. Farnsworth. *Weiner's Herbal: The Guide to Herb Medicine*. New York: Stein and Day, 1980; 152.

[252] Yaniv, Zohara, and Uriel Bachrach. *Handbook of Medicinal Plants*. New York: Food Products ; Haworth Medical, 2005; 106.

[253] Morton F. Julia, *Atlas of Medical Plants of Middle America: Bahamas to Yucatan.* Springfield, Illinois: Charles C Thomas Publisher, 1981; 671- 672.

Chapter 4: Antitussive

Plants that Suppress or Relieve Coughing

The cough may be nonproductive or productive of sputum. Suppression of the cough or periodic drainage of the sputum is necessary. Expectorants are agents which facilitate coughing in productive cough by thinning the sputum. Some of the Plants have expectorant property. Some can increase the secretion in the respiratory tract. Some can dilate the bronchial smooth muscles and relieve the tracheal spasms caused by pilocarpine, acetylcholine and histamine.

Phlegm includes sputum, goiter, scrofula and cholesterol deposits. If it is found in the lung, it will produce cough, asthma, emphysema, tracheitis and bronchiectasis. If the phlegm is stagnant in body, it will produce goiter, scrofula, chronic lymphadenitis, convulsions, CVA and epilepsy. The antitussives are divided into four major groups; Eliminating cold phlegm with Plants that are warm in nature; Elimination Heat Phlegm with Cleansing Plants; Antitussive and anti-asthmatic; Plants that relieve cough by moistening effect

Antitussive: Elimination of Cold Phlegm with Plants that are Warm in Nature

This group of Plants can increase the blood flow to the lung, bronchi and bronchioles. They can increase the cellular energy metabolic rate and reduce the edema in the respiratory tract. Disorders of the respiratory tract are caused by various viruses that destroy mucosal cells. The necrotic tissues can secondarily suffer from bacterial infections. Mucosas swell and show an enhanced mucus production. Hayfever is an allergic disturbance affecting the respiratory tract. This disorder is often a complex with rhinitis, tracheitis, laryngitis, pharyngitis and acute bronchitis. Rhinitis can lead to sinusitis, a painful inflammation of ethmoidal, frontal, maxilliary or sphenoidal sinuses. Otitis is a painful inflammation of the middle ear or outer ear caused by bacterial infections. A common cold must be distinguished from viral influenza. The latter disorder is characterised by high fever, intense headache, muscle pains and cough. Phytomedicines are usually applied locally (ointments, balsams or inhalations). Immunomodulatory drugs are taken orally. Monoterpenes such as memhol, generate the sensation of cooling, thus relieving the pain and discomfort of cold symptoms. Asthma is a complex disorder. It is influenced by infections, toxins and allergens that cause a chronic inflammation but also by stress and other psychosomatic factors. Bronchial hyperreactivity is intermediary to asthma bronchiale. An asthma attack starts with the release of cellular mediators from mast cells, granulocytes and macrophages, including leukonienes, prostaglandins, bradykinine, histamine and others. These compounds induce a contraction of smooth bronchial muscles, and enhance mucus and oedema formation. Treatment may include the avoidance of allergens, a specific hyposensitisation, anti-infective and psychotherapy. A symptomatic rrearment involves the application of bronchodilatory, expectorant, antitussive and anti-infl ammatory medicines.

In case of *status asthrrwticus* (severe attack) glucocorticoids and isolated alkaloids such as theophylline (broncholytic by inhibition of phosphodiesterase and histamine secretion) and atropine (sympatholytic; spasmolytic on smooth bronchial muscles) (and their derivatives) are used, Ephedrine is an indirect sympathomimeric that enhances the release of noradrenaline with bronchodilatory properties. Otherwise, plant extracts with weaker activities can be applied.

Onion

Antitussive: Elimination of Cold Phlegm with Plants that are Warm in Nature

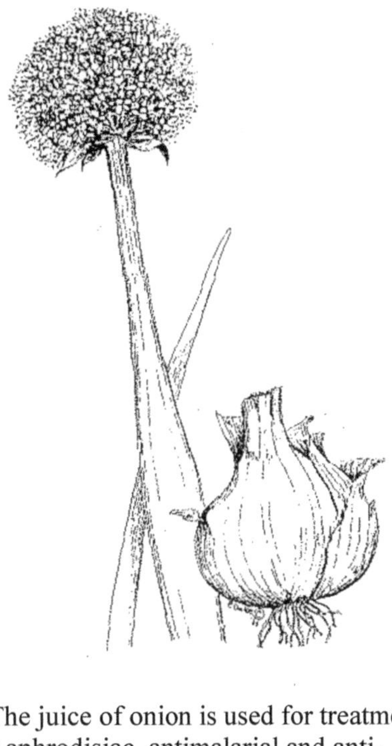

Botanical Name: Allium cepa.
Family:Alliaceae.
Region Where Grown: All regions.
Other Names: None.
Category: Elimination of Cold Phlegm with Warm Plants.
Properties: Acrid, Aromatic, Hot/Moist.
Esoteric Botanica: Tehuti.
Governing Organs: Lung, Liver.
Actions & Indications: Among the therapeutic uses of onion are hemorrhoids, rheumatism, dermatitis, abdominal pain, coughs, loss of apetite, stomach disorders, loss of weight, skin rashes, parasitic infections, leprosy, snake bites and the bite of mad dogs.[254] Onion possesses hypotensive, antidiabetic as well as major antibiotic properties.[255] Today the plant is used as a cure for more specific diseases such as dysentery, typhoid and cholera, arterio sclerosis and hypertension.
The whole plant is used as a remedy for deafness and buzzing of the ears, expels intestinal worms, treats rheumatism and neuralgia, proteinuria, coronary thrombosis, epilepsy, as a diuretic, edema and kidney stones.[256] The juice of onion is used for treatment of ophthalmia, earache and jaundice.[257] Onion is also said to possess aphrodisiac, antimalarial and anti-

---

[254] Bajaj, Yashpal Singh. *Biotechnology in Agriculture and Forestry.* Vol. 4. Berlin: Springer-Verlag, 199; 23.
[255] Oliver-Bever, Bep. *Medicinal Plants in Tropical West Africa.* Cambridge: Cambridge UP, 1986;135.
[256] Morton F. Julia, *Atlas of Medical Plants of Middle America: Bahamas to Yucatan.* Springfield, Illinois: Charles C Thomas Publisher, 1981; 75.
[257] DeFilipps, Robert A., Shirley L. Maina, and Juliette Crepin. *Medicinal Plants of the Guianas (Guyana, Surinam, French Guiana).* Washington, D.C: Dept. of Botany, National Museum of Natural History, 1997; 90.

rheumatic properties. It is also a hypoglycemic agent. The fresh bulb is taken orally as a carminative, tonic, antipyretic, hypotensive and diuretic. [258]

Cautions & Contraindications: Do not use in cases of exterior deficiency with profuse sweating. Do not use with honey when taken internally.

Major Known Ingredients: *A. cepa* is used as a vegetable and contains an essential oil (rich in allylpropyl disulphide), soluble carbohydrates, vitamins, y-glutamylpeptides, phenolic acids, flavonols, anthocyanins and oleanolic acid. The anthocyanins are 4-substituted, carboxypyranocyanidins such as 5-carboxy·-2-(3,4-dihydroxy phenyl)-3,8-dihydro pyrano-(4,3,2-de)-1- enzopyrillium (Fossen and Andersen 2003).[259] The activity (and pungent smell) is due to several sulphur-containing compounds - mainly sulfoxides, but also cepaenes (a-sulfinyldisuJfides). Sulfoxides (such *as* trans-S-(I-propenyl)L-(+)-cysteinesulfoxide, an isomero{ alliin) are present in the intact bulb, but they are converted by enzvmatic action (i.e. by alliinase) into various sulfides that spontaneously form disulfides. Thcse compounds can easily form disulfide bonds with SH-groups of proteins and thus alter their biological activities.[260]

Pharmacological & Clinical Research: The fresh juice is hypoglycemic; stimules the heart, increases systolic pressure, coronary flow and pulse volume; also stimulates intestinal and uterine muscle and promotes the flow of bile.[261] This plant is also known for its antifungal and antibacterial activity believed to be associated with sulfur-containing constituents. [262] *Allium cepa* extracts contain thiosulfmates, which inhibit mediators of bronchoconstriction (leukotriene and thromboxane).[263]

---

[258] Ross, Ivan A. *Medicinal Plants of the World: Chemical Constituents, Traditional, and Modern Medicinal Uses*. Vol. 2. Totowa, NJ: Humana, 1999; 2.

[259] Daniel, M. *Medicinal Plants: Chemistry and Properties*. Enfield, NH: Science, 2006; 90.

[260] Van, Wyk Ben-Erik., and Michael Wink. *Medicinal Plants of the World: An Illustrated Scientific Guide to Important Medicinal Plants and Their Uses*. Portland: Timber, 2004; 38.

[261] Morton F. Julia, *Atlas of Medical Plants of Middle America: Bahamas to Yucatan.* Springfield, Illinois: Charles C Thomas Publisher, 1981; 75.

[262] Yaniv, Zohara, and Uriel Bachrach. *Handbook of Medicinal Plants*. New York: Food Products ; Haworth Medical, 2005; 343.

[263] Miller, Lucinda G., and Wallace J. Murray. *Herbal Medicinals: A Clinician's Guide.* New York: Pharmaceutical Products, 1998; 196.

Garlic

Antitussive: Elimination of Cold Phlegm with Plants that are Warm in Nature

Botanical Name: Allium sativum.
Family: Alliaceae.
Region Where Grown: All Regions.
Other Names: None.
Category: Antitussive: Elimination of Cold Phlegm with Plants that are Warm in Nature.
Properties: Acrid, Hot/Moist.
Esoteric Botanica: Maat.
Governing Organs: Liver, Lung, Stomach.
Actions & Indications: It is used to relieve rheumatism, diabetes and malaria, treatment for asthma, artherosclerosis and hypertension and hyperlipidemia and peripheral vascular disorders.

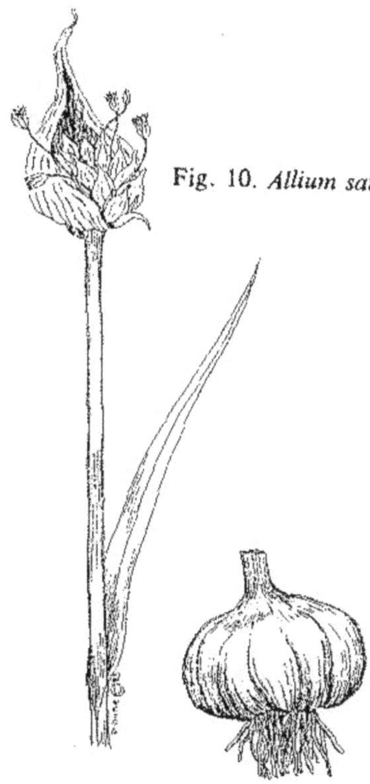

Fig. 10. *Allium sativ*

It is decoted as a diuretic, intestinal antiseptic and vermifuge.[264] It is a gastric stimulant, expectorant and carminative.
Garlic is consumed raw to strengthen the lungs.
Boiled and eaten to alleviate intestinal gas (wind, flatulence).[265] It is juiced and used as a rubefacient, caustic, vesicant or disinfectant in treating deafness, manage scabrous conditions, callouses on the feet, infected swellings and rheumatic pains. Internally, the juice is taken as a stimulant, expectorant and diaphoretic as well as to relieve indigestion, flatulence and coughs.[266] Decoted as a diauretic, stomachache, indigestion and intestinal worms.
Cautions & Contraindications: Use with caution during pregnancy, or in cases where the normal qi is weak or where there is stomach cold from deficiency.
Major Known Ingredients: Allium Sativum contains volatile oil (containing allicin, allin, diallyl sulphide ajoene and other sulphur compounds.[267]
Pharmacological & Clinical Research: Garlic has been used in traditional medicine for over 4,000 years to treat disorders of arthritis, common cold, diabetes, malaria, and tuberculosis. The microbiologist Louis Pasteur studied the bactericidal properties of garlic. During the Second World War garlic was called

---

[264] Morton F. Julia, *Atlas of Medical Plants of Middle America: Bahamas to Yucatan.* Springfield, Illinois: Charles C Thomas Publisher, 1981; 77.
[265] DeFilipps, Robert A., Shirley L. Maina, and Juliette Crepin. *Medicinal Plants of the Guianas (Guyana, Surinam, French Guiana).* Washington, D.C.: Dept. of Botany, National Museum of Natural History, Smithsonian Institution, 2004; 6.
[266] Morton F. Julia, *Atlas of Medical Plants of Middle America: Bahamas to Yucatan.* Springfield, Illinois: Charles C Thomas Publisher, 1981; 77.
[267] Singh, A. P. *Compendia of World's Medicinal Flora.* Enfield, NH: Science, 2006; 49.

"Russian penicillin" because the Russian government turned to this ancient treatment for its soldiers when supplies of antibiotics had been exhausted. It has been shown experimentally that garlic possesses therapeutic and preventive activities against bacterial infection, atherosclerosis, high total cholesterol, and Hypertension. It also protects against free radicals and also aids in prolongation of blood coagulation time. It is ranked at the top as the strongest cancer preventive vegetable on the "Designer Foods Project".[268] Used in a cure for Guinea worm with *Allium cepa* and other ingredients.[269] It is researched as an antioxidant, cardio protective, antibacterial, anti fungal, hypolipidemic, hypertensive (allicin and extract and antiplatelet (ajoene) properties.[270] It has been investigated for use in in the prevention and treatment of cancer and atherosclerosis.[271]

Toxicity: Garlic contains allicin which is antifungul and antibacterial. Garlic is toxic to mosquito larvae and has been experimentally used to protect crops from thrips and other insect pets and fungal pathogens. It is an effective mosquito and black fly repellent.[272]

[268] Ahmad Iqbal, Aqil Farrukh and Owais Mohammad. *Modern Phytomedicine: Turning Medicinal Plants into Drugs.* Germany: Wiley-VCH Verlag GmbH & Co. KGaA, 2006; 80.

[269] DeFilipps, Robert A., Shirley L. Maina, and Juliette Crepin. *Medicinal Plants of the Guianas (Guyana, Surinam, French Guiana).* Washington, D.C.: Dept. of Botany, National Museum of Natural History, Smithsonian Institution, 2004; 5.

[270] Singh, A. P. *Compendia of World's Medicinal Flora.* Enfield, NH: Science, 2006; 49.

[271] Yaniv, Zohara, and Uriel Bachrach. *Handbook of Medicinal Plants.* New York: Food Products ; Haworth Medical, 2005; 13.

[272] Morton F. Julia, *Atlas of Medical Plants of Middle America: Bahamas to Yucatan.* Springfield, Illinois: Charles C Thomas Publisher, 1981; 76.

Daisy

Antitussive: Elimination of Cold Phlegm with Plants that are Warm in Nature

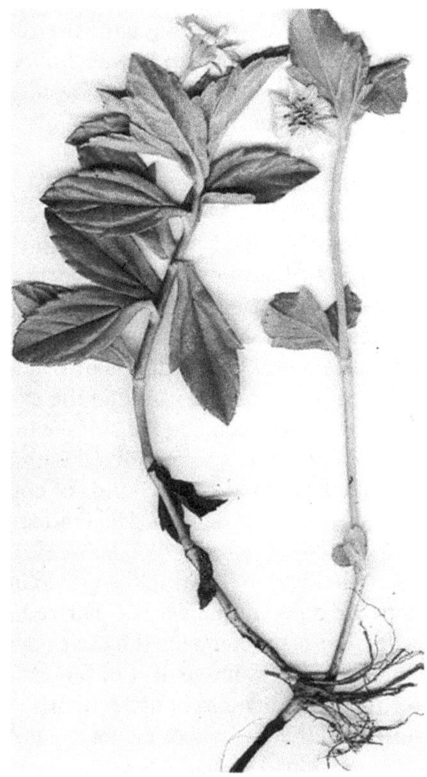

Botanical Name: Sphagneticola Trilobata.
Family: Asteraceae.
Region Where Grown: All Regions.
Other Names: Creeping Daisy, Creeping Wild Daisy, Yellow Creeping Daisy.
Category: Antitussive: Elimination of Cold Phlegm with Plants that are Warm in Nature.
Properties: Sour, Aromatic, Hot/Moist.
Esoteric Botanica: Tehuti.
Governing Organs: Liver, Lung.
Actions & Indications: Whole plant: a strong decoction is employed to treat severe chest colds.[273] Releases the exterior and disperses cold – for externally contracted wind-cold with such symptoms as fever, chills, headache, nasal congestion, cough or stifling sensation in the chest. Releases the exterior and expels wind – for exterior patterns of either wind-cold. Clears the liver and the eyes – for either wind-heat in the liver channel manifested in red, painful, dry eyes or excessive tearing, or yin deficiency of the kidneys and liver with such symptoms as spots in front of the eyes, blurry vision, or dizziness. Also for initial stages of carbuncles and boils, especially when accompanied by chills and fever. and body aches due to externally-contracted wind-cold.
Cautions & Contraindications: Not recommended for nursing mothers as the herb may lead to insufficient lactation.
Major Known Ingredients: Contains acetylenes and derivatives of kaurenic acid.

---

[273] DeFilipps, Robert A., Shirley L. Maina, and Juliette Crepin. *Medicinal Plants of the Guianas (Guyana, Surinam, French Guiana)*. Washington, D.C.: Dept. of Botany, National Museum of Natural History, Smithsonian Institution, 2004; 48.

Ironwood

Antitussive: Elimination of Cold Phlegm with Plants that are Warm in Nature

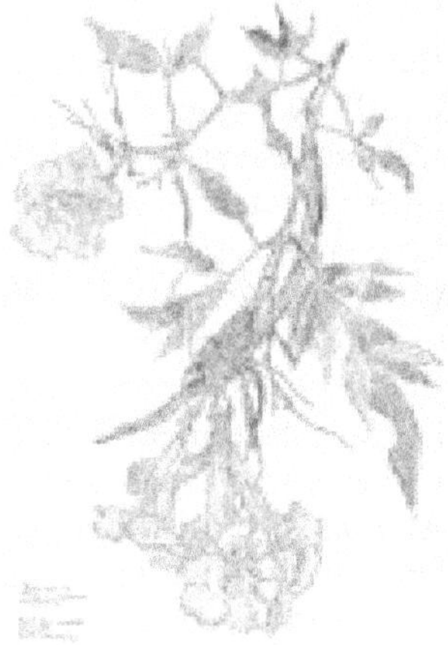

Botanical Name: Tabebuia Capitata.
Family: Bignoniceae.
Region Where Grown: Cuyuni-Mazaruni.
Other Names: Greenheart. Akawaio: Arauin, Arawnig. Arawak: Hakia. Macushi: Ranoi. Wapishana: Konawadranup.
Category: Antitussive: Elimination of Cold Phlegm with Plants that are Warm in Nature.
Properties: Sour, Aromatic, Hot/Moist.
Esoteric Botanica: Maat.
Governing Organs: Liver, Lung, Large Intestine, Heart.
Actions & Indications: Stem: Decoction of the bark used as an external wash for a febrifuge. Releases the exterior and disperses wind-heat – for patterns of wind-heat with fever, headache and cough. Clears the head and eyes and benefits the throat – for patterns of wind-heat with sore throat, red eyes and headache. Vents rashes – used in the early stages of rashes (e.g. measles) to induce the rash to come to the surface to speed recovery.
Whole plant: In a decoction mixed with honey to relieve coughing. Stops coughing and c alms wheezing – used quite broadly for many kinds of cough disorders caused by either heat or cold, depending on the combination. Because the herb is moist in nature, it is especially useful for externally-contracted dry cough.
Stem: Dried bark of the trunk is grated and applied as a plaster for a remedy for leishmaniasis, and plaster is changed daily until ulcer is cicatrized; Clears heat, relieves fire toxicity and cools the blood – for warm-febrile diseases accompanied by extreme heat or heat signs and for very high fevers at the nutritive or blood level with reckless movement of blood. Fire toxins may be either severe fevers or pustulate damp-heat sores (boils, carbuncles or appendicitis). Invigorates the blood and breaks up blood stasis – for blood stasis disorders in the lower abdomen such as dysmenorrhea, amenorrhea, palpable masses, lochioschesis and pain due to blood stasis. Also used for blood stasis obstructing the chest with chest or epigastirc pain, a well as soreness in the ribs or hypochondria due the constrained liver qi with blood stasis. Relieves toxicity, kills parasites and stops itching – applied topically for scabies, ringworm, and yin furuncles, as well as for damp festering sores, ulcers and carbuncles. Also alleviates itching associated with these types of disorders.
Bark used against fever. Alexiteric; bark used as an antidote to snake poison and manchineel poison. wood used in a sudorific decoction.
Cautions & Contraindications: Do not use during pregnancy or in cases of yin deficiency with heat signs. Not appropriate for internal use.
Major Known Ingredients: Plant contains lapachol, a naphthoquinone having antitumor activity on rat carcinosarcoma.

Okra

Antitussive: Elimination of Cold Phlegm with Plants that are Warm in Nature

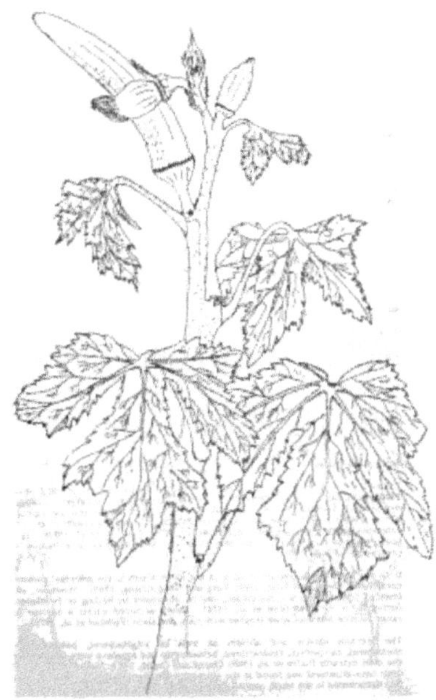

Botanical Name: Abelmoschus Esculentus.
Family: Malvaceae.
Region Where Grown: All Regions.
Other Names: Ochra, Ochro, Okra. Musk, Musk Ochro, Vegetable Musk Plant.
Category: Antitussive: Elimination of Cold Phlegm with Plants that are Warm in Nature.
Properties:Acrid, Cool/Dry.
Esoteric Botanica: Sebek.
Governing Organs: Liver, Large Intestine, Stomach.
Actions & Indications: Leaf: Absesses, boils, carbuncles, fistulas, ulcers, sudorifics, cancer tumors, gonorrhea, stomachics and carminatives.
Crushed in water for treating disturbances of childbirth and as an emollient mucilage.
Flower: Infusion to treat phlegm in mucous membranes of chest.
Fruit: Juice of young fruit used to treat chest colds, and as eyedrops. Fruit crushed with the young leaves and used to wash hair and to treat dandruff. [274]Young fruit in a remedy placed on bloody ulcers. Decoction for problems of womb or uterus. Boiled in milk for treating rheumatism. Pulp for sore eyes.
Leaf: Applied to forehead to control violent headache; febrifuge; anti-inflammatory; decoction of leaves and green fruit in a bath to ease childbirth. Seed: Stimulant and antispasmodic properties are useful in treating snakebite. Crushed seeds in oil are rubbed on a fever patient as a sudorific. Musk-scented seeds are used as a masticatory for dental cavities and bad breath. Seed also use as infusion as a cephalic, stomachic and antispasmodic and for inducing itch.
Major Known Ingredients: Seed-oil contains farnesol, ambrettolic acid and the lactone ambrettolide. Petals contain the flavonol cannabiscitrine and cyanidine glycoside.
Pharmacological & Clinical Research: Anti-tumor activity against sarcoma 180 in mice was shown by peptidoglycans obtained from the related species Hibuscus manihot in a root extract. Quercetin 3-robinobioside, quercetin 3-glucoside, quercetin, hypericin and myricetin were isolated from Abelmoschus manihot flowers which are used in the treatment of chronic bronchitis and toothache.

---

[274] DeFilipps, Robert A., Shirley L. Maina, and Juliette Crepin. *Medicinal Plants of the Guianas (Guyana, Surinam, French Guiana)*. Washington, D.C.: Dept. of Botany, National Museum of Natural History, Smithsonian Institution, 2004; 169.

Antitussive: Elimination of Heat Phlegm with Cleansing Plants

Plants that eliminate heat phelgm can lower the blood pressure and decrease the blood flow to the lung, bronchi and bronchioles. They can increase the immunity of the body and the energy metabolic rate of the tissues.

Physic Nut

Antitussive: Elimination of Heat Phlegm with cleansing Plants

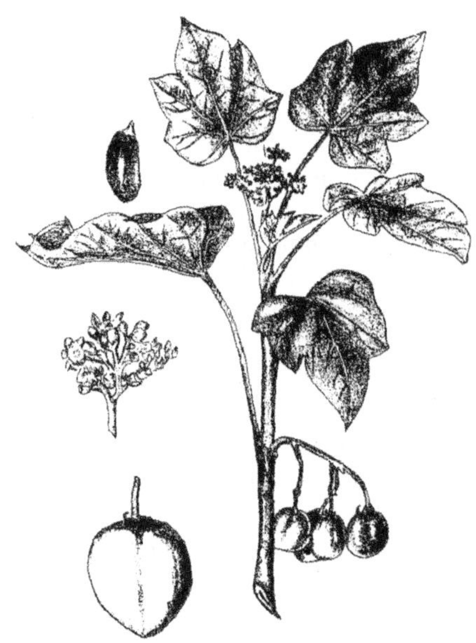

Botanical Name: Jatropha Curcas.
Family: Euphorbiaceae.
Region Where Grown: Mahaica-Berbice.
Other Names: None.
Category: A ntitussive: Elimination of Heat Phlegm with Cleansing Plants .
Properties: Sweet, Acrid, Cold/Moist.
Esoteric Botanica: Auset.
Governing Organs: Stomach, Lung, Heart, Liver.
Actions & Indications: Extracts are used in folk remedies for cancer. Reported to be abortifacient, anodyne, antiseptic, icatrizant, depurative, diuretic, emetic, hemostat, lactagogue, narcotic, purgative, rubefacient, styptic, vermifuge and vulnerary. Physic nut is a folk remedy for alopecia, anasarca, ascites, burns, carbuncles, convulsions, cough, dermatitis, diarrhea and dropsy.[275]
Latex: Dental analgesic when swabbed a tooth-cavity. Leaf: Cataplasm for neuralgia, fever, wounds, headaches, swellings; foot-rub for sand fleas.
Leaf used for abcesses, coughs and colds, heart problems, pain, sores and toothaches. Clears heat and transforms phlegm – relieves heartburn and is used as a febrifuge and in cases of constipation and diarrhea.[276] Many types of cough, chiefly chronic cough, cough with signs of fire due to yin deficiency, cough with slight sputum that is difficult to expectorate or cough with blood-streaked sputum. It is most effective in treatments for reduced appetite and a stifling sensation in the chest and upper abdomen.

---

[275] Yaniv, Zohara, and Uriel Bachrach. *Handbook of Medicinal Plants*. New York: Food Products ; Haworth Medical, 2005; 254.
[276] Morton F. Julia, *Atlas of Medical Plants of Middle America: Bahamas to Yucatan.* Springfield, Illinois: Charles C Thomas Publisher, 1981; 448.

Leaf and Fruit: Decoction for abdominal disorders, rheumatism, ulcers and swellings.[277] Reduces phlegm and softens areas of hardness – for various kinds of nodules in the neck or a sensation of fullness and obstruction in the chest caused by phlegm. Promotes urination and reduces swelling. Oil is emetic, purgative; grated in poultice for abscesses.
Cautions & Contraindications: Do not use in cases of nausea and vomiting caused by stomach cold or cold food stagnation.
Major Known Ingredients: Seed contains the toxalbumin curcine. Seeds have a depressant action on the central nervous system. Per 100 g, the seed is reported to contain 6.6 g H20, J8.2 g protein, 38.0 g fat, 33.5 total carbohydrate, 15.5 g fiber, and 4.5 g ash. Leaves, which show antileukemic activity, contain a!pha-amynn, beta-sitosterol, stigmasterol, and campesterol, 7-keto-beta-sitosterol, sigma-5ene-beta, 7-alpha-diol, stigmast-5ene-3-beta, 7-beta-diol. Leaves contain isovitexin and vitexin. From the drug (nut?) saccharose, raffinose, stachyose, glucose, fructose, galactose, protein, and an oil, largely of oleic and linoleic-acids; curcasin, arachidic-, linoleic, myristic-, stearic-acids.[278]
Pharmacological & Clinical Research: Four antitumor compounds, including jatropham and Jatrophone, are reported from other species of *Jatropha.* Homeopathically used for cold sweats, colic, collapse, cramps, cyanosis, diarrhea and leg cramps.[279]
Toxicity: The bark contains a steroidal sapogenin. The sap is irritating to the skin and toxic internally.[280] Poisonous seeds can cause death due to the toxalbumin, curcin. The poisoning is irritant, with acute abdominal pain and nausea about half hour following ingestion. Diarrhea and nausea continue but are not usually serious. Depression and collapse may occur, especially in children. Two seeds are a strong purgative. Four to five seed are said to have caused death but the roasted seed is said to be nearly innocuous.[281]

---

[277] Duke, James A., and Rodolfo Vásquez. *Amazonian Ethnobotanical Dictionary*. Boca Raton, FL: CRC, 1994; 98.
[278] Yaniv, Zohara, and Uriel Bachrach. *Handbook of Medicinal Plants*. New York: Food Products ; Haworth Medical, 2005; 254.
[279] Yaniv, Zohara, and Uriel Bachrach. *Handbook of Medicinal Plants*. New York: Food Products ; Haworth Medical, 2005; 254
[280] Morton F. Julia, *Atlas of Medical Plants of Middle America: Bahamas to Yucatan.* Springfield, Illinois: Charles C Thomas Publisher, 1981; 449
[281] Yaniv, Zohara, and Uriel Bachrach. *Handbook of Medicinal Plants*. New York: Food Products ; Haworth Medical, 2005; 254.

Crabwood

Antitussive: Elimination of Heat Phlegm with cleansing Plants

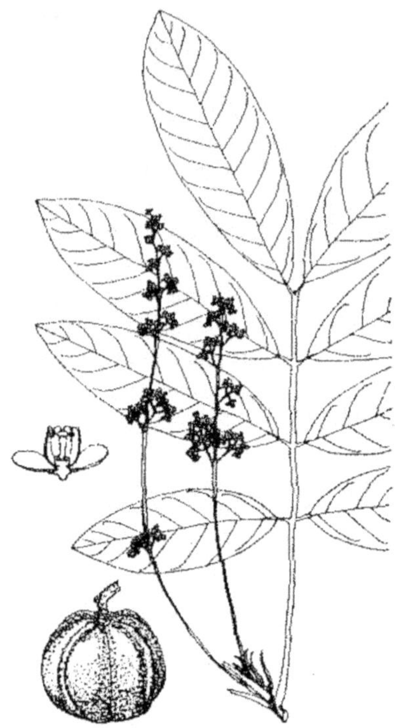

Botanical Name: Carapa Guianensis.
Family: Meliaceae.
Region Where Grown: Pomeroon-Supenaam.
Other Names: Bullet wood, Crab oil, Karapai, Caraba, Karaba.
Category: Antitussive: Elimination of Heat Phlegm with Cleansing Plants.
Properties: Bitter, Hot/Dry.
Esoteric Botanica: Heru.
Governing Organs:Heart, Lung, Spleen, Liver.
Actions & Indications: Crabwood is used primarily as an emollient and anti-inflammatory for skin rash.
Stem: Bark is macerated, left overnight in water and used for washing the skin as a medicament for chicken pox or for measles. Juice from macerated bark is used for treating eczema.
Bark decoction used to dress ulcers, cure diarrhoea and to relieve stomachache and rheumatism.[282] The bitter bark infusion is used as a febrifuge, vermifuge and as a tonic useful in herpes. Infusion used to wash dermatoses and sores (Bark used for diarrhea, malaria, burns, sores, stomachache, and wounds/cuts).[283]
Leaf: Decoction for washing wounds and persistent ulcers.
Fruit: Oil extracted from fruit is used to treat eczema, sore stomach, hacking cough, bronchial tract discomforts, lung trouble and running sores. Drop of oil and a drop of red lavender given for children's thrush. Use the oil on skin for a mosquito repellent, skin softener, to prevent colds and excess perspiration and for glossy, strong hair.
Fruit: Grated nut is mixed with palm oil and used as an analgesic for muscular aches and pain, as an anrti-fungal, as a treatment for dry skin, for sores, eczema, measles or for chicken pox. Grated nut is mixed with hot water and drunk as an anti-dysenteric. It is boiled and drunk as an anti-menorrhagic during the menstrual cycle. Grated nut is soaked overnight and drunk as an anti-diarrheal and antimalarial. Oil spread on feet to repel sand fleas. Seed-oil for a skin lotion, especially for children with thrush and dried, cracked skin and to treat pain, swelling and itching.
Seeds are ground amd the juice used as insect repellant. Seeds are ground, mixed with palm oil and used as an ointment for treating genital herpes, for treating sores, and for treating itching. Seeds are ground, oil is extracted and used as an ointment to treat swelling such as caused by mumps. Seeds are used for treating coughs and colds, wounds and cuts, sores, groin ruptures, hemorrhoids, insect bites, malaria, thrush and whooping cough. Used as soap and for treating bites, diarrhea and rhumatism.
Cautions & Contraindications: Do not use in cases of deficiency cold of the spleen and stomach, phlegm-cold or phlegm dampness.

---

[282] Morton F. Julia, *Atlas of Medical Plants of Middle America: Bahamas to Yucatan*. Springfield, Illinois: Charles C Thomas Publisher, 1981;183.
[283] Duke, James A., and Rodolfo Vásquez. *Amazonian Ethnobotanical Dictionary*. Boca Raton, FL: CRC, 1994; 40.

Major Known Ingredients: Bark contains carapine, a bitter principle soluble in alcohol and ether, insoluble in water. Carapa oil contains palmitic, stearic, arachidic, oleic, linoleic and linolenic acids. Seed contains andirobin and 7-desacetoxy-7-ketogedunin, Heartwood contains 11 B-acetoxygedunin and 6A, 11 B-diacetoxygedunin

Eucalyptus

Antitussive: Elimination of Heat Phlegm with cleansing Plants

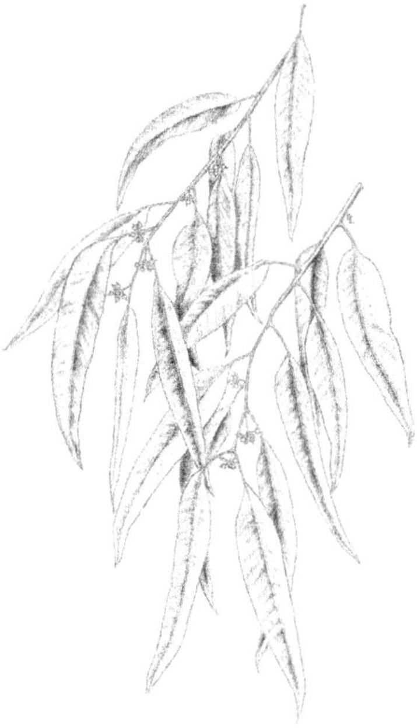

Botanical Name: Eucalyptus Camaldulensis.
Family:Myrtaceae.
Region Where Grown: E. Berbice-Corentyne.
Other Names: Red River Gum.
Category: Antitussive: Elimination of Heat Phlegm with Cleansing Plants.
Properties: Aromatic, Acrid, Hot/Moist.
Esoteric Botanica: Maat.
Governing Organs:Liver, Lung, Kidney.
Actions & Indications: Leaf: Infusion inhaled or mixed with infusion of other aromatic plants and drunk as a tea to treat colds, congestion and (less commonly) diabetes.[284] Opens the orifices and penetrates through turbidity – for closed disorders, phlegm blockages, and epidemic toxic diseases. Especially, indicated for cold disorders. Opens up areas of constraint and clears away filth – for stifling sensations, cold, fullness and pain in the chest and abdomen. Revives the spirit and unblocks closed disorders – because of its intensely aromatic penetrating nature, this substance is used for treating a wide variety of problems that impair consciousness. These include convulsions, delirium, stupor and fainting, tetanic collapse, phlegm collapse and seizures. Releases the exterior and disperses wind-heat – for patterns of wind-heat with fever, headache and cough. Clears the head and eyes and benefits the throat – for patterns of wind-heat with sore throat, red eyes & headache. Vents rashes – used in the early stages of rashes (e.g. measles) to induce the rash to come to the surface to speed recovery.
Cautions & Contraindications: Do not use in cases of exterior deficiency or yin deficiency with heat signs. Not recommended for nursing mothers as the herb may lead to insufficient lactation.
Pharmacological & Clinical Research: Eucalyptus oil is used in modern medicinal preparations as a decongestant, anti-inflammatory, vasoconstrictor and local antiseptic.[285]

---

[284] DeFilipps, Robert A., Shirley L. Maina, and Juliette Crepin. *Medicinal Plants of the Guianas (Guyana, Surinam, French Guiana)*. Washington, D.C.: Dept. of Botany, National Museum of Natural History, Smithsonian Institution, 2004; 206

[285] Morton F. Julia, *Atlas of Medical Plants of Middle America: Bahamas to Yucatan.* Springfield, Illinois: Charles C Thomas Publisher, 1981; 206.

Camphor Bush

Antitussive: Elimination of Heat Phlegm with cleansing Plants

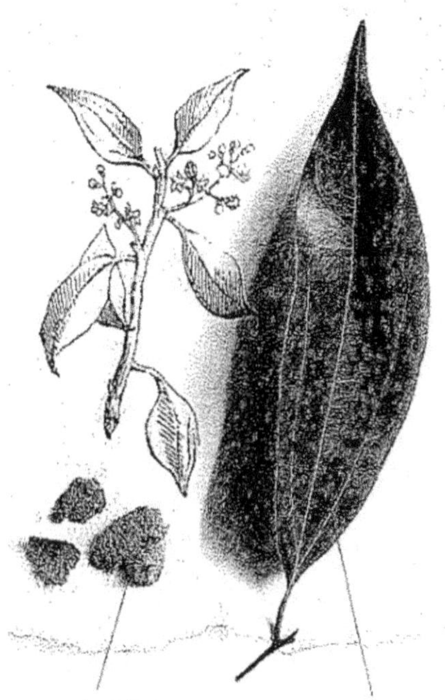

Botanical Name: Unxia Camphorata.
Family: Asteraceae.
Region Where Grown: E. Berbice-Corentyne.
Other Names: Haiwa-Balli Grass, Sand Bitters.
Category: Antitussive: Elimination of Heat Phlegm with Cleansing Plants .
Properties: Sour, Aromatic, Acrid, Cold/Dry.
Esoteric Botanica: Seker.
Governing Organs: Liver, Heart.
Actions & Indications: Camphor is a cardiac and respiratory analeptic and is also a general stimulant. The essential oil is antiseptic and is used as a pulmonary antiseptic and expectorant. It has been recommended as a mild analgesic and rubefacient for rheumatism and for pains in external use.[286] Camphor is generally used for skin care; acne, inflammation, circulation, joints and muscles: arthritis, muscular ache and pains, rhematism, sprains, respiratory; system: bronchitis, chills, cough and immune: fever, colds, flu infectious disease. Whole plant: A decoction of whole plant or of leaves is drunk as a blood purifier. [287] Clears heat, relieves fire toxicity and cools the blood – for warm-febrile diseases accompanied by extreme heat or heat signs and for very high fevers at the nutritive or blood level with reckless movement of blood. Fire toxins may be either severe fevers or pustulate damp-heat sores (boils, carbuncles, or appendicitis). Clears heat and cools the blood – for all warm-febrile diseases where heat enters the Nutritive level causing very high fever, thirst and a scarlet tongue with no coat. Also indicated in cases of hemorrhage due to heat entering the blood level.
Leaf: Leaves are macerated in alcohol and rubbed on the chest to alleviate bronchitis.
Cautions & Contraindications: Do not use in cases of cold from deficiency of the spleen or kidneys with diarrhea.
Pharmacological & Clinical research:
Toxicity: The carcinogen safrole occurs in the oil, more in the roots than in other parts. Toxic doses of camphor taken internally result in convulsions, accompanied by vertigo and mental confusion, and may lead to delirium and even to coma and death. As little as 700 mg can cause narcosis, 2000 mg inducing dulled senses, hallucinations, cramps and unconsciousness. There may be intense burning in the stomach

---

[286] Oliver-Bever, Bep. *Medicinal Plants in Tropical West Africa.* Cambridge: Cambridge UP, 1986; 4
[287] Morton F. Julia, *Atlas of Medical Plants of Middle America: Bahamas to Yucatan.* Springfield, Illinois: Charles C Thomas Publisher, 1981; 8.

accompanied by illness and nausea. Paralysis may follow, finally affecting the respiratory and vasomotor centers.[288]

Antitussive and Anti Asthmatic

The antitussive and anti-asthmatic group of Plants can inhibit the excitory state of the respiratory center, and cough reflex. They can dilate the bronchi and the respiratory tract.

Boyari

Antitussive and Anti Asthmatic

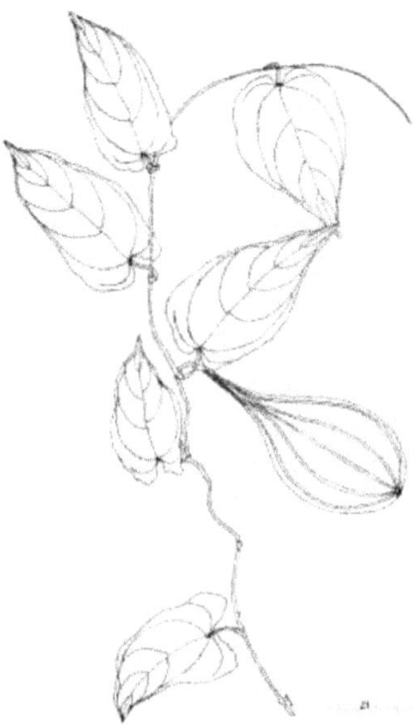

Botanical Name: Aristolochia Daemoninoxius.
Family: Aristolochiaceae.
Region Where Grown: Potaro-Siparuni.
Other Names: Pauisima.
Category: Antitussive: Anti-Asthmatic.
Properties: Sour, Hot/Moist.
Esoteric Botanica: Maat.
Governing Organs: Liver, Spleen, Kidney, Large Intestine.
Actions & Indications: Whole plant: Antispasmodic; used for tuberculosis, bronchitis, severe coughs, bowel problems, dyspepsia and indigestion.[289] Expels phlegm and stops wheezing – for wheezing with coughing and copious sputum. Depending on the other plants used, it can treat cold or hot phlegm. Stops coughing and wheezing, redirects the qi downward, and dissolves phlegm – for coughing and wheezing with copious phlegm. Especially useful when exhalation is more labored than inhalation and when there is a stifling sensation in the chest.
Stem: Used as abortive, contraceptive; and for female sterility, fever and stomachache.
Leaf: Decocted with other plants for sweating out a fever; decoction for a female oral contraceptive and abortifacient.
Cautions & Contraindications: Do not use in cases of excess. Use with caution whenever there is viscous sputum that is difficult to expectorate. This herb should not be taken in large quantities or long-term. Symptoms of overdose include headache, fever, tremors, irritability and dyspnea.
Major Known Ingredients: Juniper camphor, a sesquiterpene lactone, has been isolated from this species, and delay of oestrus in female mice can be caused by chemicals in the plant.[290]

---

[288] Yaniv, Zohara, and Uriel Bachrach. *Handbook of Medicinal Plants*. New York: Food Products ; Haworth Medical, 2005; 126.
[289] DeFilipps, Robert A., Shirley L. Maina, and Juliette Crepin. *Medicinal Plants of the Guianas (Guyana, Surinam, French Guiana)*. Washington, D.C.: Dept. of Botany, National Museum of Natural History, Smithsonian Institution, 2004; 38.
[290]Ibid., p, 38.

Ruku

Antitussive and Anti Asthmatic

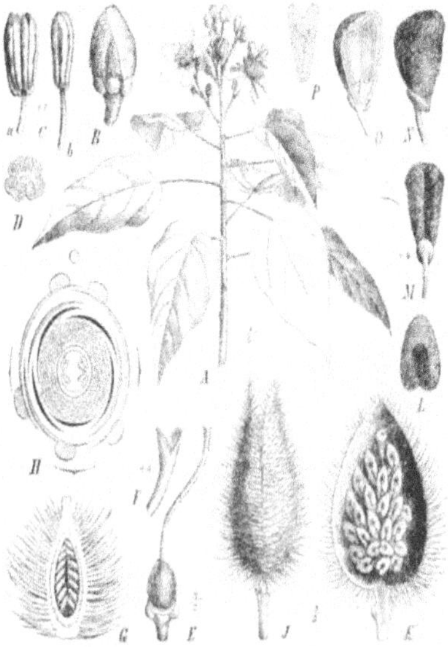

Botanical Name: Bixa Orellana.
Family: Bixaceae.
Region Where Grown: U. Takutu-U. Essequibo.
Other Names: Bixa. Bija. Rucu. Roucou.
Category: Antitussive: Anti-Asthmatic, astringent (stop diarrhea)
Properties: Sweet, Cold/Moist.
Esoteric Botanica: Auset.
Governing Organs: Stomach, Small Intestine, Heart.
Actions & Indications: Whole plant: This plant is used primarily as a diuretic, purgative, in treatment for gonorrhea, diarrhea, hemorrhoids, jaundice and emmenagogue.[291] It is also administered in cases of pleurisy, asthma and labored breathing, influenza and venereal diseases, dysentery and fever.[292]
Stem: Young shoots applied locally on abscesses. Sap from bark and crushed leaves for skin rashes; bark decoction for malaria; angina, asthma.
Leaf: The leaves are used for bronchial infections jaundice, dysentery and tumors. The pulp is used a haemostatic, antidysenteric, diuretic, febrifuge as well as epilepsy and skin diseases.[293]
Fruit: Fruit is used for flavoring food, especially curry, as well as used to rub the skin to prevent sores. The seed oil is used for treating leprosy. The gum is used gonorrhea and liver problems. Roots are antiperiodic and antispasmodic.[294]
Cautions & Contraindications: Do not use in cases Spleen deficiency or loose stool.
Major Known Ingredients: The red pulpy seed coat contains a group of pigments, with bixin, a sesterpene (having a carotenoid skeleton) amounting to 70-80%. Other pigments present are orellin, methyl bixin, β-carotene, cryptoxanthin, lutein and zeaxanthin. Tsobixin is the trans-form of the unstable naturally occurring cis-bixin, The seeds yield protein (17%), carbohydrates (14%), mucilage (4.5%,), a fixed oil, an essential oil, oleoresin, phytosterols and alkaloids. The oleoresin which amounts to l% of the seed contain all-E-geranyl geraniol (57%), farnasyl acetone, geranyl octadecanoate and volatile oil contains ishwarone (30%), ά-pinene, β-pinene, etc. The dried leaves yield a gum and an essential oil (similar to that of seeds) consisting of a sesquiterpcne, bixaghanene, ellagic acid, flavones such as apigenin, luteolin along with their

---

[291] Morton F. Julia, *Atlas of Medical Plants of Middle America: Bahamas to Yucatan.* Springfield, Illinois: Charles C Thomas Publisher, 1981; 572.
[292] Castner, James L., S. Lee. Timme, and James A. Duke. *A Field Guide to Medicinal and Useful Plants of the Upper Amazon.* Gainesville, FL: Feline, 1998; 27.
[293] Daniel, M. *Medicinal Plants: Chemistry and Properties*. Enfield, NH: Science, 2006; 141.
[294] Ibid., p, 141.

bisulphab and glucosides, isoscutellarien, bixorellin and a steroidal sapogenin. Tl roots contain a triterpene acid, tomentosic acid.[295]
Pharmacological & Clinical Research: The red pulp for coloring purposes has been assayed for vitamin A activity with the conclusion that it contains 1,000 to 2,000 I.U. Vitamin A per gram of oily extract. The leaf oil is rich in the uncommon tetracyclic sesduiterpene hydrocarbon ishwarane.[296]
Toxicity: The seed contains a toxic alkaloid.

[295] Ibid., p, 140
[296] Morton F. Julia, *Atlas of Medical Plants of Middle America: Bahamas to Yucatan.* Springfield, Illinois: Charles C Thomas Publisher, 1981; 572.

Jumbie Tree

Antitussive and Anti Asthmatic

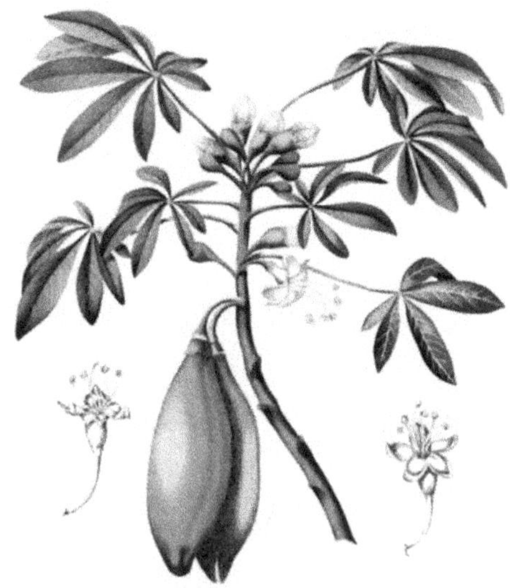

Botanical Name: Ceiba Pentandra.
Family: Bombacaceae.
Region Where Grown: U. Takutu-U. Essequibo.
Other Names: Cotton Silk. Kapok.
Category: Antitussive: Anti-Asthmatic.
Properties: Sour, Aromatic, Hot/moist.
Esoteric Botanica: Maat.
Governing Organs: Liver, Large Intestine, Lung
Actions & Indications: Primarily used as an emetic and a diuretic,[297] and decocted for its febrifuge properties. Releases the exterior and disperses cold – for externally contracted wind-cold with such symptoms as fever, chills, headache, nasal congestion or cough.
Leaf: Juice from bruised young branches in a preparation to treat asthma and dissolving phlegm; to smoothe rectal inflammation (hemorrhoids) and treat gonorrhea.[298] Leaves are decoted as a diuretic. Moistens the lungs and stops coughing – for both acute and chronic cough. Leaves stewed for a gonorrhoea remedy. Stops coughing and wheezing and drains heat from the lungs – for coughing and wheezing due to lung heat. Used in disorders where lung heat obstructs the downward movement of lung qi, preventing water from moving and cutting off perspiration.
Bark: Bark is used as a febriguge,[299] diuretic and antispasmodic and to leg ulcers
Cautions & Contraindications: Do not use for yin deficiency with heat signs
Major Known Ingredients: Leaf contains quercetin, camphorol, caffeic acid, resin and 10.82% tannin and is known to have a curarelike action on the nerves of an experiemental animal.[300]

[297] Castner, James L., S. Lee. Timme, and James A. Duke. *A Field Guide to Medicinal and Useful Plants of the Upper Amazon.* Gainesville, FL: Feline, 1998. 34.
[298] DeFilipps, Robert A., Shirley L. Maina, and Juliette Crepin. *Medicinal Plants of the Guianas (Guyana, Surinam, French Guiana).* Washington, D.C.: Dept. of Botany, National Museum of Natural History, Smithsonian Institution, 2004. 56.
[299] Castner, James L., S. Lee. Timme, and James A. Duke. *A Field Guide to Medicinal and Useful Plants of the Upper Amazon.* Gainesville, FL: Feline, 1998; 34.
[300] Morton F. Julia, *Atlas of Medical Plants of Middle America: Bahamas to Yucatan.* Springfield, Illinois: Charles C Thomas Publisher, 1981; 542.

Antitussive Plants that Relieve Cough by Moistening Effect

This group of plants has moistening effect and can regulate the electrolyte balance . External cough is caused by the dry weather and affection of flu. Internal cough is due to depletion of fluid in the lung with symptoms of dry throat with no mucous, thin blood sputum. If the kidney is affected, there is heat sensation in the hands and feet, steaming sensation in the bone and night perspiration.

Moco-Moco

Antitussive Plants that Relieve Cough by Moistening Effect

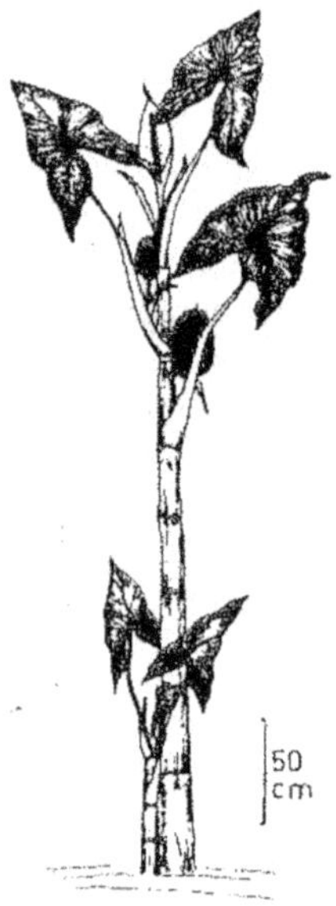

Botanical Name: Montrichardia Arborescens.
Family: Araceae.
Region Where Grown: Barima-Waini.
Other Names: Moka-Moka, Moku-Moku, Muccomucco, Mmucka-Mucka.
Category: Antitussive: Plants that Relieve Coughing by Moistening Effect.
Properties: Bitter, Hot/Dry.
Esoteric Botanica: Heru.
Governing Organs: Heart, Kidney, Lung, Liver.
Actions & Indications: For diabetes, tuberculosis, thrush, and colds.
Sap: Used to treat coughs and colds.
Stem: Contains the leakage of lung qi and stops coughing – for chronic cough and wheezing due to lung deficiency or lung and Kidney deficiency. Warms the middle and expels cold – for warming the spleen and stomach both in conditions of excess due to externally-contracted cold, as well as cold from deficiency due to insufficiency of the yang qi. Symptoms include loose stools, nausea and vomiting, loss of appetite and abdominal pain. Enriches the stomach yin and generates fluids – for dry tongue and mouth and severe thirst due to insufficient stomach yin, or for treating wasting and thirsting disorder.
Juice for remedying sting of stingray, warts.
The young, sap-filled, *leafless* shoots are roasted and applied to scorpion stings. Sap is possibly used for pulmonary phthysis and as an aphrodisiac. Used to treat stingray bites and for wounds and cuts.
Stem and Leaf: The finely ground tops of plants are stuffed into the nostrils to stop nosebleed.

Leaf: For eyelid inflammation; sap is hemostatic, used to enlarge the penis; hypertension, rheumatism. Leaf is placed on vesicles to promote discharge. Astringent; tied over sore eyes. The boiled leaves are used in baths for remedying skin conditions. Used in treatment of diabetes and tuberculosis.[301]

Cautions & Contraindications: Do not use in cases of internal heat excess and stagnation, or in unresolved exterior disorders.

Major Known Ingredients: Components of stem and leaf include steroidal saponins.

[301] DeFilipps, Robert A., Shirley L. Maina, and Juliette Crepin. *Medicinal Plants of the Guianas (Guyana, Surinam, French Guiana)*. Washington, D.C.: Dept. of Botany, National Museum of Natural History, Smithsonian Institution, 2004; 29.

Chapter 5: Digestive

Plants that Increase Digestion

The digestive plants can increase the digestion of fat, protein and carbohydrates. Some of them contain lipase and protease. Some can enhance the appetitie by increasing the secretion of gastric acid, digestion and evacuation.

Bush Rope Bowrialli

Plants that Increase Digestion

Botanical Name: Aristolochia.
Family: Aristolochiaceae (Birthworth).
Region Where Grown: Potaro-Siparuni.
Other Names: Boe-Ari, Bush Rope Bowrialli.
Category: Digestive Plants.
Properties: Sour, Hot/Moist.
Esoteric Botanica: Maat.
Governing Organs: Liver, Spleen, Lungs
Actions & Indications: Plant is used for gastritis, toothache, [302] asthma, bronchitis, coughs, fever
Stem: Scraped in an infusion for indigestion; for epigastric or abdominal pain and distention or indigestion with focal distention or gas; for epigastric or abdominal pain and distention or indigestion with focal distention or gas, for spleen or stomach stagnation with such symptoms as lack of appetite, epigastric or abdominal pain or distention, nausea, and vomiting. Stem also used for making 'bitters.'[303] Also, shredded and smoked in a cigarette to treat coughs and asthma - for chronic cough, wheezing from deficiency, asthma or consumptive coughs with blood-streaked sputum.

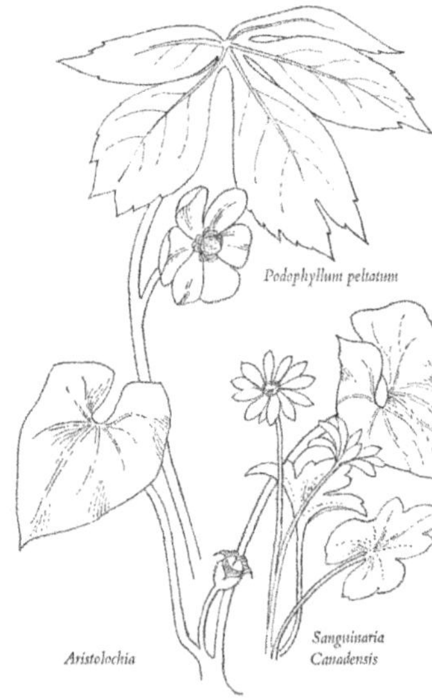

Cautions & Contraindications: Use cautiously if pregnant. It is also categorized as an abortifacient.

[302] Duke, James A. and Rodolfo Vásquez. *Amazonian Ethnobotanical Dictionary*. Boca Raton, FL: CRC, 1994; 24.
[303] DeFilipps, Robert A., Shirley L. Maina, and Juliette Crepin. *Medicinal Plants of the Guianas (Guyana, Surinam, French Guiana)*. Washington, D.C.: Dept. of Botany, National Museum of Natural History, Smithsonian Institution, 2004; 39.

Incense Tree

Plants that Increase Digestion

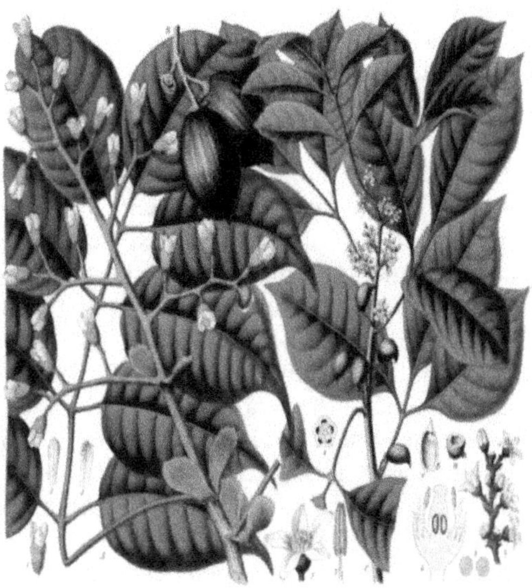

Botanical Name: Protium Guianense..
Family: Burseraceae.
Region Where Grown: Potaro-Siparuni.
Other Names: Haiawa.
Category: Digestive Plants.
Properties: Sour, Hot/Moist.
Esoteric Botanica: Tehuti.
Governing Organs: Liver, Stomach, Lungs
Actions & Indications: Bronchitis, asthma, chest pain, cough, phthysis and ulcers.
Sap is used to purge the stomach.[304]
Stem: Yields a resin which is burned as a mosquito repellent or used for remedying coughs. Alcoholic tincture of the aromatic resin is used as a topical application for ulcers, phthisis; to relieve asthma. Tonifies the Lung qi and augments the kidney essence – for wheezing due to deficiency of the lungs and kidneys. Especially useful between acute attacks or for consumption with night sweats, emaciation and debility as well as chronic cases of wheezing and cough, as in asthma.
Stem: Bark yields a resinous material which hardens on contact with air, and is put in water; the liquid is drunk to remedy chest afflictions, bronchitis and asthma.
Cautions & Contraindications: Use with caution over prolonged periods. Do not use alone for heat from yin deficiency.
Major Known Ingredients: Mix the resin into a red body paint which also has Humiria balsamifera var. floribunda, Arrabidaea chica and/or Genipa americana as ingredients, and rub the paint onto a child's head to prevent sickness caused by evil spirits.

[304] DeFilipps, Robert A., Shirley L. Maina, and Juliette Crepin. *Medicinal Plants of the Guianas (Guyana, Surinam, French Guiana)*. Washington, D.C.: Dept. of Botany, National Museum of Natural History, Smithsonian Institution, 2004; 62.

Tamarind

Plants that Increase Digestion

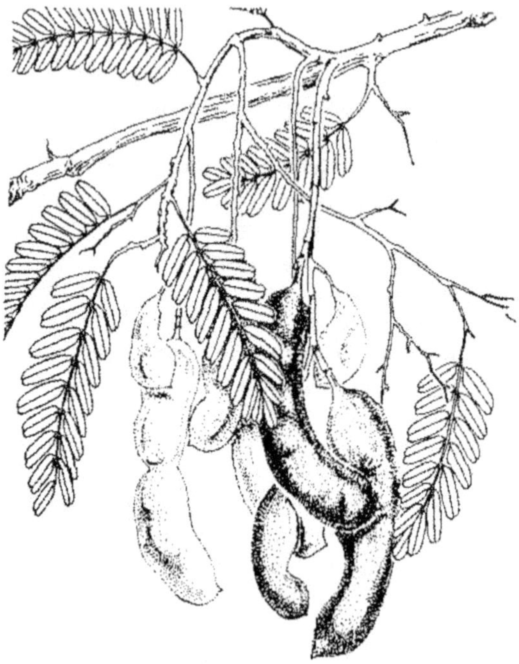

Botanical Name: Tamarindus Indica.
Family: Caesalpiniaceae.
Region Where Grown: All Regions.
Other Names: None.
Category: Digestive Plants.
Properties: Sour, Cold/Dry.
Esoteric Botanica: Seker.
Governing Organs: Liver, Large Intestine, Spleen, Lungs, Kidney .
Actions & Indications: Primarily used for laxative,[305] fevers, vermifuge, bleeding dysentery and malaria,[306] aperient, diuretic, cold and diabetes.
Leaf: Decoction or infusion for a coolant and for bathing sores or to bathe persons suffering from measles or allergies; in a rash and scabies remedy. Most of all, leaves are used for worms and gastrointestional disorders.[307] Leaf and Flower: A sweetened tea drunk by children for measles and in a preparation as a malaria remedy.
Fruit: Syrup of ripe fruit is drunk for keeping digestive organs in good condition for an aperient, as well as for a cough medicine and to remedy chest colds; pulp as a laxative. [308]
Flesh of fruit eaten to cure fevers and control gastric acid. The fruit pulp is carminative, digestive, laxative, antiscorbutic and antibilious.[309]
Flower: Decoction of flower buds used to remedy children's bedwetting and urinary complaints. Leaves and flowers are antibilious and cooling and used for constipation, dyspepsia, flatulence and urinary infection.[310]
Bark: Decoted for asthma and amenorrhea.[311]

---

305 Yaniv, Zohara, and Uriel Bachrach. *Handbook of Medicinal Plants*. New York: Food Products ; Haworth Medical, 2005; 178.

306 Bastien, Joseph William. *Healers of the Andes: Kallawaya Herbalists and Their Medicinal Plants*. Salt Lake City: University of Utah, 1987; 156.

307 Morton F. Julia, *Atlas of Medical Plants of Middle America: Bahamas to Yucatan*. Springfield, Illinois: Charles C Thomas Publisher, 1981; xvi.

308 DeFilipps, Robert A., Shirley L. Maina, and Juliette Crepin. *Medicinal Plants of the Guianas (Guyana, Surinam, French Guiana)*. Washington, D.C.: Dept. of Botany, National Museum of Natural History, Smithsonian Institution, 2004; 75.

309 Ibid., p. 210.

310 Ibid., p. 210

311 Morton F. Julia, *Atlas of Medical Plants of Middle America: Bahamas to Yucatan*. Springfield, Illinois: Charles C Thomas Publisher, 1981; xvi.

Cautions & Contraindications: Use with caution in cases of spleen or stomach deficiency without food stagnation and in cases with acid regurgitation.
Major Known Ingredients: Plant contains pyrazines and thiazoles; seed contains polyoses; bark yields proanthocyanidin and hordenine. The ripe pulp contains up to 10.86% or as much as 15.23% of tartaric acid, acetic, citric,malic and succinic acids, sugars and pectin. The seed is high in tannin.[312]

[312] Morton F. Julia, *Atlas of Medical Plants of Middle America: Bahamas to Yucatan.* Springfield, Illinois: Charles C Thomas Publisher, 1981; 351.

Papaw

Plants that Increase Digestion and Appetite

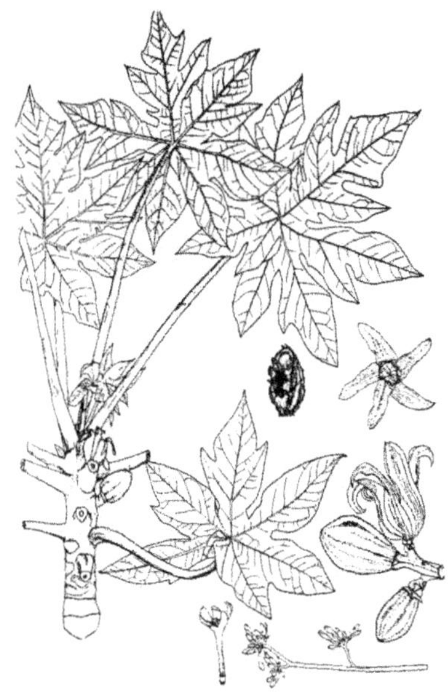

Botanical Name: Carica Papaya.
Family: Caricaceae.
Region Where Grown: Barima-Waini.
Other Names: Papaya.
Category: Digestive Plants.
Properties: Sour, Hot/Moist.
Esoteric Botanica: Tehuti.
Governing Organs: Liver, Spleen.
Actions & Indications: Papaw is rich in vitamin C and is use as a vermifuge, to induce abortion, to initiate menstruation and induce labor, treat wounds and infections.[313] The plant is used as a diuretic, anthelmintic and treat bilious conditions. Dried fruit decotion is taken orally for gall bladder and liver conditions and for disorders of fat digestion and dyspepsia.[314]
Infusion of root-bark used as an aphrodisiac; macerated root employed in gonorrhoea treatment. Decoction used externally for abdominal stricture, also drunk for the same purpose.
Root is boiled and the water drunk as an antidiarrheal, as an antimalarial or as a treatment for intestinal worm infection.
Bark: Used for diarrhea.
Leaf: As a meat tenderizer. Green leaves cooked for a tertiary malaria remedy; for irregular bowel movement in children. For high blood pressure and painful womb; smoked for asthma.
Flower: Infusion for laryngitis and bronchitis. In milk and butter for an appetite stimulant. Used to treat venereal disease.
Fruit: Sap (milky latex) is drunk in water for intestinal colic, worms in intestinal mucous membranes, and children's chlorosis. Sap is drunk for a mild digestive and anthelmintic, and to treat sunburn-caused reddish patches; latex for dyspepsia, gastritis and gastroenteritis. Infusion of young, latex-filled, green fruit as a children's vermifuge; juice to dissolve warts, hypertension and diabetes.[315]

---

[313] Castner, James L., S. Lee. Timme, and James A. Duke. *A Field Guide to Medicinal and Useful Plants of the Upper Amazon.* Gainesville, FL: Feline, 1998; 32.
[314] Ross, Ivan A. *Medicinal Plants of the World: Chemical Constituents, Traditional, and Modern Medicinal Uses*. Vol. 2. Totowa, NJ: Humana, 1999; 91
[315] DeFilipps, Robert A., Shirley L. Maina, and Juliette Crepin. *Medicinal Plants of the Guianas (Guyana, Surinam, French Guiana)*. Washington, D.C.: Dept. of Botany, National Museum of Natural History, Smithsonian Institution, 2004; 77.

Latex locally applied for toothache. Immature fruit is boiled and eaten as an anti-hypertensive. The dried latex of the Papaya is marketed under the names papayotin, papain or papoid, and is given to treat dyspepsia and gastric catarrh.[316]
Seed: Eaten as a children's vermifuge, anthelmintic, laxative; to increase visual acuity.
Cautions & Contraindications: Use with caution in cases of extreme qi deficiency.
Major Known Ingredients: Latex contains the protein-degrading (proteolytic) and mucolytic enzymes papain and chymopapain. Plant contains hydrocyanic acid, carpaine, terpene hydrocarbons, terpene alcohols, cyanogenic glycosides. The milky sap of the unripe *fruit* yields a complex proteolytic enzyme, papain, which is not destroyed by heating. The crude papain consists of two crystallized enzymes, papain and chymopapain, as well as tryptophan, tyrosine and cysteine, which all seem to be part of the crude enzyme preparation. The ellzyme has peptidase, coagulase (acting on milk casein), amylase, pectase and lipase action. Vitamins and traces of an alkaloid have also been found in the latex. This alkaloid from the pyridine group, called carpaine, has also been reported in other parts of the plant and particularly in young leaves (0.28%). The seeds contain, apart from fixed oils, carbohydrates, etc., carpasemme (a benzylrhiourea), benzyl senevol and a glucoside.[317]
Pharmacological & Clinical Research: Digestive ferment, papain, has an anticoagulant effect. Intravenous injection of a purified extract in the dog (2 mg/kg) increases prothrombin and coagulation time threefold; an anticoagulant action has been noticedon rabbits, rats and mice, the maximum effect being achieved half an hour after the injection. Standardization of the enzyme has been suggested. The maximum dose tolerated by rats and mice was found to be 50 mg/kg, while a therapeutic action was observed with doses of 1-2. mg/kg. Acute toxic effects at higher doses were similar to those observed with heparin. The enzyme is used as a digestive enzyme in dyspepsia and digestive troubles and has been successfully in peritoneal instillation to avoid adherences. [318] The enzyme chymopapain, a derivative of the latex of the Papaya, has heen used on an experimental basis by neurosurgeons to dissolve herniated ("slipped") intervertebral discs in patients complaining of back pain,[319] One in 4,000 people exposed to this treatment die of anaphylactic shock.[320] The root and leaves contain the bitter alkaloid, carpaine, which acts on the heart like digitalis but is destroyed by heat. Two new macrocyclic piperideine alkaloids, dehydrocarpaine1 & 11, have been found in the leaves in higher concentrations than carpaine.[321]
Toxicity: The 1978 report that papain was teratogenic (produced birth defects) and embryotoxic (poisonous to the embryo) in rats needs verification before it can be given much credence. [322] Recent news suggest that too much papaya might induce prostate cancer.[323] Externally, the latex is irritant, demlatitogenic, and vescicant. Internally, it causes severe gastritis. Some people are allergic to the pollen, the fruit, and the

---

[316] Weiner, Michael A., Janet Weiner, and Norman R. Farnsworth. *Weiner's Herbal: The Guide to Herb Medicine*. New York: Stein and Day, 1980; 148.
[317] Brever Bep Pliver, Medical Plants on Tropical West Africa London: Cambridge Unviversity Press, 1986; 138.
[318] Ibid., p. 138.
[319] Weiner, Michael A., Janet Weiner, and Norman R. Farnsworth. *Weiner's Herbal: The Guide to Herb Medicine*. New York: Stein and Day, 1980; 148.
[320] Duke, James A. and Rodolfo Vásquez. *Amazonian Ethnobotanical Dictionary*. Boca Raton, FL: CRC, 1994; 42.
[321] Morton F. Julia, *Atlas of Medical Plants of Middle America: Bahamas to Yucatan.* Springfield, Illinois: Charles C Thomas Publisher, 1981; 597.
[322] Foster Steven, Varro Tyler E. *Tyler's honest Herbal: A Sensible Guide to the Use of Herbs and Related Remedies*. Binghamton, NY: The Haworth Herbal Press, 2000; 280.
[323] Duke, James A. and Rodolfo Vásquez. *Amazonian Ethnobotanical Dictionary*. Boca Raton, FL: CRC, 1994; 42.

latex. Papain can induce asthma and rhinitis. Carpaine can cause paralysis, numbing of the nerve centers, and cardiac depression.[324]

[324]Duke, James A. *CRC Handbook of Medicinal Herbs*. Boca Raton, FL: CRC, 1985; 101.

Sapodilla

Plants that Increase Digestion and Appetite

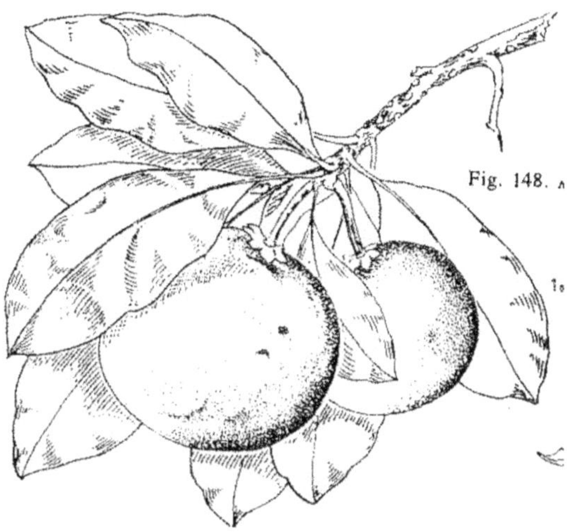

Botanical Name: Manilkara Zapota.
Family: Sapotaceae.
Region Where Grown: U. Takutu-U. Essequibo.
Other Names: Sapadillo, Sapodilla.
Category: Digestive Plants.
Properties: Salty, Cold/Moist.
Esoteric Botanica: Het Heru.
Governing Organs: Stomach, Spleen, Urinary Bladder, Kidney.
Actions & Indications: Fruit: Eaten to remedy indigestion and used for diarrhea, dysuria, diuretic.[325] Used for diarrhea. Tonifies and augments the spleen and Stomach – for spleen or stomach deficiency with such symptoms as diarrhea, fatigue, spontaneous sweating or lack of appetite.
Leaves: Decotion of leaves is used to soothe pain of rheumatism.[326]
Bark decoction is a tonic febrifuge.
Seed: Parched and/or peeled seeds are eaten to alleviate retention of urine, i.e., to stimulate release of urine. The crushed seeds are used to expel liver, bladder and kidney stones.[327]
The fatty seed is a diuretic which must be used with caution since high dosage causes dysuria. Stabilizes the essence and reserves urine – for enuresis, urinary incontinence, frequent urination, and spermatorrhea.
Cautions & Contraindications: Because this herb aids dampness, generates heat, and may readily induces fullness in the middle burner, it is contraindicated in cases of excess dampness, food stagnation, intestinal parasites, or damp-phlegm disorders with such symptoms as epigastric distention and bloating.
Major Known Ingredients: Contains the alkaloid Saponine. Its white milky sap is called *chicle,* which was the source of commercial chewing gum and the origin of the product 'chiclet'.[328] The fruit contains high amounts of tannin, a antioxidant and poly-phenolic compound. Tannins are known to have anti-parasitic, anti-bacterial, antiviral and anti-inflammatory properties. These properties make sapodilla a good remedy for hemorrhoids and diarrhea. The anti-inflammatory property of tannin present in sapodilla is helpful in treating irritating bowel disorders, enteritis, reflux-esophagitis and erosive gastritis. Sapodilla

---

325 DeFilipps, Robert A., Shirley L. Maina, and Juliette Crepin. *Medicinal Plants of the Guianas (Guyana, Surinam, French Guiana)*. Washington, D.C.: Dept. of Botany, National Museum of Natural History, Smithsonian Institution, 2004; 258.
326 Morton F. Julia, *Atlas of Medical Plants of Middle America: Bahamas to Yucatan.* Springfield, Illinois: Charles C Thomas Publisher, 1981; 659.
327 Ibid., p, 659.
328 Castner, James L., S. Lee. Timme, and James A. Duke. *A Field Guide to Medicinal and Useful Plants of the Upper Amazon*. Gainesville, FL: Feline, 1998; 78.

possess good amounts of vitamins A and C. Vitamin A helps improve vision and is also good for maintaining healthy skin and mucus membranes. It also prevents oral cavity and lung cancers. Vitamin C provides the resistance against harmful radical attacks and infections. Ripe sapodilla fruits are rich in minerals like iron, copper, potassium and vitamins like pantothenic acid, niacin and folate. It heals constipation and also prevents any form of cancers caused by toxins in the colon region.

Pharmacological & Clinical Research:

Toxicity: The Bark is said to contain the alkaloid sapotine. Methyl salicylate, HCN and benzaldehyde have been reported in the leaves. The seed kernel (50% of the whole seed) contains 1% saponin and 0.08% of a bitter principle, sapotinin. Ingestion of more than 6 seeds causes abdominal pain and vomiting and possess sufficient HCN to be toxic in quantity.[329]

[329] Morton F. Julia, *Atlas of Medical Plants of Middle America: Bahamas to Yucatan*. Springfield, Illinois: Charles C Thomas Publisher, 1981; 659.

Chapter 6: Warming Plants

Plants for Interior Cold

This group of plants are used for interior cold syndromes. One condition is caused by pathogenic cold acting on the spleen and stomach, leading to vomiting and diarrhea. The second kind of condition is the interior depletion of energy, leading to lowered body temperature and cold extremities.

Warming Plants: Action on the Digestive Tract

One condition is caused by pathogenic cold acting on the spleen and stomach, leading to vomiting and diarrhea. The action on the digestive tract are usually stomachic with pungent and spicy essential oils. They can increase the microcirculation and the excretion of gastric acid and protease. Thus they can evacuate gas and relax the intestinal muscles.

Fennel

Warming Plants: Action on the Digestive Tract

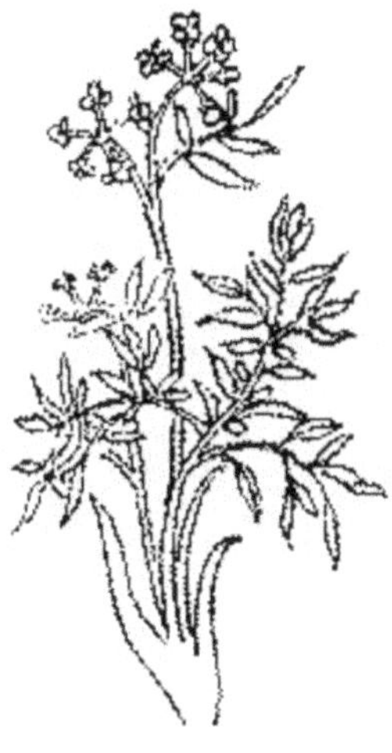

Botanical Name: Foeniculum Vulgare.
Family: Apiaceae.
Region Where Grown: Barima-Waini.
Other Names: None.
Category: Digestive: Warming Plants.
Properties: Sour, Aromatic, Cold/Dry.
Esoteric Botanica: Seker.
Governing Organs: Liver, Spleen, Small Intestine.
Actions & Indications: Fennel has a reputation for loosening phlegm and as a cough remedy as well as in other ailments, primarily as a caminative that aids in such ailments as vomiting, stomachache, flatulence/dispel gas aid digestion.[330]
Stem and Leaf: Piece of branch is cooked with other ingredients and administered periodically to children to remedy vomiting. Also occasionally used for abdominal pain and vomiting without parasites. Warms the middle burner, moves the qi and alleviates pain – for pain and distention in the epigastrum and abdomen, poor appetite and vomiting due to cold from deficiency of the spleen and stomach. Warms the middle and expels cold – for warming the spleen and stomach both in

[330] Foster Steven, Varro Tyler E. *Tyler's honest Herbal: A Sensible Guide to the Use of Herbs and Related Remedies*. Binghamton, NY: The Haworth Herbal Press, 2000; 157.

conditions of excess due to externally-contracted cold, as well as cold from deficiency due to insufficiency of the yang qi. Symptoms include loose stools, nausea and vomiting, loss of appetite and abdominal pain. Warms the middle burner, disperses cold and alleviates pain – for spleen or stomach deficiency cold with such symptoms as cold and pain in the abdomen, vomiting and diarrhea.
Leaf: Infusion for infants' stomachache.
Seed: Ingested to dispel gas. Promotes the downward movement of qi and reduces stagnation – for patterns of food stagnation and qi obstruction with such signs as epigastric and abdominal distention, regurgitation of food, and belching with acid reflux. Especially useful when these disorders are accompanied by constipation. Breaks up stagnant qi and reduces accumulation – for epigastric or abdominal pain and distention or indigestion with focal distention or gas.
Cautions & Contraindications: Use with caution in cases of yin deficiency with heat signs.
Major Known Ingredients: A large number of constituents have been identified in fennel, but its desirable stomachic and carminative properties are attributed primarily to the volatile oil that exists in the fruits to the extent of about 2 to 6 percent. This oil consists mostly (50 to 90 percent) of *trans-anethole,* with smaller amounts of fenchone (up to 20 percent), estragole, limonene, camphene, and ά-pinene. Producing essentially the same actions as the fruit, the oil has been shown to exert spasmolytic (relieves spasms) effects on smooth muscles of experimental animals. [331]
Pharmacological & Clinical Research:
Toxicity: Fennel volatile oil is quite a different matter. Quantities as small as I to 5 ml have caused not only skin irritation but vomiting, seizures and respitory problems such as pulmonary edema.[332]

[331] Ibid., p, 157
[332] Tyler's Steven Foster and Varro E. Tyler, Tyler's Honest Herbal, A Sensible Guide to the Use of Herbs and Related Remedies (The Hawthorn Herbal Press: Binghamton, 2000) p, 158

Bay Leaf

Warming Plants: Action on the Digestive Tract

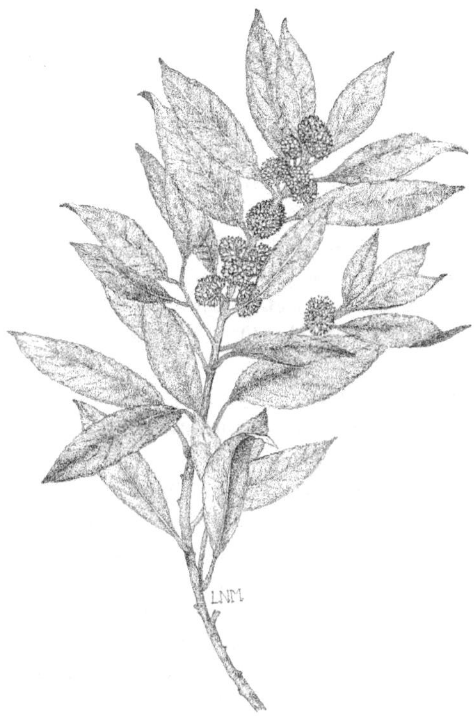

Botanical Name: Pimenta Racemosa.
Family: Myrtaceae.
Region Where Grown: Demerara-Mahaica.
Other Names: Spice, Spice-leaf. Bay tree, Wild Cinnamon.
Category: Digestive: Warming Plants.
Properties: Bitter, Hot/dry.
Esoteric Botanica: Heru.
Governing Organs: Heart, Lungs, Kidney.
Actions & Indications: Flatuence, insect repellant, skin diseases, stomach cramps, angina, (carminatives, digestive, stomachics), diarrhea and dysentery, rheumatism and toothache.
Leaf: Dried leaves made into a tea used to treat flatulence and drunk as tonic.[333] Warms the middle and expels cold – for warming the spleen and stomach both in conditions of excess due to externally-contracted cold, as well as cold from deficiency. Leaf yields an oil which is distilled and used as a mosquito repellent; for stomach pain and for skin diseases. Traditionally, the leaf oil itself is used to treat chest colds, stroke, rheumatism and toothache.
Cautions & Contraindications: Do not use in cases of yin deficiency with heat signs or the reckless movement of hot blood. Use with caution during pregnancy.
Major Known Ingredients: Leaf and fruit contain an essential oil composed mainly of the phenol eugenol, as well as methyl eugenol, isoeugenol and chavicol; many monoterpene and sesquiterpene hydrocarbons are also present[334]
Pharmacological & Clinical Research: In the essential oil, distilled from the leaf or berry, approximately 80 components have been described, including 20 monoterpenes and 19 sesquiterpenes. The major constituents are: eugenol and its derivatives, around 40%, myrcene up to 32% and chavicol up to 11%, and they contribute to the significant antiseptic and disinfectant actions of the oil). In the trade bay leaf oil (also called Myrcia oil) is used in hair lotions with minor amounts in perfumery and in food flavouring.

---

[333] DeFilipps, Robert A., Shirley L. Maina, and Juliette Crepin. *Medicinal Plants of the Guianas (Guyana, Surinam, French Guiana)*. Washington, D.C.: Dept. of Botany, National Museum of Natural History, Smithsonian Institution, 2004; 209.
Ibid., p, 209.

Warming Plants: Action on the Cardiovascular System

The action on the cardiovascular system, the depletion of vital energy condition is the same as shock.. Some cardiotonic plants can increase the blood pressure. They can also increase the tolerance of oxygen depletion in ischemic condition. Some can increase the renal blood flow, and some can increase the dilation of the peripheral skin blood vessels and cause the body to feel warmer.

Black Maho

Warming Plants: Action on the Cardiovascular System

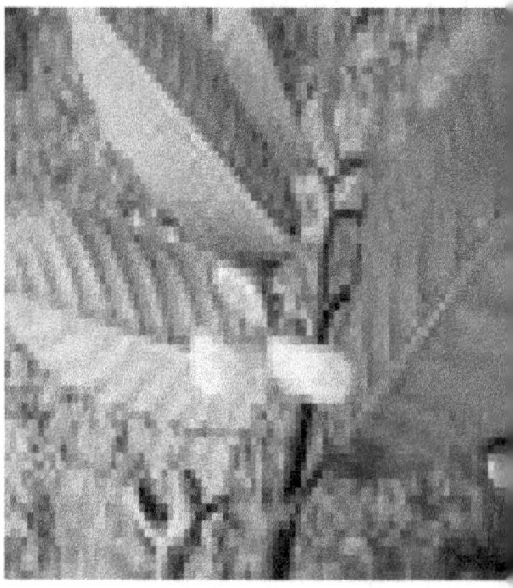

Botanical Name: Rollinia Exsucca.
Family: Annonaceae.
Region Where Grown: All Regions.
Other Names: Shirik, Iremda.
Category: Cardiovascular System; Warming Plants.
Properties: Bitter, Hot/Dry.
Esoteric Botanica: Heru.
Governing Organs: Heart, Kidney, Stomach.
Actions & Indications: Cardiac disorders, fever, hemorrhage, relieve pain and facilitate delivery, assist in childbirth.
Bark: Bark is boiled, and the water drunk for treatment of car diac disorders.[335] Tonifies the blood – for such symptoms as dizziness, sallow complexion and palpitations due to blood deficiency. Tonifies and augments the heart and spleen, nourishes the blood and calms the spirit – for insomnia, heart palpitations, forgetfulness, or dizziness due to heart and spleen deficiency. Commonly used for problems associated with an excess of pensiveness or overwork. Clears heat and soothes irritability – especially useful for restlessness, irritability, palpitations and insomnia due to heat entering the nutritive level. Can also be used in patterns of heart and kidney yin deficiency or for heart heat.
Bark also used in treatment of fever and hemorrhage. Warms the channels and stops bleeding – for cold from deficiency that may present with hemorrhage of various types, especially uterine bleeding. It is used in treating hemorrhage only if the bleeding is chronic and pale in color and is accompanied by cold limbs, ashen white face and a soggy, thin pulse.
Stem: A cold water infusion of the bark is used for washing the abdomen of women giving birth in order to relieve pain and facilitate delivery.
Cautions & Contraindications: Use with caution in cases where blood stasis is not present.

[335] DeFilipps, Robert A., Shirley L. Maina, and Juliette Crepin. *Medicinal Plants of the Guianas (Guyana, Surinam, French Guiana)*. Washington, D.C.: Dept. of Botany, National Museum of Natural History, Smithsonian Institution, 2004; 15.

Christmas Flower

Warming Plants: Action on the Cardiovascular System

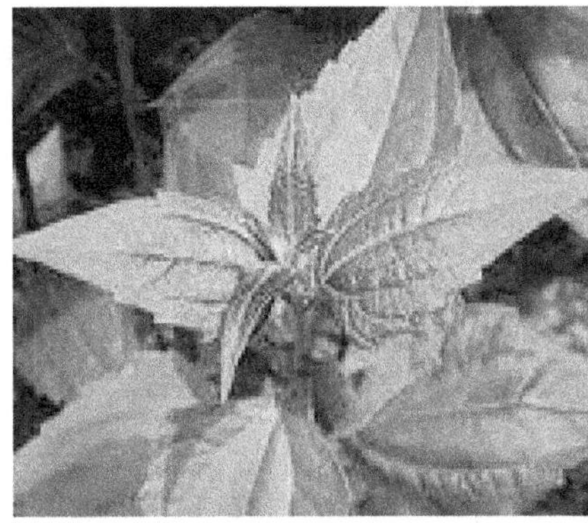

Botanical Name: Chromolaena Odorata..
Family: Aateraraceae.
Region Where Grown:
Other Names: Stink Bush.
Category: Cardiovascular System; Warming Plants.
Properties: Bitter, Hot/Dry.
Esoteric Botanica: Heru.
Governing Organs: Heart, Spleen, Liver, Small Intestine
Actions & Indications: Blood cleanser, emollient, plaster, [336] expels placenta after childbirth, fever, colds, stomach ailments and hemorroids.[337]
Stem: When the need arises for an emollient to use while extracting splinters.
Leaf: Used in a tea for cleansing the blood. Clears heat, relieves fire toxicity, and cools the blood – or warm-febrile diseases accompanied by extreme heat or heat signs, and for very high fevers at the nutritive or blood level with reckless movement of blood. Fire toxins may be either severe fevers or pustulate damp-heat sores. Cools the upward blazing of heart fire – for heat in the upper burner manifesting as Shen disturbance (irritability, insomnia, palpitations) or as mouth and tongue sores, afternoon or low-grade fevers, or malar flush. Clears heat and cools the blood – for heat entering the blood level during a warm-febrile disease manifesting as reckless blood. Also for frequent and profuse menstruation due to heat in the blood. Invigorates the blood and dispels blood stasis – for liver blood stasis patterns with amenorrhea, abdominal masses, lumps or bruises due to traumatic injury.

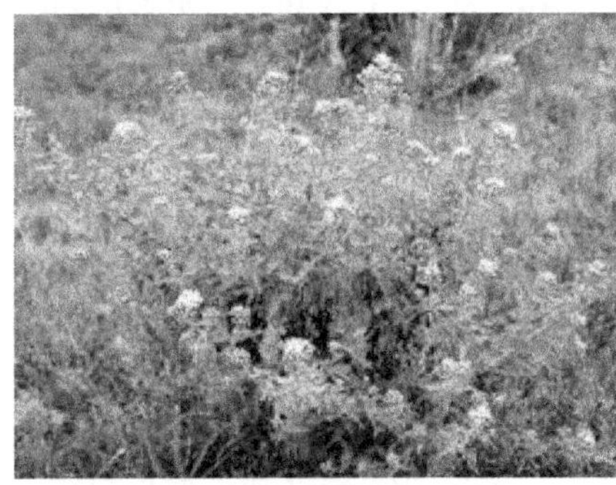

Cautions & Contraindications: Do not use in cases of spleen deficiency with dampness, yang deficiency, or in pregnant women with deficiency.
Major Known Ingredients: Seed contains alkaloids. Leaf contains cerylic alcohol, sisterol, isosakuranetine and odoratine. Oil contains sesquiterpenic acid, eupatol and anisic acid. Whole plant contains triterpenic alcohols.[338]

---

[336] DeFilipps, Robert A., Shirley L. Maina, and Juliette Crepin. *Medicinal Plants of the Guianas (Guyana, Surinam, French Guiana)*. Washington, D.C.: Dept. of Botany, National Museum of Natural History, Smithsonian Institution, 2004; 42.
[337] Morton F. Julia, *Atlas of Medical Plants of Middle America: Bahamas to Yucatan.* Springfield, Illinois: Charles C Thomas Publisher, 1981; 289.
[338] DeFilipps, Robert A., Shirley L. Maina, and Juliette Crepin. *Medicinal Plants of the Guianas (Guyana, Surinam, French Guiana)*. Washington, D.C.: Dept. of Botany, National Museum of Natural History, Smithsonian Institution, 2004; 42.

Yellow Plantain

Warming Plants: Action on the Cardiovascular System

Botanical Name: Musa Paradisiaca.
Family: Musaceae.
Region Where Grown: U. Demerara-Berbice.
Other Names:
Category: Cardiovascular System; Warming Plants.
Properties: Sweet, Cold/Moist.
Esoteric Botanica: Auset.
Governing Organs: Stomach, Lungs, Large Intestine, Spleen, Kidney.
Actions & Indications: Vermifuge, inflammation of the gums. Various parts of the plant is used to treat tuberclulosis, gout, earache, warts, bronchitis, cough, diarrhea, fever, urticaria and leishmaniasis.[339]
Root: Juice employed to treat carbuncles, swellings, fevers and as a hair tonic.[340]
Stem: Pulp of the trunk made into an infusion to soothe dysentery; liquid collected at a cut stem is an antiseptic applied to furuncles and wounds; stem used as a seat upon which a pregnant woman gives birth for a vesicatory on blistering.
Leaves: Leaves are decoted to stop diarrhea and hemorrhoids.[341]

Fig. 162. *Musa* spp. (GAV)

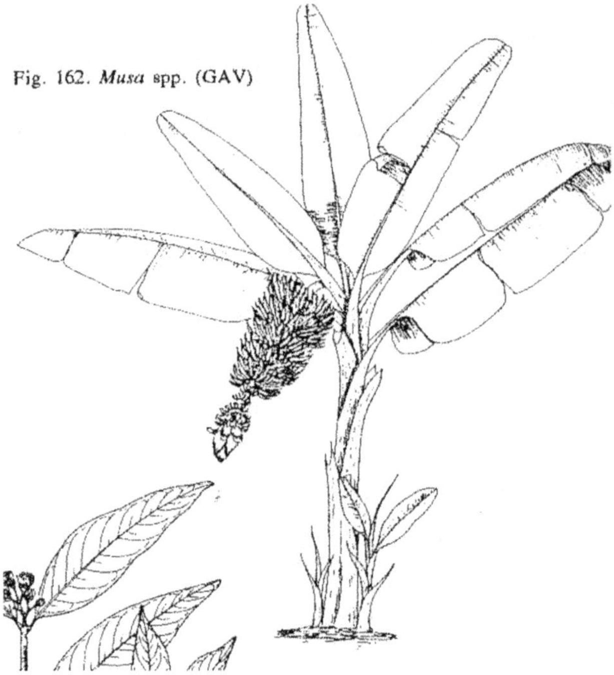

Fruit: Roasted green (unripe) fruit eaten for diarrhoea remedy. Grated green fruit in water used for chronic diarrhoea. Green fruit and its sap are astringent; sap haemostatic.
Outer skin (peel) considered an abortive. Peeled, sliced fruit placed on forehead to relieve heat of a headache. Fruit used to treat epilepsy.
Cautions & Contraindications: Do not use for cold disorders, during pregnancy or excessive menstruation, or for yin deficiency with excessive sweating.

---

[339] Duke, James A. and Rodolfo Vásquez. *Amazonian Ethnobotanical Dictionary*. Boca Raton, FL: CRC, 1994; 120.
[340] DeFilipps, Robert A., Shirley L. Maina, and Juliette Crepin. *Medicinal Plants of the Guianas (Guyana, Surinam, French Guiana)*. Washington, D.C.: Dept. of Botany, National Museum of Natural History, Smithsonian Institution, 2004; 201
[341] Morton F. Julia, *Atlas of Medical Plants of Middle America: Bahamas to Yucatan*. Springfield, Illinois: Charles C Thomas Publisher, 1981; 101.

Major Known Ingredients: Fruit contains two vasoconstrictors: norepinephrine (a chemical used to raise blood pressure) and dopamine. Fruit is rich in vitamin A. Sap of fruit contains serothine, which has an action on the long muscles. Norepinephrine is good for a weak heart.[342]
Toxicity: The seeds contain irritating rephides.[343]

---

342 2 DeFilipps, Robert A., Shirley L. Maina, and Juliette Crepin. *Medicinal Plants of the Guianas (Guyana, Surinam, French Guiana)*. Washington, D.C.: Dept. of Botany, National Museum of Natural History, Smithsonian Institution, 2004; 02

343 Morton F. Julia, *Atlas of Medical Plants of Middle America: Bahamas to Yucatan.* Springfield, Illinois: Charles C Thomas Publisher, 1981; 100

Shiny Bush

Warming Plants: Action on the Cardiovascular System

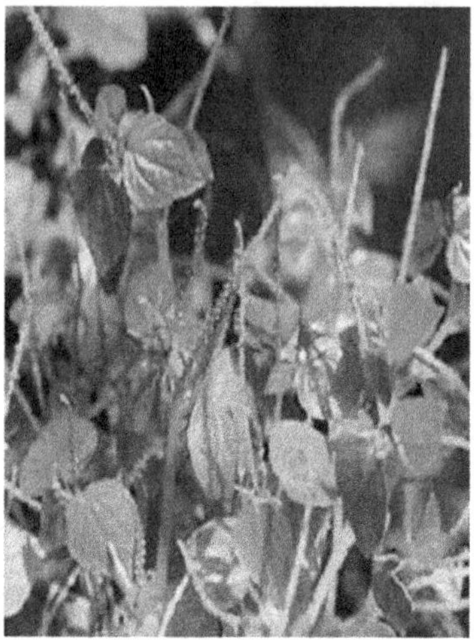

Botanical Name: Peperomia Pellucida.
Family: Piperaceae.
Region Where Grown: Demerara-Mahaica.
Other Names: Sojer Pusly, Soldier Pusley, Soldier's Purslane, Soldier-Parsley.
Category: Cardiovascular System; Warming Plants.
Properties: Sour, Cold/Dry.
Esoteric Botanica: Seker.
Governing Organs: Liver, Spleen, Heart, Kidney, Lung.
Actions & Indications: Plant is used in treatment of albuminuria, asthma, blood cleanser, bronchitis, cataract, cholague, coolant, dental analgesic, diuretic, eye diseases, gingivitis, heart problems, irritant and oral diseases. Additional uses of this plant are in treatment of syphilis and venereal diseases, urinary ailments, cholagogue, cataracts and eye infections, gingivitis and dental neuralgia, hypotension, heart problems and as a coolant.[344]
Whole plant: Infusion for cholagogue and refreshant; sap for eyedrops, eye infections.
Whole plant is also used for memorrhagia, athlete's foot, high blood pressure and headaches.[345]
Stem and Leaf: Mixed in milk for oral afflictions in general such as gingivitis and dental neuralgia; for a local vulnerary; infusion is refreshing, hypotensive, cholagogue, used to treat hypertension, heart troubles and to cool the body. Decoted to relieve abdominal pains and kidney problems.
Leaf. Used for a diuretic where it is also eaten as a salad to cleanse the blood, and used in an infusion to cure womb inflammations, rheumatism, gout and arthritis.
Juice is squeezed from the leaves into a patient's eyes to treat cataracts. Leaf is also decoted for as a tea for bronchitis and asthma, colds, coughs, influenza and diarrhea.[346]
Cautions & Contraindications: Do not usein cases of measles.
Major Known Ingredients: The plant contains apiol. The leaf extract has shown antibiotic activity.[347]

---

[344] DeFilipps, Robert A., Shirley L. Maina, and Juliette Crepin. *Medicinal Plants of the Guianas (Guyana, Surinam, French Guiana)*. Washington, D.C.: Dept. of Botany, National Museum of Natural History, Smithsonian Institution, 2004; 222.
[345] Duke, James A. and Rodolfo Vásquez. *Amazonian Ethnobotanical Dictionary*. Boca Raton, FL: CRC, 1994; 132.
[346] Morton F. Julia, *Atlas of Medical Plants of Middle America: Bahamas to Yucatan.* Springfield, Illinois: Charles C Thomas Publisher, 1981; 120.
[347] Ibid, p.120.

Teasam

Warming Plants: Action on the Cardiovascular System

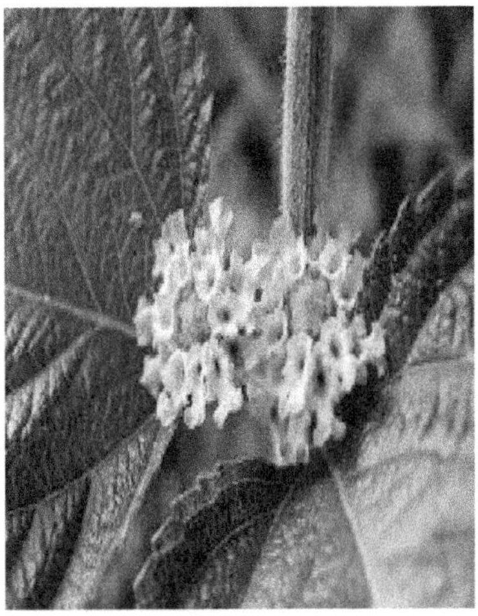

Botanical Name: Lippia Alba.
Family: Verbenaceae.
Region Where Grown: U. Takutu-U. Essequibo.
Other Names: Catmint, Colic Mint, Cullen Mint, Guinea Mint, Melissa, Oregano.
Category: Cardiovascular System; Warming Plants.
Properties: Aromatic, Sour, Hot/Moist.
Esoteric Botanica: Tehuti.
Governing Organs: Liver, Heart, Lungs, Urinary Bladder, Stomach.
Actions & Indications: Heart problems and tachycardia, influenza, fevers, stomach pain and cleanse the bladder.[348]
Leaf: A relaxant and soporific; infusion is drunk for relief of heart (cardiac) problems and to soothe tachycardia.[349] The decotion of the leaves is used as a calmant and a sedative.[350]
A decoction is further made into a tea to remedy influenza, atomachic, febrifuge and a remedy for liver complaints, dysentery, abdomincal cramps and colds.[351]
The aromatic leaves are used in herbal baths, to cure fevers and severe stomach pain, and to cleanse the bladder. tonifies the stomach – for lethargy, lack of appetite, chest and abdomine. Reduces food stagnation and harmonizes the stomach – for stomach cold with food stagnation or accumulation, with such symptoms as epigastric and abdominal fullness or distention, borborygmus and diarrhea. Especially useful in treating stagnation associated with fermented foods. Traditionally, the decoctions of the plant, alone or mixed with other plants are taken as a stomachic, to reduce fevers, for liver complaints, as an anti-spasmodic, emmenagogue and decongestant.
Cautions & Contraindications: Do not use in cases of spleen deficiency with dampness, yang deficiency, or in pregnant women with deficiency.
Major Known Ingredients: Plant contains essential oil composed principally of dihydrocarvone. Compounds also include limonene, pinene, linalol and camphor.
Pharmacological & Clinical Research: The essential oil from the leaves have demonstrated antiseptic, astringent and other health benefits. Very recently, these extracts have been shown to have anti-candida albicans activity. The plant contains 1.2% volatile oil composed of geranial (34%), neral (23.0%), caryophylle (6.0%), methylheptenone (5.8%), citronellol (5.2%), geramiol (4.1%), borneol (2.6%), caryophyllene oxide (2.5%), allo-aromadendrene (2.4%), cis-alpha-bisabolene (2.1%), germacrene D

---

[348]DeFilipps, Robert A., Shirley L. Maina, and Juliette Crepin. *Medicinal Plants of the Guianas (Guyana, Surinam, French Guiana)*. Washington, D.C.: Dept. of Botany, National Museum of Natural History, Smithsonian Institution, 2004; 283.
[349] Duke, James A. and Rodolfo Vásquez. *Amazonian Ethnobotanical Dictionary*. Boca Raton, FL: CRC, 1994; 106.
[350] Castner, James L., S. Lee. Timme, and James A. Duke. *A Field Guide to Medicinal and Useful Plants of the Upper Amazon*. Gainesville, FL: Feline, 1998; 73.
[351] Morton F. Julia, *Atlas of Medical Plants of Middle America: Bahamas to Yucatan.* Springfield, Illinois: Charles C Thomas Publisher, 1981; 745.

(2.0%), nerol (1.6%), linalool (1.1%), citronellal (0.7%), limonene (0.4%), cubenol (0.3%), transocimene (0.2%), geranyl butyrate (0.2%), eugenol (0.2%), l-octen-3-ol (0.1%) and copaene (o.1%).[352]

[352] Ibid., p. 745.

Ink Plant

Warming Plants: Action on the Cardiovascular System

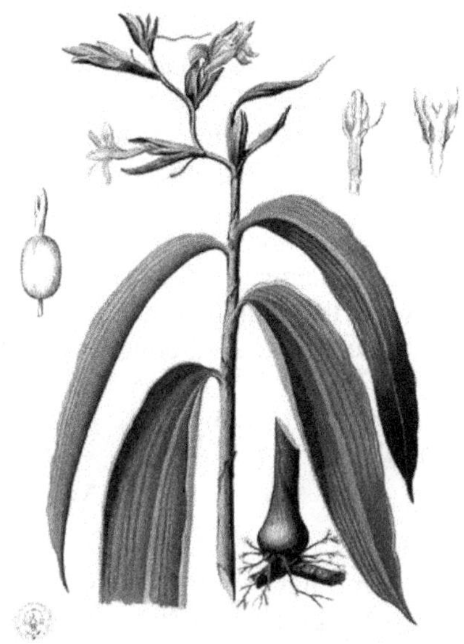

Botanical Name: Renealmia Alpinia.
Family: Zingiberaceae.
Region Where Grown: U. Takutu-U. Essequibo.
Other Names: kuruwatti, krawatee, krowatti.
Category: Cardiovascular System; Warming Plants.
Properties:Bitter, Hot/Dry.
Esoteric Botanica: Heru.
Governing Organs: Heart, Stomach, Liver, Kidney.
Actions & Indications: The plant is primarily used for people with nervous or sad tendencies.[353] Also used for dandruff, eye infections, fever, heart ailments, indigestion, nervous conditions and neuralgia, pulmonary conditions.
Root: In a tea to treat heart problems manifested by shortness of breath.[354] Tonifies the spleen and augments the qi – for spleen deficiency with shortness of breath, poor appetite, fatigue or abdominal pain.
Decoction is drunk to induce vomiting and relieve stomach pains. In a syrup with sugar for remedying chest colds.
Juice is used to treat eye diseases. Used for treating strained backs.
Stem: Shoot used for snakebite and stomachache.
Leaf: Decoction used as a fever-bath for pulmonary conditions and typhoid, and to wash hair to remove dandruff.
Leaves are used in an infusion to treat dysentery and in a herbal bath for strengthening the nerves. Used for hypertension.
Cautions & Contraindications: Use with caution for patients with untreated hypertension.
Major Known Ingredients: Leaf contains proanthocyanins.[355]

---

[353] Duke, James A. and Rodolfo Vásquez. *Amazonian Ethnobotanical Dictionary*. Boca Raton, FL: CRC, 1994; 108.
[354] DeFilipps, Robert A., Shirley L. Maina, and Juliette Crepin. *Medicinal Plants of the Guianas (Guyana, Surinam, French Guiana)*. Washington, D.C.: Dept. of Botany, National Museum of Natural History, Smithsonian Institution, 2004; 291.
[355] Ibid., p. 291.

Chapter 7: The Tonics
Plants that Tonify Vital Organs

Chronic patients are usually very weak and depleted of vital energy, blood, vital essence and vital function. Depletion of these four essence in different organs will reflect different symptoms. It is possible to have depletion of one or more factors. The tonic plants are divided into the following categories: First, they act on the CNS and sympathetic nervous system. Tonic plants can increase the cAMP, and energy metabolic rate. Tonic plants can so stimulate cellular bioelectricity. Second, they increase the specific and non-specific immunity of the body by increasing the phagocytosis of the cells. Third, they increase the adaptability and increase the resistance to the invasion of foreign bodies. Fourth, they increase the physical ability and the thinking capability of the brain. Fifth, they regulate the function of the endocrine, increase the function of the sex hormones and the adrenal cortical hormones.

Vital Energy Tonic Plants (QI)

Tonic plants have specific action on the immunity of the body. On nonspecific cellular immunity they increase the production of T-lymphocytes and prevent the loss of white blood cells caused by cyclophosphamide which is the anti tumor agent. Increase the phagocytic ability of white blood cells, the reticulo-enthdothelial system and the production of interferon. On specific humoral immunity they increase the concentration of the immunoglobulins of IgG and IgM.

They also increase the adaptability of the body. The tonics can control the activity of the adrenalin, the sudden decrease of blood pressure and excessive gastric bleeding.

They have action of the endocrine and the nervous system. The tonics can enhance the action of the adrenal cortex and prevent the degeneration of the thyroid pituitary, adrenal cortex, testis and uterus.

This group of plants also have action on metabolism. The tonics can regulate the metabolism, cholesterol, white blood cells and red blood cells. They can increase the productivity of the body at work. The tonics improve memory and mentality, dizziness, ringing in the ears and reduce stress and fatigue,

Dementia is a loss of individually acquired inrellectual capabilities (i.e. memory, concentration, learning,,. vigilance, power of judgement, spatial orientation, articulation). It also manifests as an inabilily to cope with ordinary daily problem.s or to interact properly in a professional and social context (e.g. affective disorders, such as loss of motivation emotional control or social behaviour). Severe forms of vascular (also called multiinfarct or arteriosclerotic) dementia (frequency: 10-20%) and/or degenerative dementia of the alzheimer type (50% of all demential illnesses) lead to complete loss of personality and imbecility.
The pathology of dementia is complex and includes increased vasoconstriction, deficiency of certain neurotransmitters, increased platelet aggregation and ischemia (multiinfarct free radicals, membrane defects, disorder of cerebral metabolism or progressive degeneration of neurones.

Medicinal herbs can improve quality of life or delay the progression of Alzheimer's disease by up to 1-2 years. Improvement of central cholinergic systems can be achieved through inhibition of acetylcholine esterase (e.g. by galanthamine, Ginkgo extracts or synt.hetic drugs, such donepezil, memantine, rivastigmine and tacrine). Furthermore, Ginkgo exrracts may protect membranes and neurones from death and apoptosis, improve cerebral metabolism, protect against hypoxia and ischemia, cure cerebral edemas, improve radical scavenging and haemodynamic and haemorheologifal properties of the biood (e.g. PAF antagonism).

Dizziness is the result of a disturbance of equilibrium due to the vestibular and optical senses no longer being congruent. Vertigo can be accompanied by anxiety, emesis, nausea, profuse perspiration, tachycardia, labyrinthine araxia, collapse and nystagmus. The causes of this disorder can be manifold, ranging from disturbances in the vestibule, disorder in the central nervous system, to side effects from medicines (e.g. streptomycin) or alcohol to ophthalmologic, psychiatric or orthopaedic problems. Vertigo therapy involves a treatment of any basic disorder, physical training and symptomatically by medicines.

Travel sickness
Dizziness followed by vomiting (emesis) is caused by hyperexcitation in the motoric centre of the CNS (vestibular disturbances). Medicinal plants include the tropane alkaloid scopolamine, which blocks muscarinic AChR and therefore sedates motoric and vegetative centres of the brain stem.

Ringing in the ear manifests as variable noise in rhe ears (in absence of external sources), such as whistling, buzzing, ringing or hissing sounds, often accompanied by defective or impaired hearing. Tinnitus can occur sporadically, continuously or synchronously with heartbeat or breathing. It can be caused by infection or nearly any disorder of the ear, by certain medicines (e.g. quinidine; salicylates, aminoglycoside antibiotics), by disorders of heart and circulation (e.g. hypertony; arteriosclerosis), neurodegeneration, tumours. Tinnitus can lead to insomnia, lack of concentration, anxiety, frustration, depression, headache and psychological disturbances.

Exhaution, weakness and stress comprise complex vitality problems, a decrease of psychological and physical vigilance, an increase susceptibility for infections, insomnia and buntout symptoms. It is especially common in elderly people. Treatment can be regarded as adaptogens that work against exhaustion, weakness and stress. The pharmacology of the mostly complex extracts is not well understood. It has been speculated that adaptogens might have corticomimetic and neuromodulatory effects and that they stimulate cellular metabolism.

Wild Star Apple

Vital energy Tonic Plants

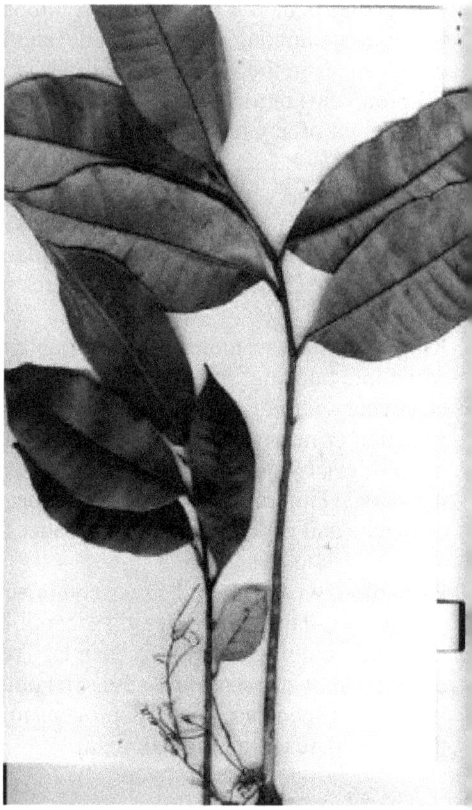

Botanical Name: Couma Guianensis.
Family:Apiaceae.
Region Where Grown: Potaro-Siparuni.
Other Names: None.
Category: Nervous System: Tonic Plants.
Properties: Bitter, Hot/Dry.
Esoteric Botanica: Heru.
Governing Organs: Heart, Spleen, Large Intestine.
Actions & Indications: The plant is used as a remedy for diarrhea.
Stem: Latex which flows from the incised trunk is ingested as a diarrhoea remedy.[356] Tonifies the kidneys, binds up essence, and stops diarrhea – for various discharges due to kidney deficiency. Also used for daybreak diarrhea due to spleen and kidney deficiency. Binds up the Intestines and stops diarrhea – for unremitting chronic diarrhea or dysenteric disorders. Also used for blood in the stool. Binds up the Intestines and stops diarrhea.
latex functions as an antidiarrhoeic.
Cautions & Contraindications: Do not use in cases of internal heat excess and stagnation or in unresolved exterior disorders.

[356] DeFilipps, Robert A., Shirley L. Maina, and Juliette Crepin. *Medicinal Plants of the Guianas (Guyana, Surinam, French Guiana)*. Washington, D.C.: Dept. of Botany, National Museum of Natural History, Smithsonian Institution, 2004; 20.

Matchwood

Vital energy Tonic Plants

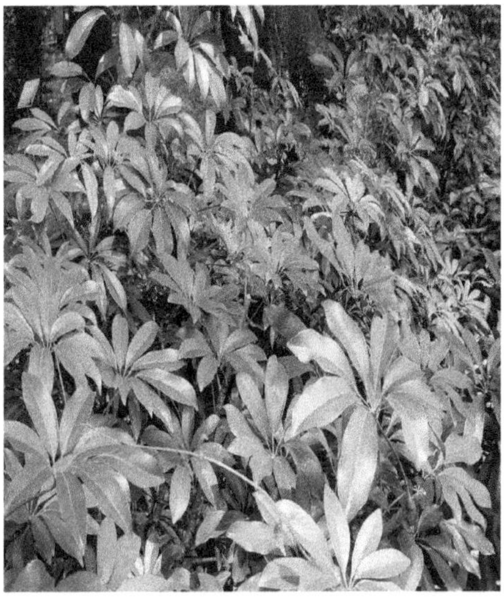

Botanical Name: Schefflera Decaphylla.
Family: Araliaceae.
Region Where Grown: E. Berbice-Corentyne.
Other Names: Karohoropornai. Puna. Morototo.
Category: Nervous System: Tonic Plants.
Properties: Acrid, Cool/Dry.
Esoteric Botanica: Sebek.
Governing Organs: Lung, Spleen, Liver, Heart, Large Intestine.
Actions & Indications: Treats abscess. Bark used to treat scorpion bite, sores and wounds and cuts.
Stem: Sap of inner bark for treating abscesses; boiled bark for relief of itching skin;
Inner bark and leaves prepared in a decoction for malaria and other fevers.
Root: Strongly tonifies the source qi – for extreme collapse of the qi or abandoned conditions that manifest in shallow respiration, shortness of breath, cold limbs, profuse sweating and a minute or weak pulse. May be used alone for this condition after severe blood loss. Tonifies Lung qi – for wheezing, shortness of breath, and dyspnea caused by Lung qi deficiency. Strengthens the spleen and tonifies the stomach – for lethargy, lack of appetite, chest and abdominal distention, diarrhea or even prolapse in severe cases. Tonifies Heart qi and calms the shen – for such symptoms as shortness of breath, anxiety, palpitations, forgetfulness and insomnia
Cautions & Contraindications: Do not use in cases of yin deficiency with heat signs, heat excess, or in the absence of significant qi deficiency. Also contraindicated in cases of Liver yang rising, or hypertension.
Major Known Ingredients: Chemical tests confirm that the root contains the same active saponins as Chinese ginseng (*Panax ginseng*), panaxatriol, panaxadiol, other panoxisides, panoquilon, panaxin, ginsenin, protopanaxadiol, protopanaxtriol, panacene, panaxynol, panaenic acid, panose, dammarane, glucose, fructose, maltose, sucrose, nicotinic acid, riboflavin and thiamine
Pharmacological & Clinical Research: Central nervous effect: Matchwood has a particular set of effects on the central nervous system, particularly the higher centers. It enhances both stimulatory and inhibitory processes. Normally, the use of matchwood is stimulating and increasing wakefulness. However, in large dosages, it has a sedative effect. Different reports state the excitatory effect of the herb is either greater or lesser than caffeine. It controls the inhibitory effect of morphine on the conditioned reflexes. Peripheral nervous system. A small dose of matchwood has a muscarinic effect on the peripheral nervous syem, while a large dose has a nicotinic effect. Preparations of matchwood exhibit inotropic effects similar to those of cardiac glycosides on toad heart specimens as well as dog, cat and rabbit hearts in situ. Matchwood has many anti-stress properties. It prevents weight changes in adrenals, thymus, spleen and thyroid of mice that were stressed.

Toxicity: Matchwood has very low toxicity. The LD50 for intravenous injection in mice is 16.5mg/kg. Humans given 100ml of a 3% tincture showed a mild degree of unrest. With 200ml symptoms of overdose appeared, including, systemic rash, pruritus, vertigo, headache, fever, and in several cases, hermorrhage, one case of fatality was reported after ingesting a single dose of 500ml of the tincture.

Sorrel

Vital energy Tonic Plants

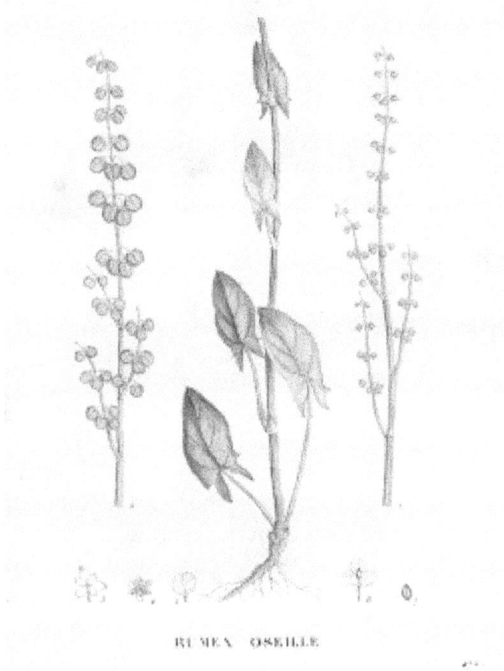

Botanical Name: Urena Lobata.
Family: Malvaceae.
Region Where Grown: Cuyuni-Mazaruni.
Other Names: Lorey, Roselle.
Category: Nervous System: Tonic Plants.
Properties: Sour, Hot/Moist.
Esoteric Botanica: Tehuti.
Governing Organs:Liver, Spleen, Kidney.
Actions & Indications: Beneficial to the liver and kidneys.[357]
Whole plant: Loss of appetite, common cold, catarrh of upper respiratory tract and stomach.
Flower employed in a gargle and used to remedy angina and aphthae.
Leaf: Leaves are decoted as a remedy for dyspepsia, palpatations. Stomache, influenza, colds, cough, tuberculosis and urinary burning.[358]
Emollient: Leaves are boiled to make a tea and used to remedy urinary tract problems, morning sickness and colds.
Root: Infusion of the root is drunk as a depurative and an emollient, angina and oral ulcers.[359] Used as a remedy for gastritis, dysentery, hepatitis, pleurisy, pulmonary ailment, nephritis, intestinal catarrh, gonorrhea and urinary ailments.[360]
Cautions & Contraindications: Do not use in cases of phlegm-fire or dampness in the middle burner.
Major Known Ingredients: The plant acids (15 - 30% in the calyx) include citric, malic and tartaric acids and others which together give sorrel drinks a pleasant and refreshing acid taste. The anthocyanin constituents colour the sorrel tea wine-re, reach about 1% content in the calyx, and, they are mainly the glycosides of delphinidin and cyanidin. Other flavonoids as well as mucilage polysaccharides and pectins also are known in the aqueous extracts of sorrel. Sorrel tea acts as a mild laxative, when it is taken in large amounts, because of the constituent acids which are difficult to absorb.

---

[357] Morton F. Julia, *Atlas of Medical Plants of Middle America: Bahamas to Yucatan.* Springfield, Illinois: Charles C Thomas Publisher, 1981; 356.
[358] Ibid., p. 540.
[359] DeFilipps, Robert A., Shirley L. Maina, and Juliette Crepin. *Medicinal Plants of the Guianas (Guyana, Surinam, French Guiana).* Washington, D.C.: Dept. of Botany, National Museum of Natural History, Smithsonian Institution, 2004; 174.
[360] Morton F. Julia, *Atlas of Medical Plants of Middle America: Bahamas to Yucatan.* Springfield, Illinois: Charles C Thomas Publisher, 1981; 541.

Pharmacological & Clinical Research: Preliminary tests have suggested the presence of anti-hypertensive constituents in the plant while polysaccharide constituents seem to possess useful properties for dermatological or cosmetic applications

Pineapple

Vital energy Tonic Plants

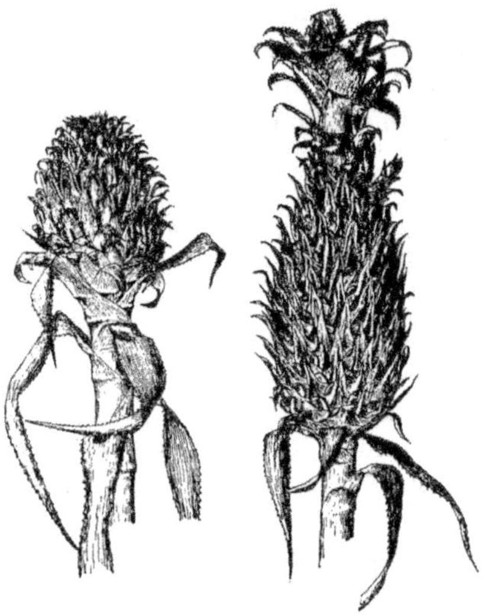

Botanical Name: Ananas Comosus.
Family: Bromeliaceae.
Region Where Grown: Cuyuni-Mazaruni.
Other Names: None.
Category: Nervous System: Tonic Plants.
Properties: Sour, Cold/Dry.
Esoteric Botanica: Seker.
Governing Organs: Liver, Spleen, Large Intestine, Spleen.
Actions & Indications: Leaf: Used for fractures, abortifacient, aperients, indigestion, sore throat,
Fruit: The fruit, peel or juice is used in folk remedies for corns, tumors and warts. Reported to be abortifacient, cholagogue, dcpurative, diaphoretic, digestive, discutient, diuretic, ecbolic, emmenagogue, estrogenic, hydragogue, intoxicant, laxative, parasiticide, purgative, refrigerant, styptic and vermifuge. Pineapple is a folk rcmedy for bladder ailments, fever, gonorrhea, hypochondria, kidney stones, parturition, scarlet fever, scurvy, sores, sprains and venercal disease
Fully ripe fruit is eaten to cure indigestion and eaten with salt as an aperient. Fruit is grated, soaked in water, sweetened with sugar and used as a beverage or tonic.
Used as abortive. The immature, green fruit is eaten by women to abort a fetus less than one month old. An antiedemic substance has been reported from the rhizome. Many pharmacological effects are attributed to bromelain: burn debridement, antiinflammatory action, smooth muscle relaxation and stimulation of muscle contractions contractions.
Leaf: Sweetened leaf decoction drunk for venereal diseases. Juice of the leaves consumed for constipation, hiccups and worms. Juice of ripe fruit regarded as antiscorbutic, cholagogue, diaphoretic, refrigerant and useful in jaundice. Young vegetative buds are used for respiratory ailments.[361]
Cautions & Contraindications: Because this substance aids dampness, generates heat, and may readily induces fullness in the middle burner, it is contraindicated in cases of excess dampness, internal dampness, fullness in the middle with vomiting, phlegm-heat cough, or childhood nutritional impairment with food accumulation.
Major Known Ingredients: Per 100 g the fruit (s reported to contain 47 to 52 calories, 85.3 to 87.0 g H20, 0.4 to 0.7 g protein, 0.2 to 0.3 g fat, 11.6 to 13.7 g total carbohydrate, *OA* to 0.5 g fiber, 0.3 to 0.4 gash, 17 to 18 mg Ca, 8 to 12 mg P, *O.S* mg Fe, I to 2 mg Na, 125 to 146 mg K, 32 to 42 fLg beta-carotene equivalent, 0.06 to 0.08 mg thiamine, 0.03 to 0.04 mg riboflavin, 0,2 to 0.3 mg niacin, and 17 to 61 (to 96) mg ascorbic acid.1 Cultivars may contain 1 to 5% citric acid (wild forms up to 8.6%), ca. 3.5% invert

[361] Duke, James A. *CRC Handbook of Medicinal Herbs*. Boca Raton, FL: CRC, 1985; 36.

sugars, 7.5% saccharose, approaching 15% at maturity. Also reported are vanillin, methyl-n··propyl ketone, n-valerianic acid, isocapronic acid, acrylic acid, L(_.)-malic acid, beta-methylthiopropionic acid methyl ester (and ethyl ester), 5-hydroxytryptamine, quinic acid-l A-di-p-coumarin (my translation). The aromatics from the essential oils of the fruit include methanol, ethanol, ll-propanol, isobutanol, n-pentanol, ethyl acetate, ethyl-n-butyrat, methylisovalerianate, methyl-n-capronate, methyl-n-caprylate, n-amyl-n-capronate, ethyl lactate, methyl-beta-methylthiolprapionate, ethyl-beta-methylthiolpropionate, and diacetyl, acetone, formaldehyde, acetaldehyde, furfural, and 5-hydroxy-2-methylfurfurol.'·' Steroid fractions of the lower leaves possess estrogenic activity,. [362]

Pharmacological & Clinical Research: Available studies show that bromelain has anti-infiammatory, anti-ocdemic, antiplatelet aggregation and flbrinolytic activities, There is evidence that a small percentage of orally administered bromelain Inay be absorbed into the bloodstream and lymph system. There appears to be sufflcient clinical evidence that bromelain is effective in the treatment of post-operative and post-traumatic swelling.[363] Ethanol (95%) extract of unripe fruit, at a dose of 200 mg/kg, and water extract at a dose 100 mg/kg, were equivocal when administered orally to rats. The petroleum ether extract, at a dose of 150 mgjkg, was inactlveAC01 %. Young fruit juice, administered intragastrically to the pregnant mouse at a dose of 0.2 rol/animal, was active. Dosing was done on day 2 and 4 of pregnancy.[364]

Toxicity: Workers who cut up pineapples have their fingerprints almost completely obliterated by pressurc and the keratolytic effect of bromelain (calcium oxalate crystals and citric acid wcre excluded as the cause). The recurved hooks on the leaf margins can painfully injure one. Ethyl acrylate, found in the fruits, produced sensitisation in 10 of 24 subjects "by a aximisation test." Ethylacrvlate is used in creams, detergents, food, lotions, perfumes and soaps. In "therapeutic doses", bromelain may cause nausea, vomiting, diarrhea, skin rash and menorrhagia. Watt and Breyer-Brandwijk state unusual toxic symptoms following ingestion of the fruit, heart failure with cyanosis and ecchymoses, followed by collapse and coma and sometimes death. The unripe pineapplc is also said to be poisonous causing violent purgation. [365]

---

[362] Ibid., p, 36

[363] Van, Wyk Ben-Erik., and Michael Wink. *Medicinal Plants of the World: An Illustrated Scientific Guide to Important Medicinal Plants and Their Uses*. Portland: Timber, 2004; 56.

[364] DeFilipps, Robert A., Shirley L. Maina, and Juliette Crepin. *Medicinal Plants of the Guianas (Guyana, Surinam, French Guiana)*. Washington, D.C.: Dept. of Botany, National Museum of Natural History, Smithsonian Institution, 2004; 58

[365] Duke, James A. *CRC Handbook of Medicinal Herbs*. Boca Raton, FL: CRC, 1985; 37.

Stinking Toe

Vital energy Tonic Plants

Botanical Name: Hymenaea Courbaril.
Family: Caesalpiniaceae.
Region Where Grown: Pomeroon-Supenaam .
Other Names: Locust.
Category: Nervous System: Tonic Plants.
Properties: Bitter, Dot/Dry.
Esoteric Botanica: Herukhuti.
Governing Organs: Heart, Kidney, large Intestine, Liver, Stomach, Small Intestine, Heart, Lungs
Actions & Indications: This plant has been used in folk medicine for various ailments including back pain (lumbago), diarrhea and dysentery, hysteria, vermifuge, antipyretic, aphodisiac, biliousness, blood cleanser, carminative and fatigue.

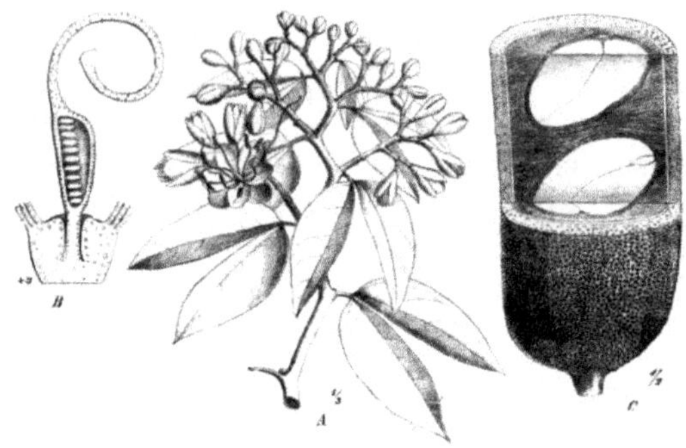

Bark is boiled and used as a blood cleanser and for fatigue tonic. Tonifies the kidneys and fortifies the yang – for deficient kidney yang patterns with such symptoms as fatigue, impotence, cold extremities, lightheadedness, tinnitus, soreness and weakness in the lower back and knees, and frequent, copious, clear urination and to treat coughs and colds.
Bark of trunk is depurative and antipyretic.[366] Resin exuding from bark used for treating fresh wounds. Also used as a cicatrizant and for pulmonary infections and for dysentery. Decocted bark tea is for upset stomach.Bark decoction or infusion for a carminative, vermifuge, purgative, dysentery and diarrhea.[367]
Purges accumulation and guides out stagnation – for heat in the stomach and intestines with constipation. This substance moistens dryness and softens hardness. Bark used as aphrodesiac to tonify the kidneys and fortifies the yang – for deficient kidney yang patterns with such symptoms as impotence, male or female infertility, premature ejaculation, frequent urination, urinary incontinence, irregular menstruation, cold and painul lower abdomen and a weak and sore back
Cautions & Contraindications: Do not use in patients with either damp-heat or heat from yin deficiency.
Major Known Ingredients: Resin contains copalic acid and other diterpenes.[368]

---

[366] DeFilipps, Robert A., Shirley L. Maina, and Juliette Crepin. *Medicinal Plants of the Guianas (Guyana, Surinam, French Guiana)*. Washington, D.C.: Dept. of Botany, National Museum of Natural History, Smithsonian Institution, 2004.;70.
[367] Ibid., p, 70.
[368] Ibid., p, 70.

Passion Flower

Vital energy Tonic Plants

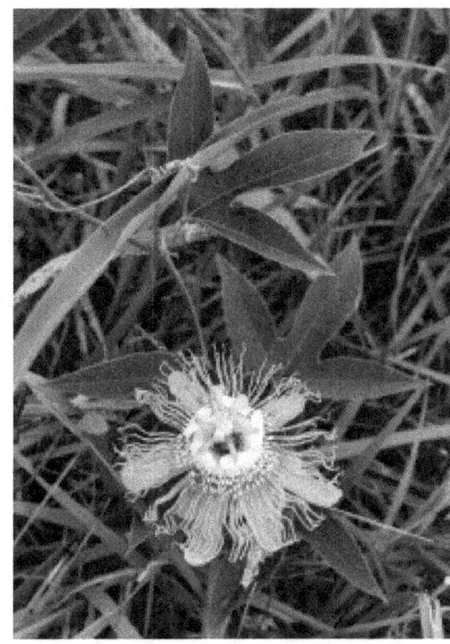

Botanical Name: Passiflora Glandulosa.
Family: Passifloraceae.
Region Where Grown: Pomeroon-Supenaam.
Other Names: Baby Semitoo, Mis-Mis, Wild Semitoo, Bimititokan.
Category: Nervous System: Tonic Plants.
Properties: Sour, Cold/dry.
Esoteric Botanica: Seker.
Governing Organs: Liver, Spleen, Small Intestine, Lungs
Actions & Indications: Passion flower has sedative, hypnotic and anti-spasmodic activity, as shown in animal studies. [369] Traditional uses for this plant includes, gonorrhoea and kidney stones, eyewash to soothe conjunctivitis, emollient for sores, cuts and bruises.
Whole plant: Sap rubbed on skin to treat gonorrhoea and kidney stones.[370]
Stem: Bark is rasped and placed inside aperture of penis as treatment for gonorrhoea .
Sap extracted from crushed stems used as an eye wash to soothe conjunctivitis.
Leaf: Leaves are used as an emollient for sores, cuts and bruises.
Fruit: Juice contains Vitamin C. Fruits are soaked in water and used for making a tonic. It is also used for anxiety.[371] Also used as an ingredient in a curative herbal bath.The entire fresh plant is boiled and the liquid given to children as an anthelmintic. A decotion of the dried plant is drunk as a treatment for chest colds and coughs.
Cautions & Contraindications: Do not use in cases of exterior excess, qi stagnation, damp obstruction, food stagnation, yin deficiency with heat signs, or skin lesions either in their early stages or where there is heat toxin.
Major Known Ingredients: Flavonoids, including chrysoenol, apigenin, isovitexin, vitexin, 2-xylosylvitexin, 2-xylosylisovitexin, luteolin-7-beta D glucose, kaempferol, luteolin, isoschaftoxide and vicenin were isolated from Passiflora foetida var. hispida, together with glucose, galactose and saccharose. [372] Constituents responsible for the pharmacological activity of passion flower have been the subject of ongoing research throughout most of this century. The plant does contain one or more harmala

---

369 Van, Wyk Ben-Erik., and Michael Wink. *Medicinal Plants of the World: An Illustrated Scientific Guide to Important Medicinal Plants and Their Uses*. Portland: Timber, 2004; 115.
370 DeFilipps, Robert A., Shirley L. Maina, and Juliette Crepin. *Medicinal Plants of the Guianas (Guyana, Surinam, French Guiana)*. Washington, D.C.: Dept. of Botany, National Museum of Natural History, Smithsonian Institution, 2004; 218.
371 Ibid., p, 206
372 Lachman-White, D. A., C. D. Adams, and Ulric O'D. Trotz. *A Guide to the Medicinal Plants of Coastal Guyana*. London: Commonwealth Science Council, 1992; 200.

alkloids, but their number and identity are disputed. Besides, such alkaloids generally act as stimulants, not depressants. A Polish report that both an alkaloid fraction and a flavonoid pigment fraction produced sedative elfects in mice was subsequently followed up by Japanese investigators. They were able to isolate small amounts of the pyrone derivative maltol from an alkaloid-containing extract of the plant. Maltol was found to induce depression in mice and to exhibit other sedative properties. The scientists concluded that the depressant effects of maltol, no doubt, counteracted the stimulant action of the harmala alkaloids but were not strong enough to explain the total sedative effects of the plant extract. Flavonoids including vitexin, isovitexin, isoorientin, schaftoside, and isoschaftoside have also been identified and may contribute to biological activity. Further studies areobviously necessary before the active principles of passion flower can definitely be identified.[373]

Pharmacological & Clinical Research: Flavonoids or the alkaloids in the extract. Clinical studies are required to verify such activity in human beings. In 1978, the FDA prohibited the use of passion flower in OTC sedative preparations on the grounds that it had not been proven safe and effective. The German Commission E, however, has authorized its use in the treatment of nervous unrest, citing its ability to bring about a reduction in mobility in animal experiments. The usual daily dose is 4 to 8 g. (three to six teaspoonfuls) taken as a tea in divided doses. Side effects and contraindications have not been reported.[374]

Toxicity: In 1978, the FDA prohibited the use of *passion flower* in OTC sedative preparations on the grounds that it had not been proven safe and effective.[375]

---

[373] Robbers James E. and Tyler Varro E., Tyler's Herbs of Choice: The Therapeutic Use of Phylomedicinals. London: The Haworth Herbal Press, 1999: 283 – 284.

[374] Ibid., p, 159-160.

[375] Ibid., p, 159-160.

Sugar Cane

Vital energy Tonic Plants

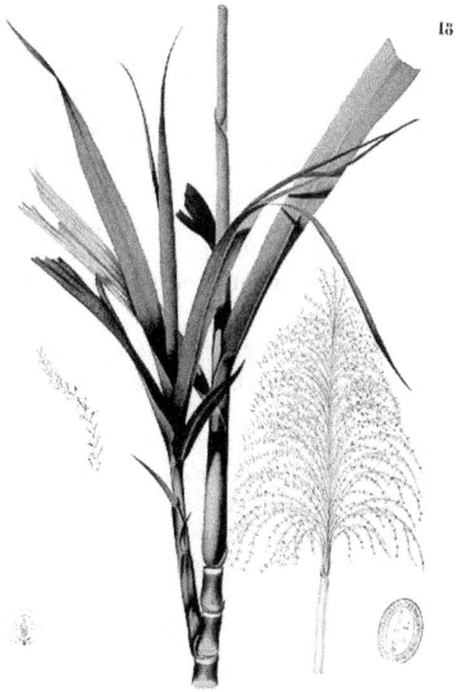

Botanical Name: Saccharum Officinarum.
Family: Poaceae.
Region Where Grown: U. Demerara-Berbice.
Other Names: None.
Category: Nervous System: Tonic Plants.
Properties: Sweet, Acrid, Cool/Dry.
Esoteric Botanica: Sebek.
Governing Organs: Lungs, Small Intestine, Spleen, Stomach
Actions & Indications: Blood cleanser, detersive, eye diseases, leucoma, rheumatism, vermifuge,
Stem: Yields finely ground sugar is used for eye diseases[376] by blowing it into a leucoma of the cornea.
Whole sugar for vermifuge. Powdered sugar for a detersive.[377] Tonifies the spleen and augments the qi for over-exertion that injures the spleen, with shortness of breath and reduced appetite
Sugar cane eaten for a blood-cleanser, digestive and to prevent dental cavities. Tonifies the middle burner qi and alleviates pain – for abdominal pain accompanied by excessive salivation, granulated sugar is sometimes placed on a scald or burn for quick relief.
Sap: Used for coughs and colds as well as to treat snakebite. Moistens the Lungs and stops coughs – for dry, nonproductive coughs with labored, slow breathing, and a weak voice due to lung deficiency.
Leaf: Decoction of young leaves is used for urinary conditions.[378]
Cautions & Contraindications: Because this substance aids dampness generates heat, and may readily induce fullness in the middle burner, it is contraindicated in cases of excess dampness, internal dampness, fullness in the middle with vomiting, phlegm-heat cough, or childhood nutritional impairment with food accumulation.

---

376 Castner, James L., S. Lee. Timme, and James A. Duke. *A Field Guide to Medicinal and Useful Plants of the Upper Amazon*. Gainesville, FL: Feline, 1998; 111.
377 DeFilipps, Robert A., Shirley L. Maina, and Juliette Crepin. *Medicinal Plants of the Guianas (Guyana, Surinam, French Guiana)*. Washington, D.C.: Dept. of Botany, National Museum of Natural History, Smithsonian Institution; 2004. 234
378 Ibid., p, 234.

Blood Tonics

The *blood tonic* plants can increase the production of peripherial white blood cells and red blood cells. There is a regeneration of the blood cells and the maturation of the reticulocyte.

Most of the *blood tonic* plants contain folic acid, vitamin B12 and vitamin A. They are good for anemia and pernicious anemia. Most of them are sedative, analgesic and anti-inflammatory. They increase the flow of blood to the coronary artery and prevent myocardial ischemia. They can relax the spasmodic muscles of the uterus. The whole root of these plants are used to regulate menstruation and blood disorders. The head of the root is hemostatic, the body is nourishing and tail is usded to invigorate the circulation of blood. Most of them can be be processed with wine to invigorate blood circulation with honey as an emollient and carbonized as hemostatic have antitumor properties. They also show possible analgesic and antimicrobial activity and contain alkaloids. Root contains coumarins.

Menstruation (occurring every *28* days) can be too frequent (polymenorrhoea), irrelgular (ohgomenorrhoea), absent (amenorrhoea), painful (dysmenorrhoea), too strong (hypermenorrhoea, menorrhagia) or "too weak (hypomenorrhoea). Uterine bleeding that is not connected with menstruation can occur during pregnancy, after birth or may be caused by inflammation, polyps or myomas. Mentrual disorder is often caused by hormonal or endocrine disturbances. Therefore, hormones or hormone mimmetics are used for therapy, such as estrogens or gestagens. Plant medicines play a role in this context. Antidysmenonhoics are medicines that reduce menstrual pains and are often spasmolytic, analgesic, astringent or aim to arrest menstrual bleeding. Other medicines (emmenagoga) induce or enhance menstrual bleeding involving a direct or indirect stimulation of the womb. The latter compounds can induce an abortion at higher concentration and should be avoided during pregnancy.

Jumbie Baby

Blood Tonics

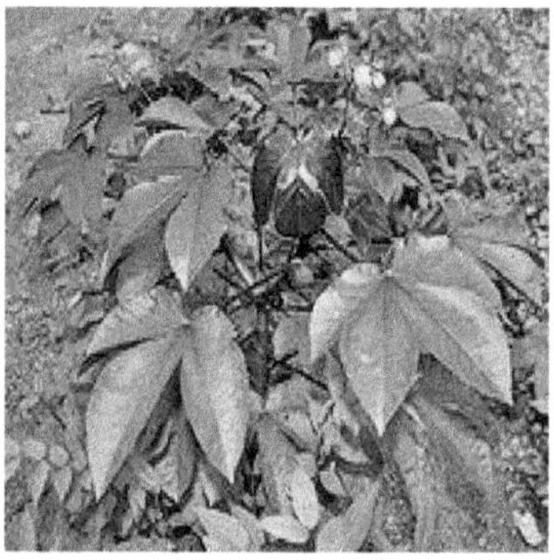

Botanical Name: Jatropha Gossypiifolia.
Family: Euphorbiaceae.
Region Where Grown: Demerara-Mahaica.
Other Names: Belly-ache bush, Wild castor oil.
Category: Nervous System: Blood Tonic Plants.
Properties: Sour, Acrid, Hot/Moist.
Esoteric Botanica: Tehuti.
Governing Organs: Liver, Heart, Stomach.
Actions & Indications: Among the ailments *Jumbie Baby* is used for are: rheumatism, cramps, beriberi, worm, scabies, stings and bites, paralysis, toothaches, and venereal disease and it may have curative qualities against pancreatic cancer,[379] cuts, inflammation, purgative and sores.
Leaf: Used for bruises, sores and swelling.

---

379 Castner, James L., S. Lee. Timme, and James A. Duke. *A Field Guide to Medicinal and Useful Plants of the Upper Amazon*. Gainesville, FL: Feline, 1998; 97.

Relieves headache – moves the qi upward and alleviates pain. Depending on other plants used, this herb may be used for headaches due to wind, heat, cold, or blood deficiency and heart problems.[380]
Administered in therapeutic baths to give good feelings, increase thinking, and improve one's outlook on life.[381] Nourishes the heart yin, augments the liver blood, and quiets the spirit – for irritability, insomnia, and palpitations with anxiety due to either blood deficiency (inability to nourish the heart) or yin deficiency (with upward- rising fire). Nourishes the heart and blood and calms the spirit – for yin or blood deficiency patterns with insomnia and irritability. Especially useful for dream-disturbed sleep. Anchors and calms the spirit – for restlessness, palpitations, insomnia or tremors, especially in patients with yin deficiency and ascendant yang. Also used for dizziness or vertigo in patients with similar patterns. Another application is treating convulsions in children caused by fear, or for fright generally.
Oil is used as a purgative.
Leaf: Infusion and poultice for a soothing emulsion to remedy inflammations and sores; relieves fire toxicity – use raw for fire toxin carbuncles, sores and lumps.
Fruit and Seed: Boiled in liquid for stomachache.
Cautions & Contraindications: Do not use in cases of high fever due to excess with an absence of sweating. Overdose may lead to indigestion or constipation.
Major Known Ingredients: Jatropholone terpenes have antitumor properties. Gossypibetiline, tetrahydrogossypibetiline, gadain and the irritant diterpenoid 12-deoxy-16-hydroxy-phorbol have been isolated

[380] DeFilipps, Robert A., Shirley L. Maina, and Juliette Crepin. *Medicinal Plants of the Guianas (Guyana, Surinam, French Guiana)*. Washington, D.C.: Dept. of Botany, National Museum of Natural History, Smithsonian Institution, 2004; 120.
[381] Castner, James L., S. Lee. Timme, and James A. Duke. *A Field Guide to Medicinal and Useful Plants of the Upper Amazon*. Gainesville, FL: Feline, 1998; 97.

Gully Root

Blood Tonics

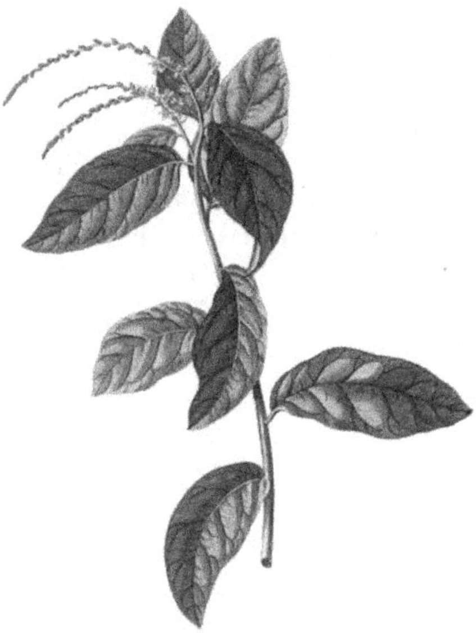

Botanical Name: Petiveria Alliacea.
Family: Phytolaccaceae.
Region Where Grown: U. Takutu-U. Essequibo.
Other Names: None .
Category: Nervous System: Blood Tonic Plants.
Properties: Salty, Cold/Moist.
Esoteric Botanica: Het Heru.
Governing Organs: Kidney, Large Intestine, Stomach, Liver, Urinary Bladder.
Actions & Indications: Female tonic, Leucorrhoea, menstruation, including menstrual cramps, flow and pain, sedative, sudorific, "female rejuvenation" and as a diuretic. Tonifies the blood and regulates the menses – for patterns of blood deficiency with such symptoms as pallid, ashen complexion, tinnitus, blurred vision and palpitations. Also very commonly used for blood deficiency associated with gynecological disorders. Nourishes the blood and regulates the menses – for blood deficiency with such symptoms as menstrual dysfunction, vaginal discharge, and uterine bleeding. Commonly used in gynecologic disorders and anticonvulsive effects[382]. The roots are antispasmodic and antipyretic; the leaf decoction, sudorific and cough suppressant, bronchitis and pneumonia. For beriberi, cramps, nerves, paralysis, rheumatism, scabies, scorpic sting, spider bites, toothache, venereal diseases and vision, calling the herb abortifacient analgesic, contraceptive, diuretic, emmenagogue, venuifuge and insecticide. Tramil all but endorses inhala of the aroma for migraine and sinusitis and using as a mouthwash for toothache. [383]
Root: For an antispasmodic, febrifuge, sedative, diuretic, emmenagogue and abortifacient. Nourishes the heart yin, augments the liver blood, and quiets the spirit – for irritability, insomnia, and palpitations with anxiety due to either blood deficiency (inability to nourish the heart) or yin deficiency (with upward-rising fire). Nourishes the heart and calms the spirit – for irritability, insomnia, forgetfulness, and palpitations with anxiety due to heart blood deficiency. Anchors, settles and calms the spirit – for emotional distress, restlessness, insomnia, palpitations, anxiety, or even seizures or mania-withdrawal due to an agitated heart and spirit. Settles the heart and calms the spirit – for symptoms associated with disturbed spirit, such as restlessness, palpitations with anxiety, insomnia, or convulsions.
Roots used for an analgesic to remedy toothache. Root has the odor of onion.
Leaf: Sudorific, depurative; in a decoction for a dry cough. Used for fevers.
Powdered leaves used in a treatment for ulcerated wounds and as an insecticide to prevent itching.
Cautions & Contraindications: Do not use in cases of yin deficiency with heat signs. Use with caution in cases of diarrhea or bloating due to damp obstruction.

---

[382] Duke, James A. and Rodolfo Vásquez. *Amazonian Ethnobotanical Dictionary.* Boca Raton, FL: CRC, 1994; 133.
[383] Ibid., p, 134.

Major Known Ingredients: Leaf extracts show possible analgesic and antimicrobial activity and contain alkaloids. Root contains coumarins. Plant has garlic odor and contains trithiolaniacin (which is also found in the onion), potassium nitrate and isoarbonnol.

Vital Essence Plants

The plants in this section contain curare which aids in control of muscles essential in respiration and assists lactating mothers with milk production.

Porter-Bush

Vital Essence Plants

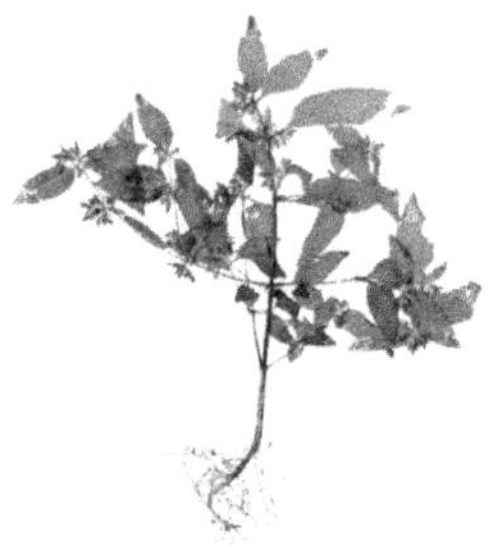

Botanical Name: Eleutheranthera Ruderalis.
Family: Asteraceae.
Region Where Grown: E. Berbice-Corentyne.
Other Names: Twelve o'clock.
Category: Nervous System: Vital essence Plants.
Properties:Sour, Hot/Moist.
Esoteric Botanica: Maat.
Governing Organs: Liver, Heart, Liver, Kidney.
Actions & Indications: Whole plant: Decoction is drunk to enhance milk production by lactating and nursing mothers; for high blood pressure. Drains liver heat and pacifies liver yang – for liver fire and liver yang rising patterns with such symptoms as headache, irritability, red eyes, and dizziness. This herb is highly useful in treating many types of headache, not just those from liver yang rising or liver fire. Recently used for hypertension associated with liver yang rising, coronary heart disease and to reduce cholesterol. Promotes the movement of blood and invigorates the channels – in the upper part of the body this herb promotes lactation and in the lower part it unblocks menstruation due to blood stasis. This herb promotes lactation by clearing the channels.
Cautions & Contraindications: According to some texts, long-term use of this herb may injure the kidneys.

Devildoer

Vital Essence Plants

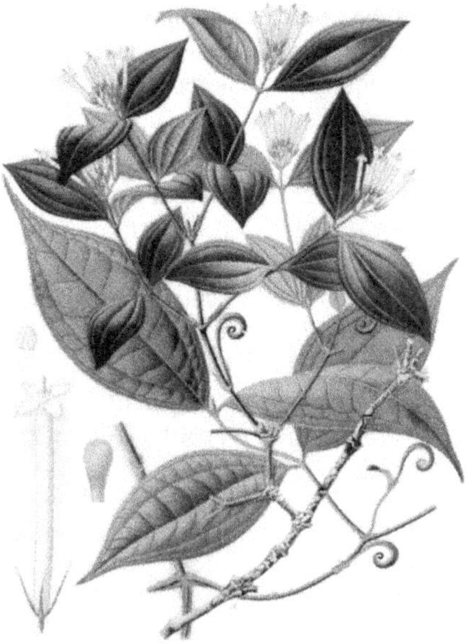

Botanical Name: Strychnos Cogens.
Family: Loganiaceae.
Region Where Grown: E. Berbice-Corentyne.
Other Names: Common Devildoer, White devildoer, Black Devildoer, Bush-rope.
Category: Nervous System: Vital Essence Plants.
Properties: Salty, Cold/Moist.
Esoteric Botanica: Het Heru.
Governing Organs: Kidney, large Intestine, Liver
Actions & Indications: Used for leucorrhoea and as a aphrodisiac.
Bark decoction used to treat fever. Releases the exterior and disperses cold – for exterior cold patterns with such symptoms as chills, fever, headache and body aches and pains.
Stem: A tonic prepared from the bark is used as an aphrodisiac and to treat leucorrhoea and loss of libido.[384]
Tonifies the kidneys and fortifies the yang – for deficient kidney yang patterns with such symptoms as fatigue, impotence, cold extremities, lightheadedness, tinnitus, soreness and weakness in the lower back and knees and frequent, copious, clear urination. Augments the kidney and tonifies the yang – for impotence and sore and weak lower back and lower extremities from kidney yang deficiency. Tonifies the kidneys and strengthens the yang – for deficient kidney yang patterns with such symptoms as impotence, spermatorrhea, urinary incontinence, posturinary dripping and cold pains in the lower back and knees.
Cautions & Contraindications: Do not use in deficient yin patterns with heat signs.
Major Known Ingredients: Contains alkaloids with a curare-like action including diaboline, henningsanine, condensamine and erichsoniine. Erichsoniine seems to be neither toxic nor biologically active.
Pharmacological & Clinical Research: Plant contains diaboline, a weak alkaloid having a mixture of the action of strychnine and curarine, but without a curare-like action. Weakly curarizing alkaloids in Strychnos diaboli include diaboline and desacetyldiaboline and macrophylline. As of 1954 it was reported that this plant contains at least two alkaloids, one of which has a weak curare-like action, i.e., able to paralyze the peripheral nerves
Toxicity: Curare causes death by asphyxiation, the loss of control of muscles essential in respiration.

[384] DeFilipps, Robert A., Shirley L. Maina, and Juliette Crepin. *Medicinal Plants of the Guianas (Guyana, Surinam, French Guiana)*. Washington, D.C.: Dept. of Botany, National Museum of Natural History, Smithsonian Institution, 2004; 159.

Vital Function Plants (Yang)

The plants in this section treat such diseases as menorrhagia, vaginal hemorrhagia and menstrual pain for women and male impotence. Some contain the hormones testosterone and progesterone, which are used to revitalize men and prevent infections, i.e., used for impotence, venereal and bladder disease and syphilis. Others contain many flavonoids which variously have cardiotonic, vasodilating, spasmolytic, antiedemic, diuretic, hypotensive, anticoagulant, anti-inflammatory or antitumor properties.

Benign prostatic hypertrophy (BPH) is characterised by an increased size of the prostate caused by growth of tlbromuscular arid epithelial tissues around urethra. The frequency ofBPH increases with age and about: 70% of men above 75 have BPH, but only 30--40% of men suffer from it. Symptoms include dysuria, increased urination, urgency to urinate, especially at night (nycturia), and difficulty to urinate. Consequences of urethra constriction through BPH are decreased urine flow and pressure and urine retention in the bladder. It is tikely that BPH is caused by a decrease in testosterone production and in it's increased conversion to estradiol (by aromatasc), dihydrotestosterone (known to induce growth of prostatic epithelia) and androstandiol. BHP can be treated with phytotherapy (especially plants with phytosterols). The aim is to inhibit the proliferation of periurethral tissues and to relax urethral and prostatic muscles in order to enhance urethral flow.

Monkey Ladder

Vital Function Plants

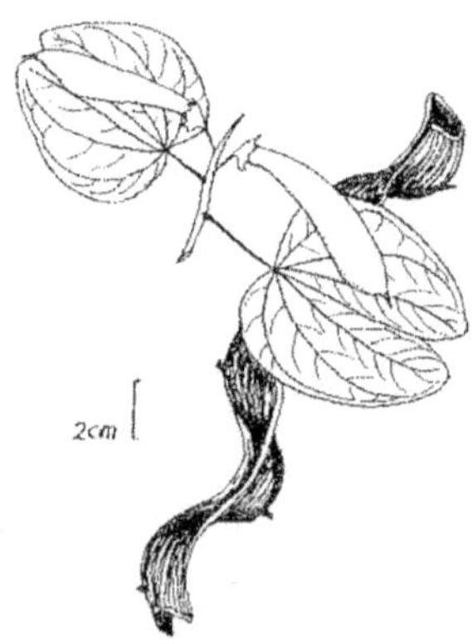

Botanical Name: Bauhinia Kunthiana.
Family: Caesalpiniaceae.
Region Where Grown: Essequibo Isl-W. Demerara.
Other Names: Turtle Steps.
Category: Nervous System: Vital Function (Yang) Plants.
Properties: Sour, Acrid, Cold/Dry.
Esoteric Botanica: Seker.
Governing Organs: Liver, large Intestine, Spleen, Kidney, Lungs.
Actions & Indications: Used for dysentery, diarrhea and as a tonic and aphrodisiac. Decoction for backache.[385]
Stems: The Stems are used to treat kidney diseases while the seeds are employed as diureties.[386]
Also used as a treatment for malaria.[387] Treats malarial disorder – for

[385] DeFilipps, Robert A., Shirley L. Maina, and Juliette Crepin. *Medicinal Plants of the Guianas (Guyana, Surinam, French Guiana)*. Washington, D.C.: Dept. of Botany, National Museum of Natural History, Smithsonian Institution, 2004; 65.
[386] Castner, James L., S. Lee. Timme, and James A. Duke. *A Field Guide to Medicinal and Useful Plants of the Upper Amazon*. Gainesville, FL: Feline, 1998; 22.
[387] Ibid., p. 29.

chronic malarial disorder with signs of qi and blood deficiency.
Root: Used for diarrhea. Wood is boiled and the water drunk as an antidiarrheal or as an antidysenteric for bloody dysentery. Decoction or infusion in wine, used as a tonic and aphrodisiac. Tonifies the kidneys and fortifies the yang – for kidney yang deficiency patterns with such symptoms as impotence, premature ejaculation, cold and painful lower back, or weak lower back and extremities.
Bark used for hemorrhages.
Flower used for coughs and colds, hemorrhage, whooping cough and tuberculosis. Stops coughing – especially cold or deficiency coughs.
Cautions & Contraindications: Do not use in cases of externally-contracted excess heat patterns or in cases of spleen deficiency with dampness and loose stools.
Pharmacological & Clinical Research: The bark is for treating "women's diseases" such as menorrhagia, vaginal hemorrhagia and menstrual pains

Congo Pump

Vital Function Plants

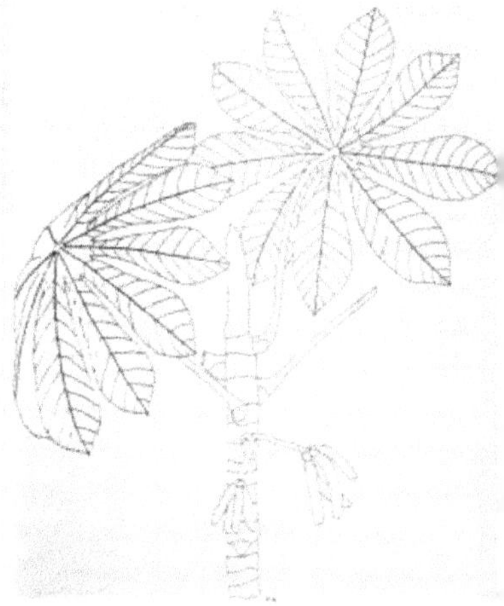

Botanical Name: Cecropia Angulata.
Family: Cecropiaceae.
Region Where Grown: Potaro-Siparun.
Other Names: Trumpet Tree, Monkey pump, Trumpeter.
Category: Nervous System: Vital Function (Yang) Plants.
Properties: Astringent, Hot/Moist.
Esoteric Botanica: Maat.
Governing Organs: Liver, Heart, Stomach.
Actions & Indications: Dried leaves are decocted for a diuretic to alleviate kidney disorders. [388] Tonifies the kidneys and fortifies the yang – for deficient kidney yang patterns with such symptoms as fatigue, impotence, cold extremities, light headedness, tinnitus, soreness and weakness in the lower back and knees.
Leaf: Diuretic tea made from the leaves is used to lessen kidney and bladder discomfort. Topically apply sap from crushed leaves to treat eye problems and use a leaf decoction to remedy fevers. Fallen leaf is boiled in water, and the liquid is drunk to calm a nervous heart. Used for heart and liver problems. Fresh green leaves are boiled and the water drunk as an antimalarial. Leaves are boiled as a tea or tonic.
Stem: Decoction of inner bark for dysentery; hot poultice of young shoots used for dressing ulcers and sores.
Stem and Leaf: A tea or decoction of the dried leaf or inner stem-bark as a antimalarial.[389]
Bark: Bark is squeezed in water for a preparation to stupefy wasps. Sap used to treat fresh cuts; juice for warts.[390] Shoot used to treat abcesses and for wounds and cuts.
Bark used to treat abcesses, wounds and cuts, and for kidney problems.
Cautions & Contraindications: Do not use in deficient yin patterns with heat signs.
Major Known Ingredients: Leaf contains many flavonoids which variously have cardiotonic, vasodilating, spasmolytic, antiedemic, diuretic, hypotensive, anticoagulant, anti-inflammatory or antitumor properties.
Pharmacological & Clinical Research: In pharmacologic assay, the leaves and stems have shown antiatherogenic and central nervous system depressant activity.[391]

---

[388] DeFilipps, Robert A., Shirley L. Maina, and Juliette Crepin. *Medicinal Plants of the Guianas (Guyana, Surinam, French Guiana)*. Washington, D.C.: Dept. of Botany, National Museum of Natural History, Smithsonian Institution, 2004; 79.
[389] Ibid., 79.
[390] Morton F. Julia, *Atlas of Medical Plants of Middle America: Bahamas to Yucatan.* Springfield, Illinois: Charles C Thomas Publisher, 1981; 144.
[391] Ibid., p. 143.

Kapadula

Vital Function Plants

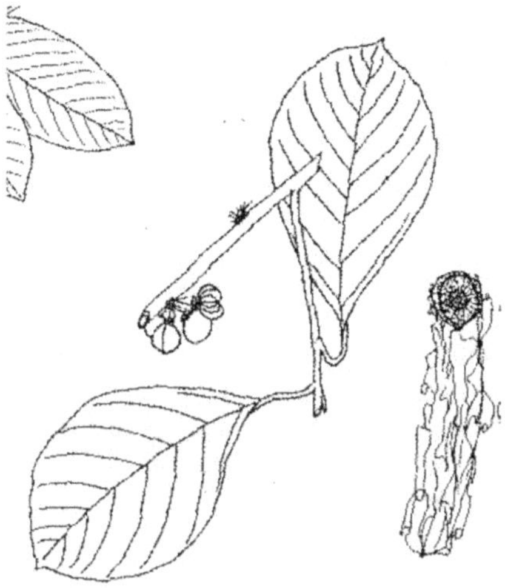

Botanical Name: Doliocarpus Dentatus.
Family: Dilleniaceae.
Region Where Grown: Potaro-Siparuni.
Other Names: Cappa-dula, kabuduli.
Category: Nervous System: Vital Function (Yang) Plants.
Properties: Acrid, Cool/dry.
Esoteric Botanica: Sebek.
Governing Organs: Lungs, Kidney, Spleen.
Actions & Indications: Whole plant: Decoction for venereal disease.
Stem: Stem and bark in an aphrodisiac tea or in an infusion when chopped and soaked in wine; Tonifies the kidneys and fortifies the yang – for deficient kidney yang impotence, low libido, frequent urination and spermatorrhea. Used in the after effects of malaria.[392]
Sap of stem drunk to relieve stricture or as a thirst quencher. Sap used as an abortive, for coughs and colds and to treat snakebites. [393]
Leaf: Used to disinfect the umbilical cord of newborn babies. Also used as a depurative.
Wood: Concentrated mixture of the wood boiled with water is used as an aphrodisiac. [394]
Dry wood boiled with water is used as a tea, a tonic or for impotence. Tonifies the kidneys and stabilizes the essence – for premature ejaculation and spermatorrhea due to unstable and deficient kidneys. Also used for excessive uterine bleeding and vaginal discharge.
Stem: Infusion in hot water for a tea to remedy diarrhea. Strengthens the spleen and stops diarrhea – for chronic diarrhea caused by weakness of the transportative functions of the spleen.
Cautions & Contraindications: Do not use in patients with either damp-heat or heat from yin deficiency. It may be drying. Do not use in patients who have difficulty urinating.

---

[392] Duke, James A. and Rodolfo Vásquez. *Amazonian Ethnobotanical Dictionary*. Boca Raton, FL: CRC, 1994; 67

[393] DeFilipps, Robert A., Shirley L. Maina, and Juliette Crepin. *Medicinal Plants of the Guianas (Guyana, Surinam, French Guiana)*. Washington, D.C.: Dept. of Botany, National Museum of Natural History, Smithsonian Institution, 2004; 110.

[394] Ibid., p, 110.

Ironweed

Vital Function Plants

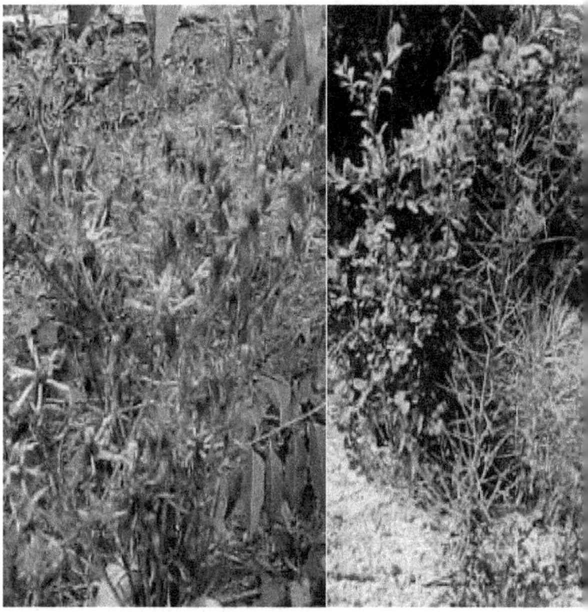

Botanical Name: Desmodium Ascendens.
Family: Fabaceae.
Region Where Grown: U. Takutu-U. Essequibo.
Other Names: Ironweed, Sweetheart, Weak-back, Watch Backdam, Watchman.
Category: Nervous System: Vital Function (Yang) Plants.
Properties: Hot/Moisty Acrid.
Esoteric Botanica: Maat.
Governing Organs: Liver, Heart, Stomach.
Actions & Indications: Whole plant: Decoction used to strengthen the kidneys and back, and to treat nervous conditions and eczema.[395] Tonifies the kidneys and fortifies the yang – for kidney yang deficiency patterns with such symptoms as impotence, premature ejaculation, cold and painful lower back or weak lower back and extremities.
Whole plant: Decoction used to treat coughs and colds and to reduce blood-sugar level.
Used for cramps (babies), stomachache, pain, fever, hemorrhage, heart problems, impotence, menstruation, and to prevent miscarriage. Tonifies the kidneys and fortifies the yang – for impotence, urinary incontinence, and nocturnal emission from deficient kidney yang.
This herb may be used for infertility from either a cold womb (women) or cold essence (men). Cold essence can manifest as low sperm count, malformed sperm, etc
Leaf: Used for hair loss.
Cautions & Contraindications: Do not use in deficient yin patterns with heat signs. This herb is hot and toxic. Long-term use is not recommended.

---

395 DeFilipps, Robert A., Shirley L. Maina, and Juliette Crepin. *Medicinal Plants of the Guianas (Guyana, Surinam, French Guiana)*. Washington, D.C.: Dept. of Botany, National Museum of Natural History, Smithsonian Institution, 2004; 29.

Granny Backbone

Vital Function Plants

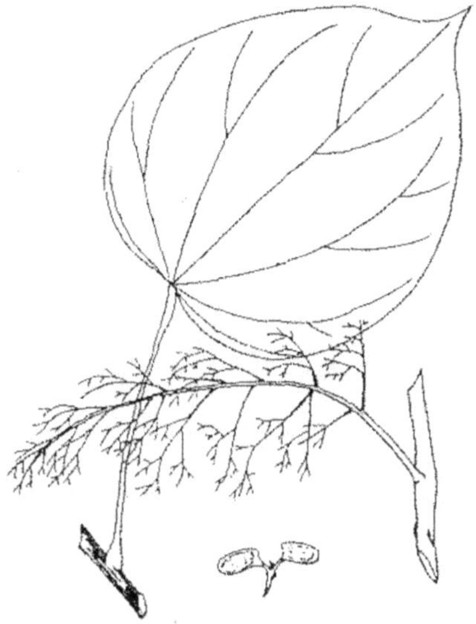

Botanical Name: Curarea Candicans.
Family: Menispermaceae.
Region Where Grown:Cuyuni/Mazaruni.
Other Names: Teteabo.
Category: Nervous System: Vital Function (Yang) Plants.
Properties: Slightly Acrid, Cool/Dry.
Esoteric Botanica: Sebek.
Governing Organs: Lungs, Kidney, liver.
Actions & Indications: Whole plant: Mixed with other plants in a tonic for pain.[396] Tonifies the liver and kidneys and augments essence – for infertility, impotence, spermatorrhea, low back pain, lightheadedness, and tinnitus from insufficiency of kidney qi and debility of the essence and blood. Tonifies the kidneys – for such symptoms as weak lower back and knees, diarrhea, tinnitus, decreased hearing, and toothache and bleeding gums from deficient kidneys. Tonifies the kidneys and fortifies the yang – for impotence, urinary incontinence, and nocturnal emission from deficient kidney yang. Drip the sap into ears for treating earache.[397]
Stem: Wood used as aphrodisiac, malaria and sores.[398]
Cautions & Contraindications: Do not use in patients with spermatorrhea, frequent urination or vaginal discharge due to heat.
Major Known Ingredients: Contains the alkaloids berberine and isochondrodendrine.
Pharmacological & Clinical Research: Menispermaceae, a group of lianas often endowed with powerful muscle relaxants, including one that is the source of the myorelaxant tubocurarine used in modern medicine, especially in open heart surgery.[399]
The menispermaceae root is also used as diuretic, emetic, resolvent (for bruises), tonic and toxic.[400]
Another species of this plant *Abuta rujescens* is used to make "curare" and is considered antimalarial,

---

[396] Robert A. DeFilipps, Shirley L. Maina and Juliette Crepin, Medicinal Plants of the Guianas (Guyana, Surinam, French Guiana), (National Museaum of Natural History, Smithsonian Institute: Washington D.C) p, 188

[397]Robert A. DeFilipps, Shirley L. Maina and Juliette Crepin, Medicinal Plants of the Guianas (Guyana, Surinam, French Guiana), (National Museaum of Natural History, Smithsonian Institute: Washington D.C) p, 188

[398] Robert A. DeFilipps, Shirley L. Maina and Juliette Crepin, Medicinal Plants of the Guianas (Guyana, Surinam, French Guiana), (National Museaum of Natural History, Smithsonian Institute: Washington D.C) p, 188

[399] James Alan Duke and Rodolfo Valquez Martinez, Amazonian Ethnobotanical Dictionary (CRC Press: Florida, 1994), p 9

[400] James Alan Duke and Rodolfo Valquez Martinez, Amazonian Ethnobotanical Dictionary (CRC Press: Florida, 1994), p 13

emmenagogue, tonic, good for kidney stones, sterility, vaginitis and weak vision.[401] This plant contains alkaloids which relax the muscular system.

[401] James Alan Duke and Rodolfo Valquez Martinez, Amazonian Ethnobotanical Dictionary (CRC Press: Florida, 1994), p29 Amazonian Ethnobotanical Dictionary, p, 13

Cockshun

Vital Function Plants

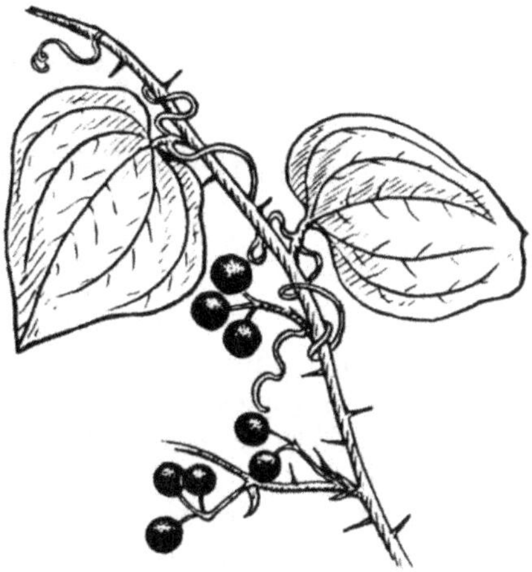

Botanical Name: Smilax Schomburgkiana.
Family: Smilacaceae.
Region Where Grown: U. Takutu-U. Essequibo.
Other Names: Spotai.
Category: Nervous System: Vital Function (Yang) Plants.
Properties: Salty, Cold/Moist.
Esoteric Botanica: Het Heru.
Governing Organs: Kidney, Spleen, Liver.
Actions & Indications: Antisyphilitic, aphrodisiac, bladder problems, dental analgesic, impotence, syphilis and venereal disease.
Root: Grated into a male aphrodisiac decoction which is both consumed as a beverage and rubbed onto the sexual organs.[402]
Tonifies the kidneys and strengthens the yang – for deficient kidney yang patterns with such symptoms as impotence, spermatorrhea, urinary incontinence, posturinary dripping and cold pains in the lower back and knees.
Stem: Antisyphilitic; maceration or decoction as a depurative.
Root used for back pain and as aphrodesiac.
Cautions & Contraindications: Do not use in patients with deficient Kidney yin with heat signs. Do not use in patients with diarrhea from Spleen deficiency or constipation from excess heat.
Pharmacological & Clinical Research: The root contains the hormones testosterone and progesterone, which are used to revitalize men and prevent infections, i.e., used for impotence, venereal and bladder disease including syphilis.

[402] DeFilipps, Robert A., Shirley L. Maina, and Juliette Crepin. *Medicinal Plants of the Guianas (Guyana, Surinam, French Guiana)*. Washington, D.C.: Dept. of Botany, National Museum of Natural History, Smithsonian Institution, 2004; 266.

Chapter 8: The Carminatives

Plants that Promotes Expulsion of flatus - Gas Generated in the Stomach or Bowels.

The carminatives all have certain kinds of essential oils which can stimulate the local sites, increase the peristalsis of the intestines and the bowel movements, evacuate gas and relieve the distention caused by overeating. The relaxation of the smooth muscles relaxing the smooth muscles of the bronchi and blood vessels, and the tension of the respiratory skeletal muscles. They can also increase the secretion of bile and regulate the smooth muscles of the liver, bile duct, breast, uterus and the digestive tract. They can also increase the hepatic blood flow to the liver. The essential oils are also used in certain analgesic ointments to alleviate bronchial troubles and in other medicines. Nutmeg oils are anti-oxidant agents and they also exhibit strong antimicrobial and insecticidal properties.

The stagnation of Qi flow means the abnormal function of the smooth muscles of the blood vessels, the intestines and the skeletal. Any stagnation of flow in the body/organs/channels will lead to local pain, distention or oppression.

The regulatory action on the digestive tract is both excitatory and inhibitory on the smooth muscles of the intestines. Inhibitory action on the alimentary tract reduce the tension of the intestinal tubules. They are used for regurgitation, hiccough, diarrhea, abdominal pain and other hyperactive symptoms. The excitatory action on the alimentary tract can enhance the contraction of the GI-Tubules and increase the secretion of gastric juice. They are also used for indigestion, abdominal distention, constipation and other hypo-active symptoms.

Anise

Remove Stagnation of the Digestive Tract

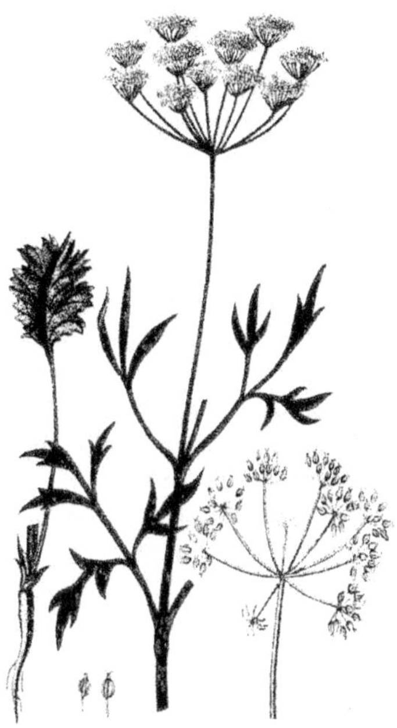

Botanical Name: Pimpinella Anisum.
Family: Apiaceae.
Region Where Grown: Barima-Waini.
Other Names:None.
Category: Caminatives.
Properties: Astringent, Hot/Moist.
Esoteric Botanica: Maat.
Governing Organs: Liver, Stomach, Heart.
Actions & Indications: Reported to be abortifacient, antiseptic, antispasmodic, aperient, apbrodisiac, aromatic, balsamic, carminative, diaphoretic, digestive, diuretic and expectorant. It is also fungicidal, lactagogue, pectoral, stimulant, stomachic, sudorific and tonic. Anise is a folk remedy for asthma, bronchitis, cancer, cholera, colic, cough, dropsy, dysmenorrhea, epilepsy, gall bladder, halitosis, indigestion, insomnia, lice, migraine, nausea, nephrosis, neuralgia, purperium, scabies, stomach and stones.[403]
Whole plant: As a carminative and vermifuge. This is a relatively strong and effective herb.
Flowers are boiled and the water is drunk for treating stomachache. Absorbs acidity and alleviates pain – used calcined for excessive stomach pain with a sour taste in the mouth.
The fruit and the oil are a traditional remedy {or catarrh of the respiratory tract (colds and tlu, cough, bronchitis) and also for dyspeptic complaints (indigestion, flatulence, colic). At high doses, the oil is antiseptic and antispasmodic and has been used as a stimulating liniment against ectoparasites. Many cough remedies and other medicinal products contain aniseed extract or aniseed oil not only for its medicinal properties (antitussive, expectorant) but also to improve the flavour and taste.[404]
Seed: Dry seeds are boiled and the water is drunk for wind (gas) pain.
The fresh bulb is taken orally as a carminative, tonic, antipyretic, hypotensive and diuretic. [405]
Cautions & Contraindications: Do not use in cases of yin deficiency with heat signs, heat excess, or in the absence of significant qi deficiency. Also contraindicated in cases of liver yang rising or hypertension.
Major Known Ingredients: Per 100 g, anise seed is reported to contain 337 calories (1412 kJ), 9.5 g H20, 17.6 g protein, 15.9 g fat, 50.0 g total carbohydrate, 14.6 g fiber, 7.0 gash, 646 mg Ca, 440 mg P, 37 mg Fe, 170 mg Mg, 16 mg Na, 1441 mg K, and *5.3* mg Zn. Fresh leaves, used in garnishes and salads, may contain 8 to 9 mg vitamin C per 100 g. Simple coumarins (6,7-furocoumarins) and acetylinic compounds have been reported. Anetho!-glycol, creosol, anethol, acetaldehyde, isoamylamine, umbelliferone, bergaptene, isopimpinellin, isobergaptene, and sphondin, flavonoids: quercetin-3-gJucoronide, rutin,

---

403 Duke, James A. *CRC Handbook of Medicinal Herbs*. Boca Raton, FL: CRC, 1985; 375.
404 Van, Wyk Ben-Erik., and Michael Wink. *Medicinal Plants of the World: An Illustrated Scientific Guide to Important Medicinal Plants and Their Uses*. Portland: Timber, 2004; 240.
405 Ross, Ivan A. *Medicinal Plants of the World: Chemical Constituents, Traditional, and Modern Medicinal Uses*. Vol. 2. Totowa, NJ: Humana, 1999; 3.

luteolin 7-glucoside, isoorientin, isovitexin, and apigenin 7-glucoside. [406] Anethole has documented expectorant, antispasmodic and antimicrobial activities. The carminative effect is less pronounced than with other oils (caraway, fennel). Distinct expectorant activity is linked to the ability of anethole to stimulate cilial movement of the bronchial epithelium.[407]

Pharmacological & Clinical research: Anise enjoys considerable reputation as a medicine in coughs and pectoral affections. In hard, dry coughs where expectoration is difficult, it is of much value. It is greatly used in the form of lozenges and the seeds have also been used for smoking, to promote expectoration. The volatile oil, mixed with spirits of wine forms the liqueur anisette, which has a beneficial action on the bronchial tubes and for bronchitis and spasmodic asthma. Anisette, if administered in hot water, is an immediate palliative. For infantile catarrh, aniseed tea is very helpful. It is made by pouring half a pint of boiling water on two teaspoonsful of bruised seed. This, sweetened, is given cold in doses of one to three teaspoonsful frequently. The stimulant and carminative properties of anise make it useful in flatulency and colic.[408]

Toxicity: Its major component, anethole, can cause dermatitis (erythema, scaling, and vesiculation). Anethole has two isomers, the cisisomer 15 to 38 times more toxic than the trans isomer. Like fennel oil, anise oil contains compounds that can be aminated in vivo resulting in a series of three dangerous hallucinogenic amphetamines. Anethole used to flavor toothpaste has produced contact sensitivity, according to reports. Aniseed is reported to have caused cheilitis and stomatitis. Anethole (l-methoxy-4-propenylbenzene) is a major component of the essential oils of bitter fennel, anise, star anise, et a1. Anethole is a moderate acute toxin with an oral LD of 2090 mg/kg in rats. Bitter fennel oil, with an oral LD_{50} of 4.52 mc/kg in rats, is irritant when applied to the skin. Rats fed a diet containing 0.25% anethole for one year showed no ill effects, while those receiving 1.0% anethole for 15 weeks had microscopic alterations of the hepatocytes. Anethole and the essential oils of anise and fennel significantly stimulated hepatic regeneration in rats. [409]

---

[406] Duke, James A. *CRC Handbook of Medicinal Herbs*. Boca Raton, FL: CRC, 1985; 375.

[407] Van, Wyk Ben-Erik., and Michael Wink. *Medicinal Plants of the World: An Illustrated Scientific Guide to Important Medicinal Plants and Their Uses*. Portland: Timber, 2004; 240.

[408] Morton F. Julia, *Atlas of Medical Plants of Middle America: Bahamas to Yucatan.* Springfield, Illinois: Charles C Thomas Publisher, 1981; 43.

[409] Duke, James A. and Rodolfo Vásquez. *Amazonian Ethnobotanical Dictionary*. Boca Raton, FL: CRC, 1994; 375.

Cacao

Remove Stagnation of the Digestive Tract

Botanical Name: Theobroma Cacao.
Family: Sterculiaceae.
Region Where Grown: Demerara-Mahaica.
Other Names: None.
Category: Caminatives.
Properties: Sweet, Acrid, Aromatic, Cold/Moist.
Esoteric Botanica: Auset.
Governing Organs: Stomach, Spleen, Liver.

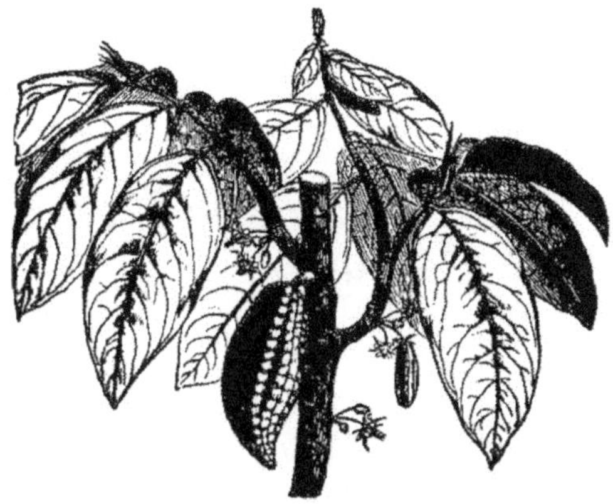

Actions & Indications: Analgesic, anemia, antirhematic, anti diarrhea and emollient. Used as cardiotonic, diuretic and in modem medicine as antiasthmatic.[410] Casao acts on the respiratory tract.
Leaf-bud: Infusion used with incense to treat diarrhoea.
Fruit: Infusion of dry pods used to decrease leprosy spots. Treats malarial disorder – for chronic malarial disorder with signs of qi and blood deficiency.
Seed: Infusion of baked seed-membranes is drunk for remedy in anemia.
Major Known Ingredients: Cocoa butter contains glycerides, and its sterols include ergosterol, sitosterol and stigmasterol. Seed alkaloids include caffeine and the diuretic theobromine. Seed phenolic compounds include coumarin, esculetine and catechol. Leaf contains genistic acid, an antirheumatic and analgesic.[411] The seeds contain 45 to 50% fatty oil. Their essential oil contains about 50% linalool; also alipharic acids and various esters. Leaves, roots and seeds contain the alkaloids caffeine and theobromine is toxic to horses in doses exceeding five grams per day. The antitumor activity of the root bark is attributed to its tannin content.[412]
Pharmacological & Clinical Research: Chocolate constitutes a significant dietary source of theobromine. Hot cocoa, for example, prepared from instant mix provides approximately 60 mg of theobromine and 4 mg of caffeine per serving. Chocolate contains less caffeine per serving than coffee (0.4 - 1.2 % of caffeine in cocoa), but may still have significant amounts, depending on the preparation. For example, milk chocolate contains up to 15 mg of caffeine per ounce, but dark chocolate can contain'up to 35 mg per ounce.[413] Theobromine is richer in nitrogen than caffeine, which contains only 28 percel nitrogen. Regarding its

---

[410] Duke, James A. and Rodolfo Vásquez. *Amazonian Ethnobotanical Dictionary*. Boca Raton, FL: CRC, 1994; 169.
[411] DeFilipps, Robert A., Shirley L. Maina, and Juliette Crepin. *Medicinal Plants of the Guianas (Guyana, Surinam, French Guiana)*. Washington, D.C.: Dept. of Botany, National Museum of Natural History, Smithsonian Institution, 2004; 275.
[412] Morton F. Julia, *Atlas of Medical Plants of Middle America: Bahamas to Yucatan.* Springfield, Illinois: Charles C Thomas Publisher, 1981; 556 – 557.
[413] Spinella, Marcello. *The Psychopharmacology of Herbal Medicine: Plant Drugs That Alter Mind, Brain, and Behavior*. Cambridge, MA: MIT, 2001; 79.

physiological effects, it is most probable that, similar to caffeine in coffee, theobromine is one of the most important components of cocoa. The decomposition products of theobromine, on the other hand, have been studied several times. They are so similar to those of coffee that on this basis alone, physiologically in terms of metabolism, a close affinity may be assumed between these two substances.[414]

---

[414] Bibra, Baron Ernst Von, *Plant Intoxicants: A Classic Text on the Use of Mind Altering Plants.* Vermont: Healing Arts Press, 1995; 68.

Nutmeg

Regulate the Action on the Digestive Tract

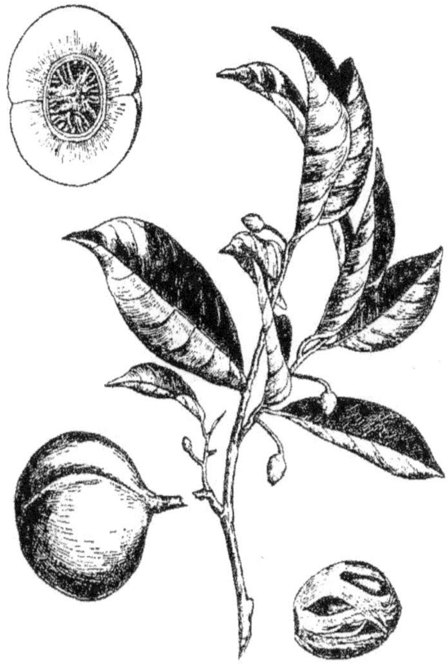

Botanical Name: Myristica Fragrans.
Family: Myristicaceae.
Region Where Grown: Demerara-Mahaica.
Other Names: Mace, Nutmeg.
Category: Caminatives and Stomachic.
Properties: Astrigent, Aromatic, Hot/Moist.
Esoteric Botanica: Maat.
Governing Organs: Liver, Stomach, Heart.
Actions & Indications: Nutmeg is a carminative used against indigestion and other stomach problems. Nutmeg stimulates production of gastric juice, promoting digestion, increasing appetite, relieving intestinal spasm and flatulence.[415]
Fruit: A piece is chewed to alleviate stomachache.
Seed: The seeds are employed as an excitant and stimulant. The seed decoction is drunk as a treatment for asthma and even for malaria. Sufferers from a stroke keep a piece of nutmeg seed in their mouths, and this is expected to ward off further attacks.
Major Known Ingredients: Medicinally, the nutmeg is said to have stimulant, carminative and astringent properties. Its hallucinogenic properties are ascribed to the aromatic ethers myristicin, elemicin and safrole. The red pigment in mace is mainly lycopene, identical to the red colourant in tomato. The seed contains mainly trimyristin and essential oils. The seeds are used medicinally. The odor is aromatic, the taste strongly pungent. The seeds contain 3.6 % of a volatile oil comprising 60-80 % d-camphene, 8 % d-pinene, 8 % dipentene, 6 % d-linalol, 0.6 % safrole, 0.2 % eugenol, isoeugenol, d-borneol, I-terpineol, geraniol, and 4 % myristicin ($C_{11}H_{12}O_3$).[416]
Pharmacological & Clinical Research: More recent work has indicated that myristicin may not be the only factor in nutmegs responsible for these psychotic or hallucinogenic activities. Continuing research is bringing forth evidence that factors in untmegs have a widespread effect on the sympathetic nervous system of the body and that they may also antagonize the action of prostaglandins which are among the most important constituents of the body. [417]
Toxicity: Doses exceeding one teaspoon take effect within 2 to 5 hours, producing timespace distortions, feelings of unreality and sometimes visual hallucinations accompanied by dizziness, headache, illness and rapid heartbeat. The"carcinogen" safrole, responsible for the banning of sassafras, also occurs in nutmeg. The oral LD_{50} for safrole in rats is 1950 mg/kg body weight, with major symptoms including ataxia,

[415] Keys, John D. *Chinese Herbs: Their Botany, Chemistry, and Pharmacodynamics*. Rutland, VT: C.E. Tuttle, 1997; 140.
[416] Ibid., p, 140.
[417] Thomsom, William A. R., M.D., *Herbs that Heal*. New York: Charles Scribner's Sons, 1976; 124.

depression, and diarrhea, death occurring in 4 to 5 days. With rats, dietary safrole at levels of 0,25, 0.5, and 1 % produced growth retardation, stomach and testicular atrophy, liver necrosis, biliary proliferation and primary hepatomas. Research on myristicin, which occurs also in black pepper, carrot seed, celery seed and parsley, the psychoactive and hallucinogenic properties of mace, nutmeg and purified myristic is still onn going. It has been hypothesized that myrisiticin and elemicin can be readily modified in the body to amphetamines. The oral LD_{50} for nutmeg oil in rats, mice, and hamsters is 2600, 4620 and 6000 mg/kg, respectively.[418]

[418] Duke, James A. and Rodolfo Vásquez. *Amazonian Ethnobotanical Dictionary*. Boca Raton, FL: CRC, 1994; 320.

Mangrove

Regulate the Action on the Digestive Tract

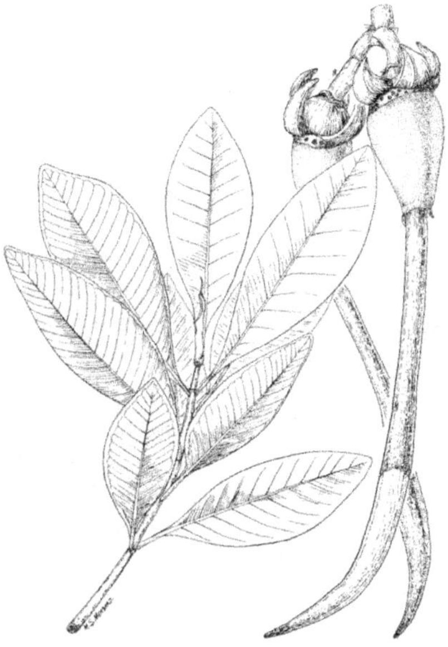

Botanical Name: Rhizophora Mangle.
Family: Rhizophoraceae.
Region Where Grown: Barima-Waini.
Other Names: Mangero, Konopo, Red Mangrove.
Category: Caminatives.
Properties: Astringent, Sour, Hot/Moist.
Esoteric Botanica: Tehuti.
Governing Organs: Liver, Spleen, Urinary Bladder, Heart.
Actions & Indications: Root: Used to treat diarrhea.
Strengthens the spleen and tonifies the stomach – for lethargy, lack of appetite, chest and abdominal distention, diarrhea, or even prolapse in severe cases.
A bark decoction is used to treat frequent dysentery, diarrhea, micturition and bladder diseases.
Bark is febrifuge, astringent, rich in tannin, used in a decoction for haemorrhages and in gargles to remedy angina. Decotion is taken to stop spitting of blood from lungs, trachea or bronchi.[419]Tonifies heart qi and calms the spirit – for such symptoms as shortness of breath, anxiety, palpitations, forgetfulness and insomnia.
Cautions & Contraindications: It is contraindicated in cases of excess dampness, food stagnation, intestinal parasites or damp-phlegm disorders with such symptoms as epigastric distention and bloating.
Toxicity: The dry bark contains 10 to 40% tannin. The aerial roots contain10.5% tannin.[420]

---

[419]DeFilipps, Robert A., Shirley L. Maina, and Juliette Crepin. *Medicinal Plants of the Guianas (Guyana, Surinam, French Guiana)*. Washington, D.C.: Dept. of Botany, National Museum of Natural History, Smithsonian Institution, 2004; 615.
[420] Ibid., p, 615.

Bully Tree

Regulate the Action on the Digestive Tract

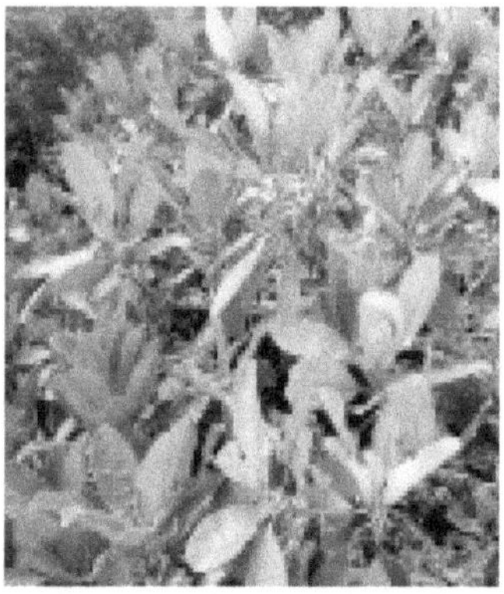

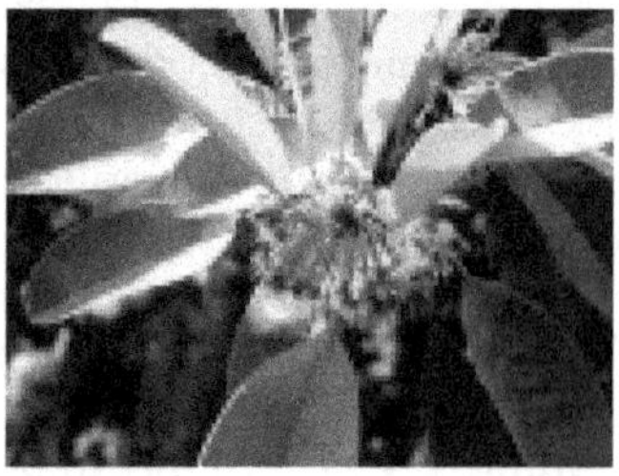

Botanical Name: Manilkara Bidentata.
Family: Sapotaceae.
Region Where Grown: Pomeroon-Supenaam.
Other Names: Beefwood, Bulletwood.
Category: Caminatives.
Properties: Sour, Cold/Dry.
Esoteric Botanica: Seker.
Governing Organs: Liver, Spleen, Small Intestine.
Actions & Indications: Whole plant: Latex used as an effective cure for dysentery. Clears heat and dries dampness – for damp-heat in the middle burner (stomach or intestines) manifesting as diarrhea or dysenteric disorder, or for vomiting and/or acid reflux due to stomach heat. Drains damp-heat, especially from the lower burner – for such problems as thick yellow vaginal discharge, urinary tract infections, STDs, foul-smelling diarrhea or dysenteric disorder. Drains damp-heat from the liver and gallbladder channels – for damp-heat in the upper portion of the gallbladder channel with such symptoms as red, swollen sore throat and eyes, swollen and painful ears or sudden deafness. Also for damp-heat in the liver or gallbladder channels (especially the lowe r parts) with such symptoms as jaundice, pain, swelling or dampness in the genital area or foul-smelling vaginal discharge and itching.
Stem: A clyster is used for "carabisi sickness".
Bark is used to treat "buck sickness" and used also as emetic. Promotes the movement of qi and promotes urination – for damp leg qi and symptoms of damp-phlegm malarial disorders. Can also treat other malarial disorders.
Resinous Gum: Gum from the cut in the trunk is decoted and taken as a remedy for "strain in the testicles or men's swollen glands.[421]
Cautions & Contraindications: Do not use in cases of spleen or stomach deficiency with diarrhea.

[421] Morton F. Julia, *Atlas of Medical Plants of Middle America: Bahamas to Yucatan.* Springfield, Illinois: Charles C Thomas Publisher, 1981; 617.

Negro-Broom

Regulate the Action on the Digestive Tract

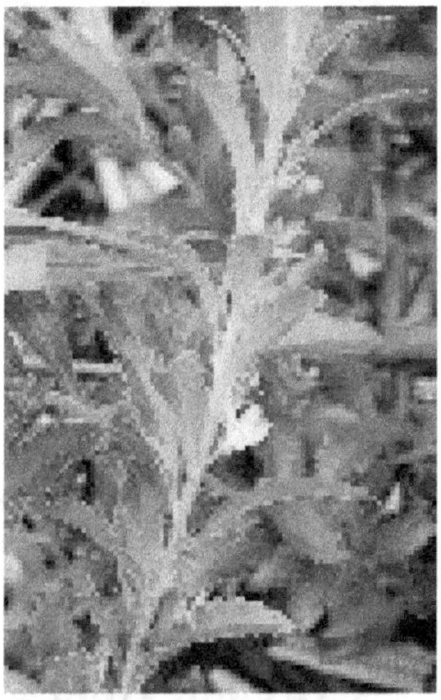

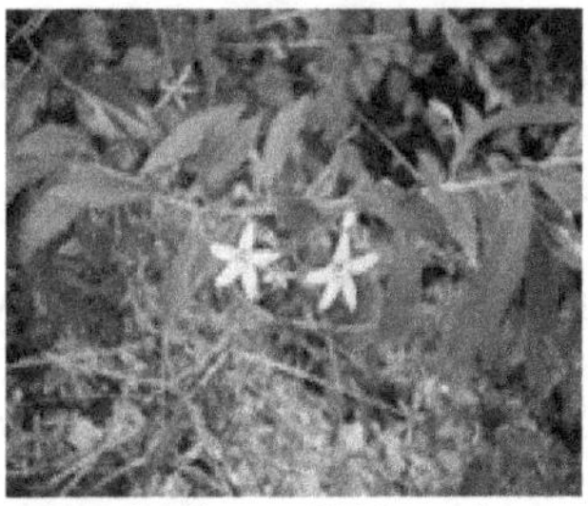

Botanical Name: Capraria Biflora.
Family: Scrophulariaceae.
Region Where Grown: Demerara-Mahaica.
Other Names: Huyara, Negro-broom, Wild tea.
Category: Caminatives.
Properties: Acrid, Warm, Hot/Moist.
Esoteric Botanica: Maat.
Governing Organs: Liver, Spleen, Kidney, Gall Stones.
Actions & Indications: Infusion is also drunk for a calming effect, tonic, digestive and cholagogue.[422]
Whole plant: Infusion is drunk for a calming effect, tonic, digestive and cholagogue; infusion has an antispasmodic action, especially after a violent purgative; Saline decoction for a vermifuge. [423]
Young plant is pulverised and mixed with soft grease and sugar in a poultice which is applied to hard boils to bring them to a point.
Stem and Leaf: Infusion for colic, diuretic and antiperiodic.
Leaf: Crushed leaves are salted and moistened in rum or vinegar and applied in a row as a cataplasm on the forehead to treat violent headache. Decoction of crushed leaves or of young shoots used for an eyewash. Infusion used as a cholagogue, refreshant and tea. Used in treatment of gallstones and menstrual pain, pelvic inflammation and reheumatic disorders.
Pharmacological & Clinical Research: "The antinflammatory effects of leaves of *Capraria biflora* L. were investigated. The aqueous extract 10% was administered at different doses in two models of inflammation: the carrageenin-induced paw edema in rats and the peritonitis induced by carrageenin in mice. In two tests, the dose of 200 mg kg-1 of the extract showed anti-inflammatory activity like indometacin and the effect was dose dependent. It is possible that the antiimflammatory effect of this plant may obbey to more than one mechanism and that the flavonoids could be involved in it."[424]

---

[422] Morton F. Julia, *Atlas of Medical Plants of Middle America: Bahamas to Yucatan.* Springfield, Illinois: Charles C Thomas Publisher, 1981; 260.
[423] Ibid., 260.
[424] Acosta, Sulay loy, Muro, Liliana Vicet, Sacrerio Arelys Lopez, Monteagudo, Geidy Lorenzo, Pena, Ania Reinosa and Okwei, Samuel Narku, *Anti-inflammatory Effects of an Aqueous Extract of Capraria Biflora L.,* Santa Clara Cuba: Departmento de Farmacia, Facultad de Quimica y farmacia, Universidad Central De las Villas, Carretera a Camajuani Km 5, Acta Farm. Bonaerense 22, 2003; 53-5.

Chapter 9: Blood Stasis

Plants for Coagulation & Blood Regulation

Blood stasis is generally caused by bleeding, stagnation of energy flow, asthenia of energy, pathogenic heat or cold factors or external trauma. Any blockage in circulation (especially microcirculation) causing inflammation, abnormal growth, fibroid, metabolic or autoimmune disorders can be relieved by eliminating blood stasis.

The plants of this section are divided into two groups imflammatory: they are used for angina, atherosclerosis and rheumatoid arthritis and hemostatic plants which can shorten the process of coagulation by increasing the number of platelets and throbin. They can also shorten the bleeding time, construct the local blood vessels, improve the function of the membranes of the blood vessels, increase the resistance of the capillaries, decrease vascular permeability and inhibit fibrinolysin.

Invigorating Blood Circulation and Removing Blood Stasis

Plants for coagulation and blood regulation affect circulation and regulate the metabolism of the cardiac muscles, reduce the oxygen consumption, reduce heart beat, prevent ischema condition, dilate the coronary artery, increase the blood flow in the artery and cardiac muscle.

Some of the plants can even lower blood pressure by dilating the blood flow to the peripherial blood vessels in the brain and kidney, inhibit the agglutination of the platelets, increase the activity of plasmin (fibrinolysin) reduce fibrin stabilizing factors, prevent the formation of thrombus and enhance thrombolysis, lower blood cholesterol and prevent the formation of altherosclerosis by improving local circulation, permeability of the capillaries and increase phagocytosis.

Others inhibit the growth of the cancer cells by increasing the monocytes and phagocytes,inhibit the formation of collagen and regulate the metabolism of the connective tissues. For soft tissue injury, the plants can increase the phagocytosis of the monocytes and macrophages, increase the regeneration of blood cells and the repair of the soft tissues. Effects on the immune system helps to regulate the function of the humoral and cellular immune system, inhibit the abnormal growth of the tumor cells and tissues which are effective for conditions such as nephritis, scleroderma, newborn hemolytic anemia, nodular periarteritis and systemic lupus erythematosus.

Cardiac rhythm disturbance is treated by isolated alkaloids, such as quinidine, ajmaline and sparteine inhibit Na^+, channels and exhibit anti-arrhythmic effects in that they influence the conduction system. Atropine reduces the influence of the vegetative nerve system by blocking mAChR. Other phytochemicals influence the factors that have brought about cardiac rhythm disturbances, such as hypoxia, blood flow or metabolic imbalances.

Chapter 9: Plants for the Coagulation & Blood Stasis

Angina pectoris is a coronary disorder caused by ischemia; it occurs in irregular attacks, accompanied by intense pains and feeling of constriction and anxiety. Angina pectoris is usually treated with nitrates, beta blockers and calcium antagonists.

Circulatory disorders such as peripheral vena-occlusive arterial disease occur when peripheral veins and arteries become obstructed or narrower because of arteriosclerotic deposits or inflammation of arterial walls, circulation of peripheral organs, such as legs, is reduced. As a consequence muscles and other tissues are no longer optimally supplied witb oxygen, so that physical efforts become difficult and painful. The aim is to improve blood flow by dilatation of blood vessels and increase of cardiac output and the control of prostacyclin and thromboxane formation in arteries and thrombocytes.

Hypertension is characterised by a blood pressure above 140/90 mm Hg. Causes arc often difficult to define. Hypotension is defined by a blood pressure below 105/60 mm Hg and can be caused by physiological or hormonal imbalances and blood loss. Common treatment approaches for hypertension includes reducing salt (NaCI) and alcohol intake, nicotine abstinence and increasing physical activity. Medicinal treatment involves the application of diuretic, sympathetic, vasodilarative drugs of ACE inhibitors, Ca-antagonists and aldosterone antagonists. Phytotmedicine can provide diurectic, sympathetic and vasodilatative drugs that can be useful in mild forms of hypertension. The alkaloids reserpine, rescinnamine and serpentine (which inhibit the reuptake of noradrenaline into presynaptic vesicles) have been used to treat severe forms of hypertension. Hypotension can be improved by physical exercise and plant extracts with stimulating properties, such as purine alkaloids (caffeine) or vasoconstricting activities (e.g. ergot alkaloids, ephedrine).

Manicole

Invigorate Blood Circulation and Remove Blood Stasis

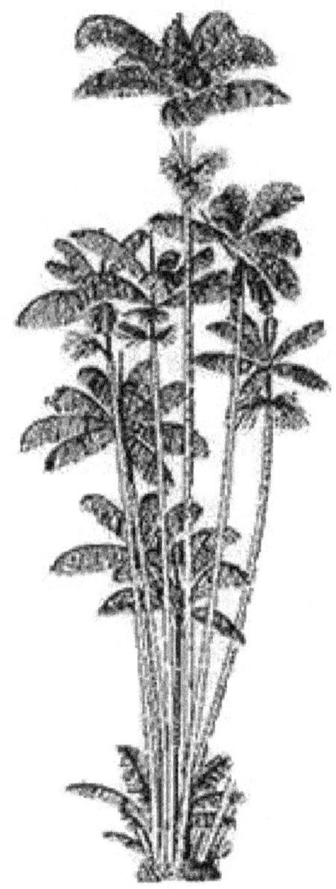

Botanical Name: Euterpe Oleracea Martius.
Family: Arecaceae.
Region Where Grown: Pomeroon-Supenaam.
Other Names: Manaka, Acai.
Category: Plants that Coagulate and regulate by Invigorating blood and Remove Stasis.
Properties: Acrid, Hot/Moist, Sour.
Esoteric Botanica: Tehuti.
Governing Organs: Liver, Heart, Spleen.
Actions & Indications: Ethnobotanists have recorded no less than twenty-two different uses for all parts of the tree.
The oil: From the fruit is used to treat diarrhea; an infusion of the root is used for jaundice and to build the blood.
Grated fruit Rind: Used as a topical wash for skin ulcers.
Fruit seeds: Crushed and prepared in an infusion for fevers.
Decoction of the root: Used for malaria, diabetes, hepatitis and jaundice, hair loss, hemorrhages, liver and kidney diseases, menstrual pain and muscle pain.
Sap applied to cuts as haemostatic. Used to treat hemorrhage, clears heat and cools the blood – for all warm-febrile diseases where heat causes very high fever and thirst. Also indicated in cases of hemorrhage due to heat entering the blood level. For scorpian bites and in the treatment of wounds and cuts.[425]
Heart is dried, pulverised and used in a plaster to cicatrize open cuts; liquid extracted from warm palm-heart is patted on an open wound. Overeating of heart or pith causes diarrhoea.
Leaf: Decoction for fever.
Seedling: Infusion of whole seedling used to treat shot wounds from hunting.
Stem: The palm cabbage is roasted and applied to soothe the pain of scorpion stings; juice from roasted palm cabbage should be drunk simultaneously. Also used as cold water infusion of wood used as an external wash for a contraceptive;
Fruit: Used in a savory, violet-colored beverage drunk as a refreshant.
Major Known Ingredients: Phenols occur in the heart of palm. The fruit liquid, called simply acai or *vinho de acai* (although it's not alcoholic or fermented) is not really that nutritious in comparison to many other fruit juices. The nutrient content analyzed is 1-4% protein, 7-11% fats, 25% sugar, 0.05% calcium, 0.033% phosphorous, and 0.0009% iron. It also has some sulphur, traces of vitamin B1 and some vitamin A and E. It also delivers 88 to 265 calories per 100 grams, depending on the preparation method. The dark

[425] DeFilipps, Robert A., Shirley L. Maina, and Juliette Crepin. *Medicinal Plants of the Guianas (Guyana, Surinam, French Guiana)*. Washington, D.C.: Dept. of Botany, National Museum of Natural History, Smithsonian Institution, 2004; 36.

purple color of the fruit is due to the polyphenolic compounds present. One of the main plant chemicals getting a lot of attention in acai, is a compound called anthocyanin. Anthocyanins are a group of flavonoids widely distributed in plants and lending a red to purple color to fruits like grapes, blackberries, and raspberries. As a well known antioxidant, anthocyanin-rich foods and fruits have been marketed as cancer preventative and anti-aging products. Anthocyanins have also been studied as novel sources of natural food colorings and dyes. The anthocyanin in acai however is highly unstable and degrades easily in the presence of heat, humidity, as well as in the presence of enzyme actions of other chemicals in the fruit. This makes acai fruit highly perishable; it readily changes in color, taste and anthocyanin content with even short term (12 hours) refrigerated storage.

In addition to the standard vitamins and minerals found in most fruits, the main plant chemicals in acai fruit include epicatechin, p-hydroxy-benzoic acid, gallic acid, (+)-catechin, protocatechuic acid, ellagic acid, p-coumaric acid, ferulic acid, vanillic acid, cyaniding and pelaronidin 3-glucoside.[426]

Pharmacological & Clinical Research: The antioxidant capacities of 11 commercial and non-commercial samples of Euterpe oleracea Mart (açaí) fruit pulp were studied with the total oxidant scavenging capacity assay in a modified and automated version against three reactive oxygen species. The antioxidant capacities of all purple açaí samples were found to be excellent against peroxyl radicals, good against peroxynitrite and poor against hydroxyl radicals compared with common European fruit and vegetable juices recently analysed. In all cases the correlation between sample concentration and antioxidant capacities was non-linear. The antioxidant capacities against all three reactive oxygen species of the fruit pulp from one white açaí variety were very low. The phenolic compounds in purple açaí fruit pulp were identified by high-performance liquid chromatography-mass spectrometry and the two major anthocyanins, cyanidin-3-glucoside and cyanidin-3-rutinoside, were quantified by high-performance liquid chromatography-visible spectrometry. The contributions of the anthocyanins to the overall antioxidant capacities of the fruit were estimated to be only approximately 10%. Obviously, compounds not yet identified, are responsible for the major part of the antioxidant capacities of the açaí fruit pulp.[427]

[426] "Tropical Plant Database." *Wealth of the Rainforest*. Web. 14 Mar. 2012. <http://www.rain-tree.com/plants.htm>.
[427] Rodriques RB, Lichtenthaler R., Maria JG, Papagiannopoulous M., Fabricius H., and Marx F. "Total Oxidant Scavenging Capacities of Euterpe Oleracea Mart. (Açaí) Fruits." *Pubmed Abstract PMID:16019315*

Black Sage

Invigorate Blood Circulation and Remove Blood Stasis

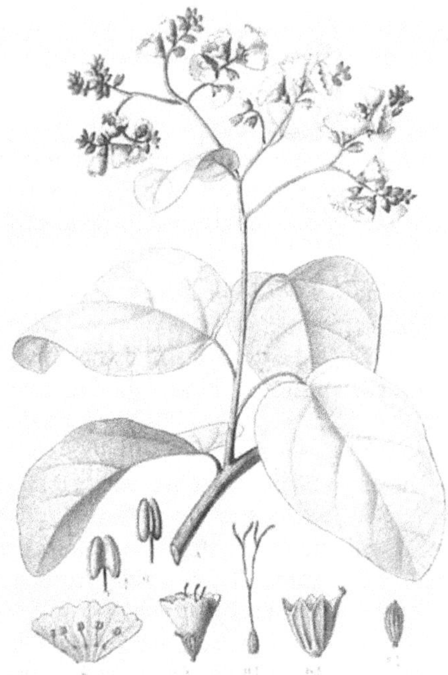

Botanical Name: Cordia Curassavica.
Family: Asteridae.
Region Where Grown: U. Takutu-U. Essequibo.
Other Names: None.
Category: Plants that Coagulate and Regulate by Invigorating Blood and Remove Stasis.
Properties: Aromatic, Acrid, Hot/Moist.
Esoteric Botanica: Maat.
Governing Organs: Liver, Spleen, Stomach.
Actions & Indications: Stem and Leaf: Infusion for a stomachic, sudorific, to treat hypertension, biliousness, breath freshener, diarrhoea and colds.[428]
Stem: Chewed to clean the teeth and destroy bad breath. Reduces and guides out food stagnation – for accumulations due to meat or greasy foods with accompanying symptoms of abdominal distention, pain, bad breath, aversion to food or diarrhea.
Leaf: Dried and boiled in a liquid drunk to control heavy menstrual flow. Macerated leaves used externally as dandruff treatment and to remedy gonorrhoea.
Boiled in a tea for a coolant - in a bath for fever. Also decoted to relieve cold, influenza, fever, pneumonia, cough and insomnia. [429]
Infusion of young leaves for grippe and as an aromatic, pectoral and stimulant. Leaves crushed and rubbed on the skin to prevent mosquito bites. Leaves used in curative herbal bath. Boiled infusion of sun-dried leaves is employed for a gonorrhoea remedy. Juice of finely crushed leaves is used for alleviating monthly stomach pains (menstrual cramps).
Cautions & Contraindications: Use with caution in cases of spleen or stomach deficiency without food stagnation, and in cases with acid regurgitation.
Major Known Ingredients: Branches and leaves show antimicrobial activity

[428] DeFilipps, Robert A., Shirley L. Maina, and Juliette Crepin. *Medicinal Plants of the Guianas (Guyana, Surinam, French Guiana)*. Washington, D.C.: Dept. of Botany, National Museum of Natural History, Smithsonian Institution, 2004; 57.
[429] Morton F. Julia, *Atlas of Medical Plants of Middle America: Bahamas to Yucatan*. Springfield, Illinois: Charles C Thomas Publisher, 1981; 714

White Clary

Invigorate Blood Circulation and Remove Blood Stasis

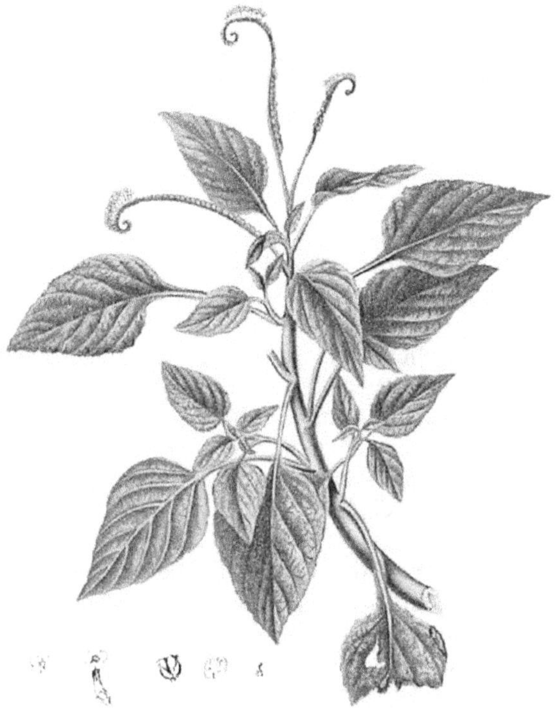

Botanical Name: Heliotropium Indicum.
Family: Boraginaceae.
Region Where Grown: E. Berbice-Corentyne.
Other Names: White Cleary.
Category: Plants that Coagulate and Regulate by Invigorating blood and Remove Stasis.
Properties: Acrid, Sour, Hot/Moist.
Esoteric Botanica: Maat.
Governing Organs: Liver, Lung, Spleen.
Actions & Indications: Use for cough, eczema, fever, leprosy, rheumatism and warts. It is also reported as a folk remedy for cancer, as a medication to induce abortions and as a treatment for scorpion stings. [430]
Whole plant: Boiled and the beverage employed as a heat rash remedy. Vents rashes – used in the early stages of rashes (e.g. measles) to induce the rash to come to the surface to speed recovery
Decoction for thrush, diarrhoea, and frequent excretion of urine.
Used for diabetes and to treat venereal disease.
Leaf: Juice to treat and soothe the pain of conjunctivitis. Clears the liver and brightens the eyes – for ascending liver fire with red, painful, or swollen eyes, or headache and dizziness. Also used for eye pain that increases in the evening due to liver deficiency, especially when the eyes are neither red nor swollen. Clears the Liver and benefits the eyes – for patterns of liver yang rising with such symptoms as headache, red and painful eyes, excessive tearing or sensitivity to light.
Leaf-juice mixed with coconut oil and small amount of salt is administered to children for colds, grippe and coughing.
Infusion for asthma, ulcers, dysentery, bronchitis, red eyes, boils, stomachic and as an antihaemorrhagic.
Flower: To control menstrual blood loss, yaws and skin ulcers.[431]
Major Known Ingredients: Contains the hepatotoxic pyrrolizidine alkaloids heliotrine and lasiocarpine. The major alkaloid indicine, shows antitumor activity.

[430] Castner, James L., S. Lee. Timme, and James A. Duke. *A Field Guide to Medicinal and Useful Plants of the Upper Amazon*. Gainesville, FL: Feline, 1998; 58.
[431] DeFilipps, Robert A., Shirley L. Maina, and Juliette Crepin. *Medicinal Plants of the Guianas (Guyana, Surinam, French Guiana)*. Washington, D.C.: Dept. of Botany, National Museum of Natural History, Smithsonian Institution, 2004; 59

Bloodwood

Invigorate Blood Circulation and Remove Blood Stasis

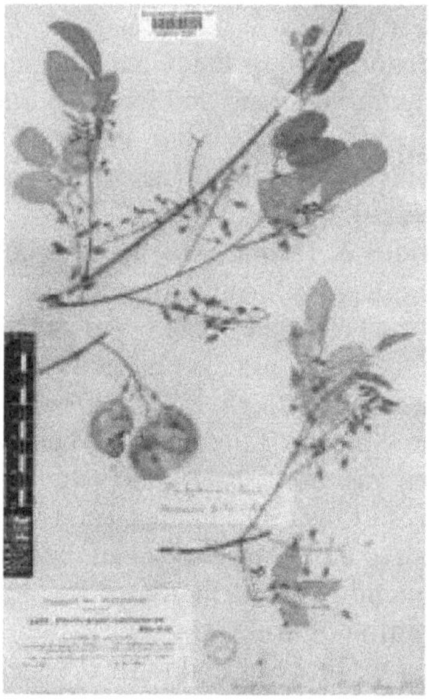

Botanical Name: Vismia Cayennensis.
Family: Clusiaceae.
Region Where Grown: All Regions.
Other Names: Orali.
Category: Plants that Coagulate and regulate by Invigorating blood and Remove Stasis.
Properties: Bitter, Acid, Hot/Dry.
Esoteric Botanica: Heru.
Governing Organs: Heart, Lung, Small Intestine.
Actions & Indications: Bark: Juice from macerated bark is applied around the groin region as an antiherpetic. [432]
Stem: Orange latex from inner bark is applied onto skin infections.
Bark: inner bark with heavy latex content in a decoction for a body-wash to treat skin rash, eye remedy, scabies and other cutaneous eruptions. Also for dermatitis and as a mouthwash for children's gum infections.
Fruit: Latex for treating yaws and leishmaniasis. Latex is used in an ointment as an antipruritic, as an anti-fungal agent or for treating scaling of the skin. Latex is used as an antiinfective agent. Latex is dropped into the eyes to cure infections.[433]
Cautions & Contraindications: Do not use during pregnancy. Use with caution in cases with blood and qi deficiency or where there is excessive menstruation.

---

[432] DeFilipps, Robert A., Shirley L. Maina, and Juliette Crepin. *Medicinal Plants of the Guianas (Guyana, Surinam, French Guiana)*. Washington, D.C.: Dept. of Botany, National Museum of Natural History, Smithsonian Institution, 2004; 90.
[433] Ibid., p, 90.

Fine-Leaf Bloodwood

Invigorate Blood Circulation and Remove Blood Stasis

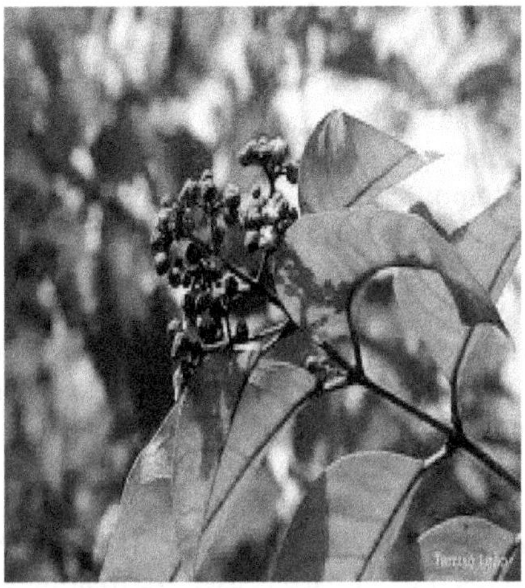

Botanical Name: Vismia Guianensis.
Family: Clusiacea.
Region Where Grown: All Regions.
Other Names: Fine-Leaf, Small-leaf.
Category: Plants that Coagulate and regulate by Invigorating blood and Remove Stasis.
Properties: Bitter, Acrid, Hot/Moist.
Esoteric Botanica: Maat.
Governing Organs: Liver, Lung, Spleen.
Actions & Indications: Dermatitis, anti herpetic, scabies, antipruritic and anti fungal, anti infective agent.[434]
Whole plant: Latex for purgative and to relieve itching, "lotta", ground itch (athlete's foot), ulcers, minor cuts and bruises. Latex is applied onto ringworm and other fungal infections for healing and is applied onto persistent sores to promote healing. Exudate used to treat ground itch, fungal infections and warts.
Bark: Juice from macerated bark is used as an anti-infective agent. Bark used to treat sores. Stem and Leaf: Boiled together and drunk for thrush.
Stem: Orange latex from inner bark is applied on skin infections.
Leaf: Boiled for intermittent fevers.
Fruit: Latex for yaws and leishmaniasis.[435]
Cautions & Contraindications: Do not use during pregnancy. Use with caution in cases with blood and qi deficiency or where there is excessive menstruation.
Major Known Ingredients: Plant contains the terpene phellandrene, flavonoids, coumarins and rodoxantin. Fruit contains ferruginin A, delta-hydroxyferruginin A and delta-y-dihydroxyferruginin A.

---

[434] DeFilipps, Robert A., Shirley L. Maina, and Juliette Crepin. *Medicinal Plants of the Guianas (Guyana, Surinam, French Guiana)*. Washington, D.C.: Dept. of Botany, National Museum of Natural History, Smithsonian Institution, 2004; 90.
[435] Ibid., p, 91.

Large-Leaf Bloodwood

Invigorate Blood Circulation and Remove Blood Stasis

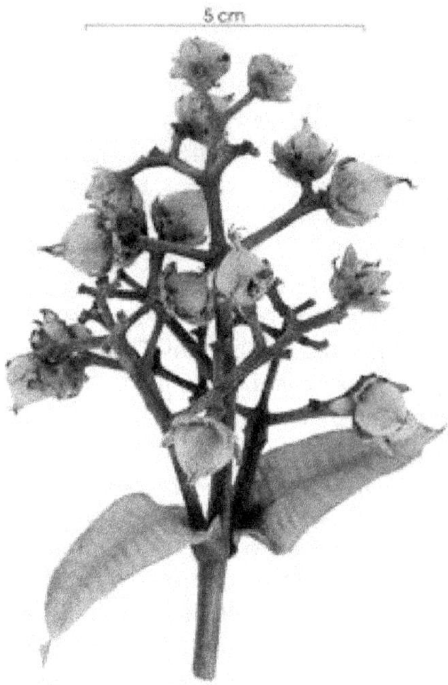

Botanical Name: Vismia Macrophylla.
Family: Clusiaceae.
Region Where Grown: All Regions.
Other Names: Bloodwood, Large-leaf bloodwood. Arawak: Orali. Patamona: why-ah-mac-yik, wouy-wey-yik, wa-ya-mak-yik.
Category: Plants that Coagulate and regulate by Invigorating blood and Remove Stasis.
Properties: Sweet, Acrid, Cold/Dry.
Esoteric Botanica: Seker.
Governing Organs: Spleen, Liver, Small Intestine.
Actions & Indications: Antidiarrheal, treatment for herpes and syphilis, yeast and fungal infections, measles, ulcers, ringworm, eczema, laws and leishmaniasis.[436]
Bark: Inner bark is boiled, and the water drunk as an antidiarrheal. Inner bark is ground into powder and inserted into the vagina as a treatment for genital herpes or as a treatment for syphilis. Macerated inner bark is used for treating yeast infections. Bark is used in the treatment of fungal infections.
Bark and Latex: Inner bark and latex are used as an anti-fungal.
Latex: Orange latex from inner bark is used to treat measles, ulcers, bush yaws, ringworm, "lotta" and many other skin infections. Latex is used as a medicament for treating genital herpes, as an anti-infective, as an ointment for treating eczema, for itching or for scaling, and also as a medicament for ringworm infection. Latex is applied to athlete's foot as a treatment for healing. It is used in the treatment of fungal infections.
Leaf: Used to treat diarrhea.
Fruit: Latex is employed in treating yaws and leishmaniasis.
Cautions & Contraindications: Do not use during pregnancy. Use with caution in cases with blood and qi deficiency or where there is excessive menstruation.
Major Known Ingredients: The fruit of *Vismia* spp. contains anthracene derivatives such as vismin, ferruginins A and B, haruganin and ferruanthrone. Amazonian *Vismia* spp. Contains vismiaquinone.

[436]DeFilipps, Robert A., Shirley L. Maina, and Juliette Crepin. *Medicinal Plants of the Guianas (Guyana, Surinam, French Guiana)*. Washington, D.C.: Dept. of Botany, National Museum of Natural History, Smithsonian Institution, 2004; 92.

Zeb Grass

Invigorate Blood Circulation and Remove Blood Stasis

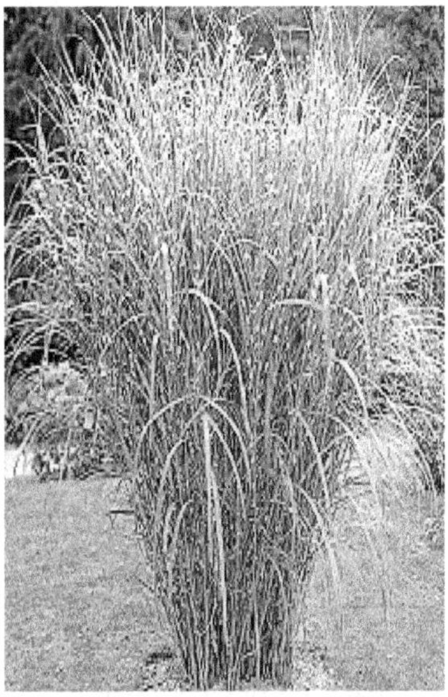

Botanical Name: Commelina Diffusa.
Family: Commelinaceae.
Region Where Grown: Barima-Waini.
Other Names: Purple Zeb Grass.
Category: Plants that Coagulate and regulate by Invigorating blood and Remove Stasis.
Properties: Sour, Acrid, Hot/Moist.
Esoteric Botanica: Tehuti.
Governing Organs: Liver, Heart, Spleen, Lung.
Actions & Indications: Stomachache, venereal disease, urinary burning and leucorrhea, gonorrhea and kidney ailments.[437]
Whole plant: Juice used in a decoction against warts; Treats corns and warts – used topically as a plaster.[438]
Infusion against hair loss, fever and biliousness. Tonifies the liver and kidneys, nourishes the blood and augments the essence – for patterns of yin or blood deficiency with such signs as thinning or graying hair, weak lower back and knees, dizziness, blurred vision, sore extremities and insomnia. This herb is commonly used as it both tonifies and preserves, and is neither cold, drying, nor too cloying. Juice is drunk for high blood pressure.
Plant is boiled and the water drunk to treat biliousness, loss of hair, kidney disease, and to cleanse womb and tubes.
Leaf: Leaves are used in a tea for cleansing the blood and treating influenza.
Whole plant: Infusion of "red" and "white" plants is used for kidney disorders. Tonifies the kidneys and fortifies the yang – for deficient kidney yang patterns with such symptoms as fatigue, impotence, cold extremities, lightheadedness, tinnitus, soreness and weakness in the lower back and knees and frequent, copious, clear urination.
Cautions & Contraindications: Do not use in cases of yin deficiency with heat signs, headaches due to liver yang rising, qi deficiency, excessive menstrual bleeding or during pregnancy.

---

[437] Morton F. Julia, *Atlas of Medical Plants of Middle America: Bahamas to Yucatan.* Springfield, Illinois: Charles C Thomas Publisher, 1981; 68-70.
[438] Ibid., p, 94.

Jamoon

Invigorate Blood Circulation and Remove Blood Stasis

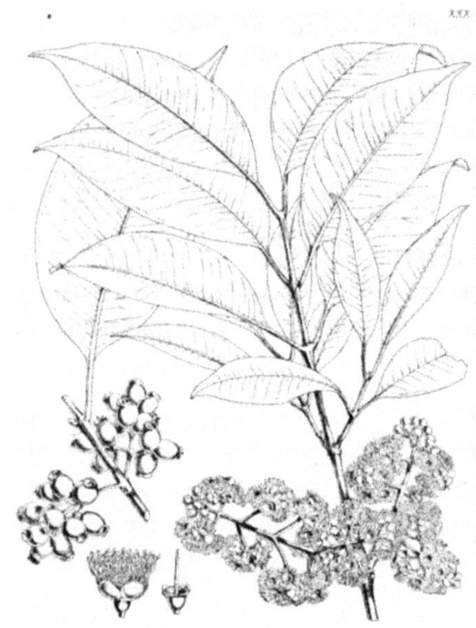

Botanical Name: Syzygium Cumini.
Family:Myrtaceae.
Region Where Grown: Demerara-Mahaica.
Other Names: None.
Category: Plants that Coagulate and Regulate by Invigorating Blood and Remove Stasis.
Properties: Acrid, Cold/Dry.
Esoteric Botanica: Seker.
Governing Organs: Liver, Spleen, Kidney, Heart, Large Intestine.
Actions & Indications: Diabetes, dysentery, indigestion, blood purifier, venereal disease, gastrointestinal ailments including stomach ulcers and reduce acidity, leuorrhea and antipyretic and anti inflammatory.[439]
Stem: Bark infusion for irregular menstruation.
For treating diarrhoea, dysentery and children's thrush. Bark used for diarrhea and to stop vomiting.
Branches employed in whitening teeth.
Leaf: Infusion for diabetes. Used to treat diarrhea.
Fruit: Used for diarrhea. Fruits are used as a beverage/tonic and wine,
Seed: Seeds are parched, pulverised and made into a coffee beverage used to treat diabetes. For children's bed-wetting. Infusion for catarrhal fever.
Seed-pits are used for regulating blood pressure, and sugar in the urine. Used to treat diabetes.
Cautions & Contraindications: Do not use in cases of yin deficiency with heat signs, headaches due to liver yang rising, qi deficiency, excessive menstrual bleeding or during pregnancy.
Major Known Ingredients: Dried seed yields a hypoglycemically active substance. Seed contains the alkaloid jambosin and jambulol. [440] The fruits and seeds of Syzygium cumini which are used as antidiabelics contain cyanidin rhamnoglucosides, galliand ellagi tannins as well as phytosterol glycosides. The seeds contain phytosterin jamboian, essential oil, galli and ellagi-tannins. Flowers and Fruits contain cyanidine-2-rhamnoglucoside. [441]

---

[439] DeFilipps, Robert A., Shirley L. Maina, and Juliette Crepin. *Medicinal Plants of the Guianas (Guyana, Surinam, French Guiana)*. Washington, D.C.: Dept. of Botany, National Museum of Natural History, Smithsonian Institution, 2004; 284.
[440] Oliver-Bever,Bep. *Medicinal Plants in Tropical West Africa*. Cambridge: Cambridge UP, 1986; 249.
[441] Ibid., p, 257.

Lionbush

Invigorate Blood Circulation and Remove Blood Stasis

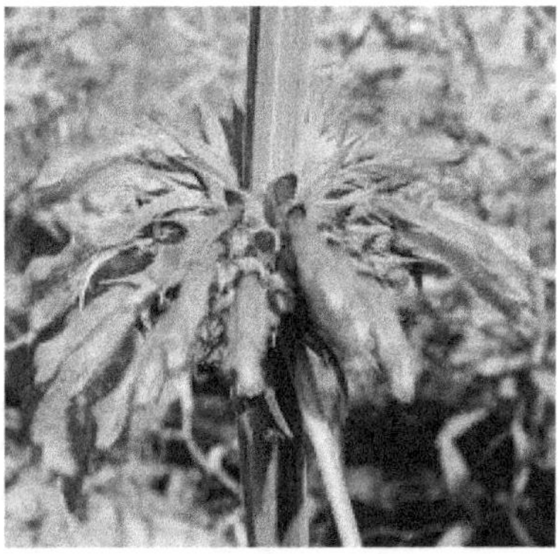

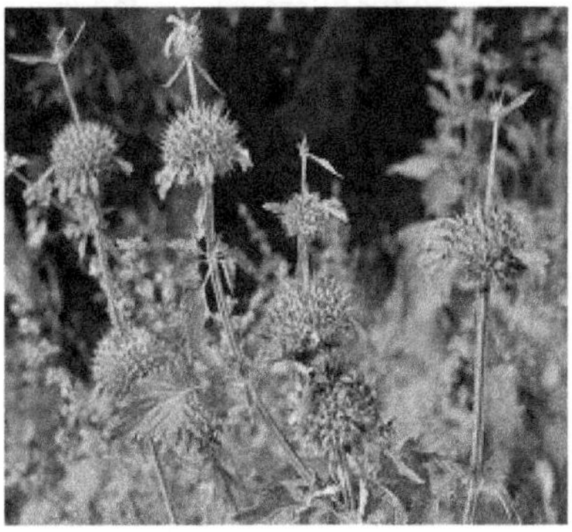

Botanical Name: Leonotis Nepetifolia.
Family:Lamiaceae.
Region Where Grown: Essequibo, W. Demerara.
Other Names: Man-Piaba.
Category: Plants that Coagulate and regulate by Invigorating blood and Remove Stasis.
Properties: Acrid, Cool/Dry.
Esoteric Botanica: Sebek.
Governing Organs: Lung, Kidney, Spleen.
Actions & Indications: Used for anthrax, antidysenteric, bed-wetting, cholagogue, diuretic, hemorrhoids (piles) and kidney ailments. Decoction is employed to clean out the uterus. It is also used as a diuretic and a tonic to strengthen the back. [442] Infusion for diarrhoea and heavy cramps.
Leaf and Flower: Used for cholagogue. Infusion as an antidysenteric. Decocted with salt or sugar in a preparation to dissolve renal calculi (kidney stones).
Leaf: Juice for thrush. In a plaster for wounds. Cooked in an infusion which is drunk to treat itches and skin diseases and yaws.
Cautions & Contraindications: Do not use during pregnancy
Major Known Ingredients: Ethanolic extract of the plant showed antitumor and possibly antimicrobial activity.
Pharmacological & Clinical Research: In Rwanda, leaves of this plant are used to treat pneumonia, anthrax and syphilis

[442] DeFilipps, Robert A., Shirley L. Maina, and Juliette Crepin. *Medicinal Plants of the Guianas (Guyana, Surinam, French Guiana)*. Washington, D.C.: Dept. of Botany, National Museum of Natural History, Smithsonian Institution, 2004; 149.

Thick-leaf Thyme

Invigorate Blood Circulation and Remove Blood Stasis

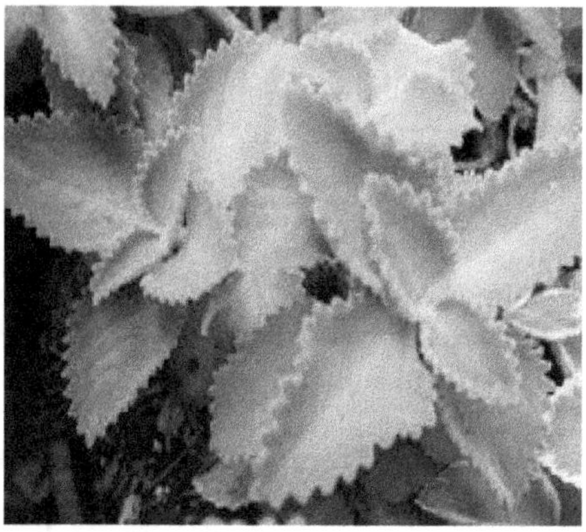

Botanical Name: Plectranthus Amboinicus.
Family: Lamiaceae.
Region Where Grown:Demerara Mahaica.
Other Names: Coarse-leaf thyme, Podina, Portuguese Thyme, Thick-leaf Thyme, Thyme.
Category: Plants that Coagulate and regulate by Invigorating blood and Remove Stasis.
Properties: Bitter, Hot/Dry.
Esoteric Botanica: Herukhuti.
Governing Organs: Heart, Liver, Spleen.
Actions & Indications: Relieve colds, digestive, kidney ailments like kidney stones, stomachache and congestive heart failure. [443]
Leaf: Juice of roasted leaves is drunk or rubbed with a pinch of salt on swellings and inflamed areas, and used for allergies. Boiled in a tea for colds, menstrual pains, labor pains, delayed labor and to aid expulsion of the afterbirth. Infusion for digestive drink.[444]
Cautions & Contraindications: Use with caution in cases of blood deficiency.
Major Known Ingredients: Medicinal, antibacterial and antiseptic properties of the plant have been attributed to extract components such as carvacrol, codeine, flavones, phenols, tannins and aromatic acids.

---

[443] Morton F. Julia, *Atlas of Medical Plants of Middle America: Bahamas to Yucatan.* Springfield, Illinois: Charles C Thomas Publisher, 1981; 757.
[444] Ibid., p, 150.

Bird-Pepper

Invigorate Blood Circulation and Remove Blood Stasis

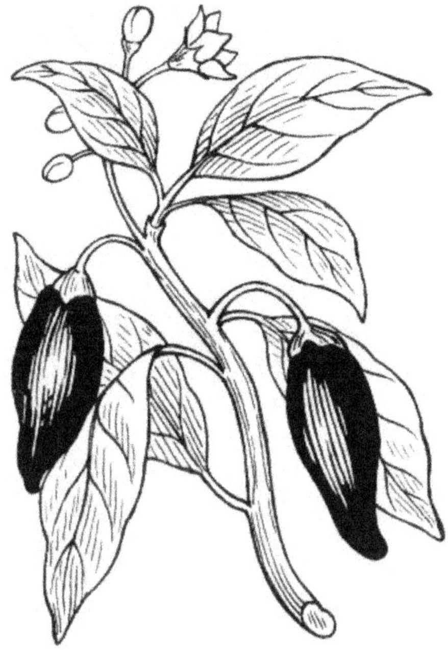

Botanical Name: Capsicum Annuum.
Family: Solanceae.
Region Where Grown: U. Takutu-U. Essequibo.
Other Names: None.
Category: Plants that Coagulate and regulate by Invigorating blood and Remove Stasis.
Properties: Acrid, Cool/Dry.
Esoteric Botanica: Sebek.
Governing Organs: Lungs, Heart, Spleen.
Actions & Indications: Externally, Capsicum Annuum is used to relieve pain of muscle tension and spasm, diabetic neuropathy and rheumatism. Cayenne is sometimes taken internally to relieve gastrointestinal disorders, although human studies have yet to confirm such uses.[445]
Alcoholism, fever, gargle, hemorroids, heart problems, indigestion, laxative, mouth sores, ulcers, arthritis and painful joints, diuretic and hemorroids.
Fruit: The conical fruit of this indigenous plant is crushed and eaten to strengthen the heart, and as a laxative.
Leaf: A preparation for cleansing the blood is made from leaves steeped in hot water. A well-known "hot" condiment. Green fruit mixed with leaves in an infusion for colds and coughs. The globular fruit of the cultivated form is eaten to stimulate digestion and strengthen the heart. Used for colds and coughs.
Fruit: Fruit infusion is considered antipyretic, tonic and vasoregulatory; the decoction used as a gargle for sore throat or pharyngitis; the tincture is applied to bugbites, mange, hemorrhoids and rheumatism.[446] The fruit is also crushed and eaten to strengthen the heart and as a laxative.[447]
Cautions & Contraindications: Topical Cayenne preparations should not be used for more two consecutive days, with a two-week break between applications.never be used on broken skin or near the eyes. When used, Cayenne preparations should not be taken with aspirin or antifungal. They should also be avoided by people who have stomach ulcers, inflammation and chronic irritable bowel, [448] gastro intestinal disease, renal disease and by those who are undergoing inhalation therapy.
Major Known Ingredients: The primary chemicals of interest are capsaicinoids, namely Capsaicin (0.0 2%) and dihydrocapsaicin. Also found are flavonoids, carotenoids (capsanthin), steroid saponins(capsicidium) and ascorbic acid or vitamin C (0.2%). Capsaicin has a valloid chemical structure.

---

[445] *PDR for Nonprescription Drugs.* Montvale, NJ: PDR Network, LLC., 2011; 424.
[446] Duke, James A. and Rodolfo Vásquez. *Amazonian Ethnobotanical Dictionary.* Boca Raton, FL: CRC, 1994; 40.
[447] DeFilipps, Robert A., Shirley L. Maina, and Juliette Crepin. *Medicinal Plants of the Guianas (Guyana, Surinam, French Guiana).* Washington, D.C.: Dept. of Botany, National Museum of Natural History, Smithsonian Institution, 2004; 268.
[448] *PDR for Nonprescription Drugs.* Montvale, NJ: PDR Network, LLC., 2011; 424.

Capsaicin is derived from Capsicum jrutescens, Capsicum annuum, or any of several other hot chili peppers of the Solanaceae family. Topical capsaicin has been used effectively to treat, among other conditions, the pain of rheumatoid arthritis, osteoarthritis, shingles, diabetic neuropathy and phantom limb pain. Capsaicin depletes substance P from peripheral nerve endings. Substance P is active in the transmission of pain impulses from the periphery to the spinal cord. Therefore, even though the source of the pain remain unchanged, the patient does not feel it.[449]
Pharmacological & Clinical Research: Decreased bioavailability of aspirin with concomitant use. Theophylline may increase absorption, resulting in toxicity; use cautiously and monitor tor side effects. [450]

---

[449] Miller, Lucinda G., and Wallace J. Murray. *Herbal Medicinals: A Clinician's Guide*. New York: Pharmaceutical Products, 1998; 100 -101.
[450] *PDR for Nonprescription Drugs.* Montvale, NJ: PDR Network, LLC., 2011; 421.

Chapter 10: Diuretic

Plants That Increase Urine Flow

The diuretics are agents which increase the rate of urine flow. There can increase glomerular filtration or decreased tubular reabsorption. The most effective diuretics influence the excretion of sodium ion rather than the water itself. Most of the diuretics Plants contain increased potassium ion and can increase the excretion of sodium ion or the output of urine.

Some of these plants are antibacterial, they inhibit the growth of bacilli in the urinary tract infections. Others are effective in treating hepathitis: Hepatitis is considered to be related to "dampness". The icteric color of the skin reveals two kinds of conditions: bright yellow is related to heat and dampness, dull yellow is related to cold and dampness. They are all cholagogue, protecting the damage of liver and gallbladder.

Some others are aromatic. Accumulation of dampness in the spleen and stomach is related to hypo-function of the digestive tract with symptoms of indigestion, loss of appetite, abdominal distention, thick and greasy tongue. The aromatic all contain essential oils which stimulate the movement of the bowels, evacuation of the food content and elimination of the cellular edema in the GI tract.

Prickly Pear

Diuretic Plants That Resolve Dampness

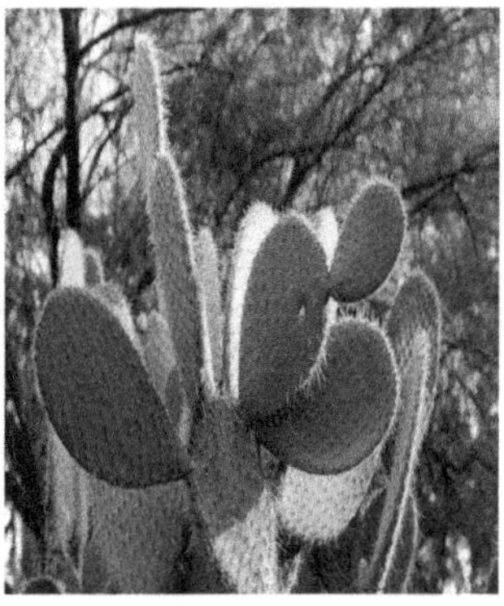

Botanical Name: Opuntia Vulgaris.
Family: Cactaceae.
Region Where Grown: U. Takutu-U. Essequibo.
Other Names: Cochineal, Scrutchineal, Prickly Pear.
Category: Diuretics: Plants that Resolve Dampness.
Properties: Sour, Hot/Moist.
Esoteric Botanica: Tehuti.
Governing Organs: Liver, Urinary Bladder.
Actions & Indications: Use as a diuretic, emollient, eye disease and infections.
Stem: Bit of stem placed in water, and the water given for dropsy.[451] Several thin slices of stem are warmed and placed in water and the water is drunk for

[451] DeFilipps, Robert A., Shirley L. Maina, and Juliette Crepin. *Medicinal Plants of the Guianas (Guyana, Surinam, French Guiana)*. Washington, D.C.: Dept. of Botany, National Museum of Natural History, Smithsonian Institution, 2004; 64.

stomach inflammations. Slices of stem applied to inflammations of the joints, skin and intestines to draw off heat. Ground stem in an infusion used for treating stomach ulcers. Small piece of stem in a glass of water is used for removing mucus from inflamed eyes.
Fruit: Diuretic.
Leaves: Boiled leaves taken for alimentary disturbance.
The joint is sliced and applied on arthritic and rheumatic places. In addition, it is the joint, not the "crushed plant" that is used as shampoo.[452]
Cautions & Contraindications: Use with caution in cases of yin deficiency.
Major Known Ingredients: Like many members of the family, these plants contain cardiac glycosides or biochemically related compounds, such as pregnane derivatives. The main active compound is a pregnane glycoside known as P57 which has powerful appetite-suppressant effects that were demonstrated in animal experiments. [453]

[452] Morton F. Julia, *Atlas of Medical Plants of Middle America: Bahamas to Yucatan.* Springfield, Illinois: Charles C Thomas Publisher, 1981; 15.
[453] Van, Wyk Ben-Erik., and Michael Wink. *Medicinal Plants of the World: An Illustrated Scientific Guide to Important Medicinal Plants and Their Uses*. Portland: Timber, 2004; 171.

Chapter 11: Anti Imflammatory

The Anti Rheumatic

The anti rheumatics include rheumatic arthritis, rheumatoid arthritis, sciatica and all kinds of muscular pain. They are caused by wind, cold and dampness factors. This group of plants can alleviate pain, increase qi and blood circulation and strengthen the tendons.

Rheumatic disorders that can be treated with phytomedicines include soft tissue rheumatism, polyarthritis, spondylitis, athrosis and gout. These disorders are complex and involve inflammation and degeneration of skeletal muscles, bones and joints, often accompanied by severe pain. Because of pain and inflammation, a symptomatic treatment is carried out by inhibiting enzymes of prostaglandin and leucotriene formation, such as cyclooxygenase, and 5-hpoxygenase (e.g. by salicylic acid, iridoid glycosides and derivatives). Another approach uses conico-mimetic substances (triterpenes, steroids, and other secondary metabolites) that induce endogenous cortisone formation and thus block the first step of arachidonic acid release, i.e. by inhibiting phospholipase *Al* and C. Immune modulatillg and immune-suppressive therapy can also be useful. 11-aditional medicine employs counter irritants drugs against *dyscrasia* as well as hydrolytic enzymes, such as papain, hromelain, ficin, pepsin, trypsin, amylases and lipases

Gout is an imbalance of uric acid, known as hyperuricemia (>6.5 mg uric acid/ 100 ml serum) is caused by disorder of the purine metabolism and leads to a precipitation of sodium urate crystals in the synovial fluid of the big toe (hallux), and less common, of the knee, tarsus, wrist and finger joints. These crystals cause an inflammation and attract leukocytes and macrophages. Macrophages are lysed when digesting the urate crystals and release lysosomal enzymes that aggravate the inflammation. In addition, leukocytes release lactic acid thar lowers the local hydrogen ion concentration and decreases the solubility of urate, thus intensifying its crystallisation. Colchicine is used to stop the vicious cycle. Colchicine binds to tubulin and thus inhibits microtubule formation and therefore the motility of macrophages (chemotaxis) which no longer aggregate in the inflamed joints. In addition, colchicine has indirect analgesic properties, as it inhibits the release of prostaglandin. Because colchicine is very toxic (lethal dose 20 mg), not more chan 8 mg should be used to treat an acute attack of gout.

This group of plants are anti-inflammatory. They have sikilar action as sodium salicylate. Some has excitory action on the hypophysis-adrenal gland system. Others are analgesic. They can increase the pain threshold in the body. They have sedative action and can looses the skeletal muscles. Yet others are diuretic. They can dilate the blood vessels and lower blood pressure.

Tulsie

The Anti Rheumatic Plants

Botanical Name: Ocimum Gratissimum.
Family: Lamiaceae.
Region Where Grown: Demerara-Mahaica.
Other Names: Jumbie-Balsam.
Category: Anti-Rheumatics.
Properties: Acrid, Bitter, Warm, Aromatic
Esoteric Botanica: Heru.
Governing Organs: Lungs, Stomach, Kidney.
Actions & Indications: This herb produces a volatile oil which has been shown to have both antimicrobial and anthelmintic properties. It is also used as a laxative to stop diarrhea. [454]
A tea made from the aerial parts is used as a treatment for chest-colds and alimentary disorders such as stomach pains caused by wind.
Juice from the leaves is dropped into the ear for relief of earache. It is also an anticeptic.
Cautions & Contraindications: Do not use with excessive sweating due to qi deficiency or yin deficiency with interior heat. Use with caution with loose, wet stools.

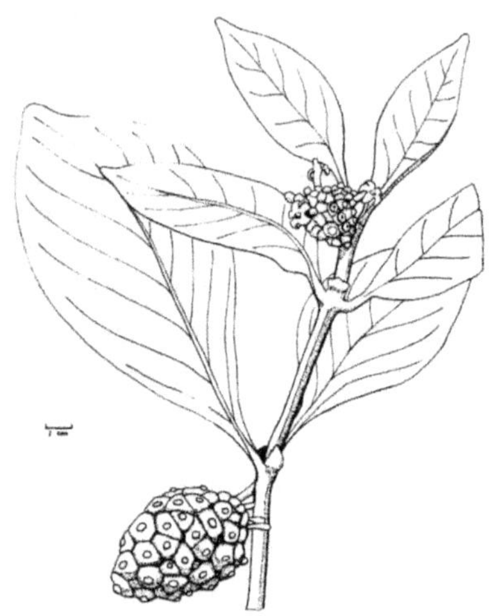

Major Known Ingredients: Methyichavicol, eugenol and other volatile oils of commercial importance have been found in this plant.
Pharmacological & Clinical Research: Extracts prepared in cold water, hot water and acetone exhibited antifungal activity. Essential oils obtained from leaves have shown marked antibacterial activity.[455]
Ocimum gratissimum leaf or the whole herb is a popular treatment for diarrhoea. The plant is rich in volatile oils which contain up to 75 per cent of thymol, the antimicrobial activity of which is well known. In fact, the antimicrobial activity of the water saturated oil had been shown to be proportional to the thymol content. In preparations where *O. gralissimum* is used as cold infusion, therefore, the antimicrobial effect of the extracted thymol is probably sufficient explanation for the antidiarrhoeal effect. However, in certain other preparations *O. gratissimum* is boiled with water to form a decoction which will contain little of the steam thymol volatile thymol. Such aqueous decoctions were shown to be devoid of antimicrobial activity, but they do not relax the guinea pig ileum and rat jejunum *in vitro.* Such decoctions could, therefore, still be effective in calming an overactive gut und thus curing diarrhoea.[456]

---

[454] Sofowora, Abayomi. *Medicinal Plants and Traditional Medicine in Africa*. Chichester, West Sussex: Wiley, 1982; 119.
[455] Lachman-White, D. A., C. D. Adams, and Ulric O'D. Trotz. *A Guide to the Medicinal Plants of Coastal Guyana*. London: Commonwealth Science Council, 1992; 199.
[456] Sofowora, Abayomi. *Medicinal Plants and Traditional Medicine in Africa*. Chichester, West Sussex: Wiley, 1982; 71.

Coconut

The Anti Rheumatic Plants

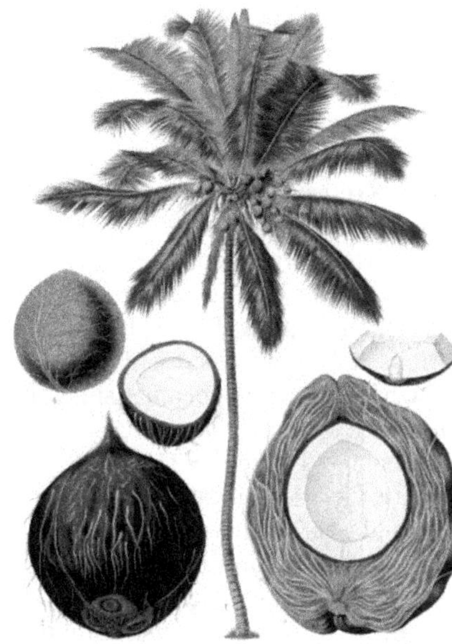

Botanical Name: Cocos Nucifera.
Family: Arecaceae.
Region Where Grown: Demerara-Mahaica Region.
Other Names: Narial.
Category: Anti-Rheumatics.
Properties: Acrid, Cool/Dry.
Esoteric Botanica: Sebek.
Governing Organs: Lung, Heart, Liver, Spleen.
Actions & Indications: Coconut is used for arthritis and painful joints, diarrhea and dysentery, emmenagogues and parturifacients, erysipelas, aphrodisiac, bladder problems, blood pressure reducer or regulator, coughs, furuncles, gout, hair growth stimulant, kidney ailments, laxative, rheumatism, skin cleansers, conditioners, lotions and softeners, ulcers and hemorrhage.
Stem: Poultice for ulcers.
Fruit: Used in treatment of hypertension.
Seed: Used as oil for skin.
Fruit and Seed: Grated coconut meat yields oil which is rubbed on babies for soft skin, also to promote hair growth and soothe furuncles. Water in fruit is drunk to clean the kidneys. Coconut fibers made into a tea for regulating blood pressure.
Seed oil used as a febrifuge, laxative and to treat grippe. Juice is drunk with molasses and sour orange to treat colds. Oil is drunk plain or mixed with salt for gout, rheumatism, coughs and colds. Also used for treating typhoid and earache.
The husk fibre decoction is used in the traditional medicine for treating diarrhea and arthritis.[457]
Cautions & Contraindications: Do not use for spleen qi deficiency or spermatorrhea, for depleted fluids due to a warm-febrile disease or for excessive urination.
Major Known Ingredients: Ripe coconut contains water, lipids, cellulose, vitamin C, riboflavin and niacin.

---

[457] Ahmad Iqbal, Aqil Farrukh and Owais Mohammad. *Modern Phytomedicine: Turning Medicinal Plants into Drugs.* Germany: Wiley-VCH Verlag GmbH & Co. KGaA, 2006; 252.

Garlic Rope

The Anti Rheumatic Plants

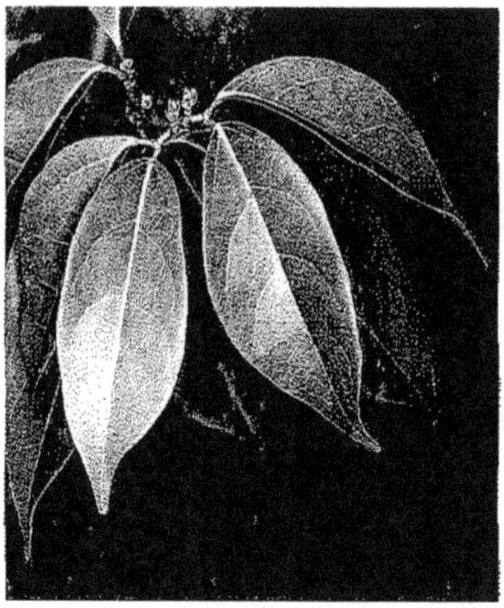

Botanical Name: Mansoa Alliacea.
Family: Bignoniaceae.
Region Where Grown: U. Takutu-U. Essequibo.
Other Names: None.
Category: Anti-Rheumatics.
Properties: Acrid, Cool/Dry.
Esoteric Botanica: Sebek.
Governing Organs: Lungs, Large Intestine, Kidney.
Actions & Indications: Used for treating aching and swollen parts of the body, arthritis, rheumatism, colds, influenza, coughs, and sore throat.[458]
Whole plant: To remedy fevers, head colds and rheumatic pain Also used as a vermifuge.
Stem and Leaf: In a decoction for baths to treat fever, influenza, rheumatism and colds.
Stem: Fragments in a decoction for an external wash to treat fatigue and lameness or lumbago. Stem in a glass of water is drunk in the last month of pregnancy for a healthy confinement.
Bark decoction for fever.
Leaf: Cold water infusion for fever. Decoction and infusion for general weakness. Wild garlic bark is used for fever, influenza and aches and pains as well as nervousness, fatigue and cramps.[459]
Cautions & Contraindications: Use with caution during pregnancy.

[458] Leeuwenberg, A. J. M. *Medicinal and Poisonous Plants of the Tropics: Proceedings of Symposium 5-35 of the 14th International Botanical Congress, Berlin, 24 July-1 August 1987*. Wageningen: Pudoc, 1987; 100

[459] Castner, James L., S. Lee. Timme, and James A. Duke. *A Field Guide to Medicinal and Useful Plants of the Upper Amazon*. Gainesville, FL: Feline, 1998; 79.

Asashi

The Anti Rheumatic Plants

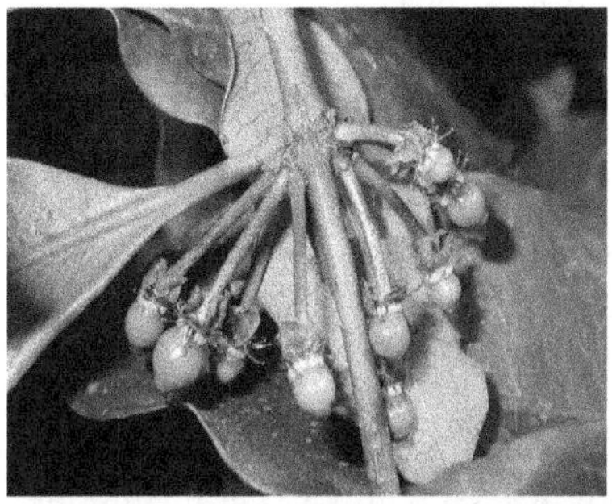

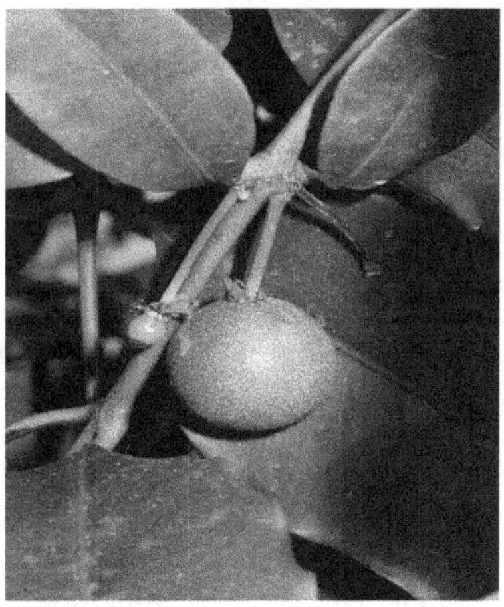

Botanical Name: Rheedia Macrophylla.
Family: Clusiaceae.
Region Where Grown: Potaro-Siparuni Region.
Other Names: None.
Category: Anti-Rheumatics.
Properties: Sweet, Cold/Moist.
Esoteric Botanica: Auset.
Governing Organs: Stomach, Spleen, Lung, San Jiao, Gall Bladder.
Actions & Indications:
Stem: Latex in a plaster for bruised muscles; inner bark is rasped into cold water and infusion drunk for stomachache and diarrhoea.
Stem and Leaf: Decoction of leaves and bark for relief of pains in the side of body;
latex for skin sores.
Leaf: Use in a decoction of boiled leaves as wash for fevers caused by eating fish and decoction poured into cracks in the skin of the foot.
Cautions & Contraindications: Use with caution in cases of damp cold or loose stools.

Pain-Killer

The Anti Rheumatic Plants

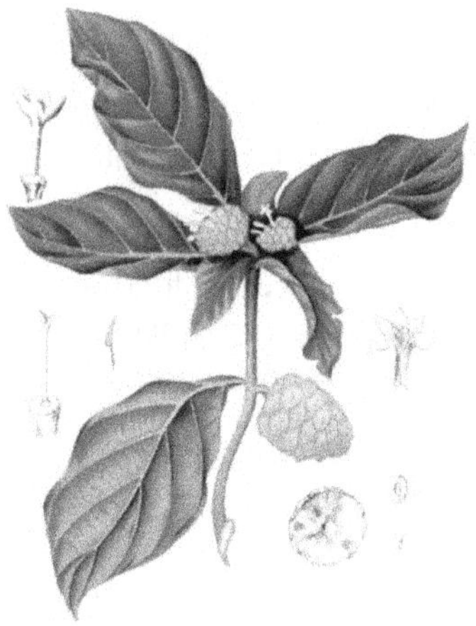

Botanical Name: Morinda Citrifolia.
Family: Rubiaceae.
Region Where Grown: Barima-Waini.
Other Names: Yaw-weed, Noni, Morinda, Indian Mulberry, Hog Apple, Canary Wood.
Category: Anti-Rheumatics.
Properties: Sweet, Cold/Moist.
Esoteric Botanica: Auset.
Governing Organs: Spleen, Heart, Kidney.
Actions & Indications. Rheumatism, arthritis, joint inflammation and joint swellings.
Fruit: Mixed with vinegar to smooth a turgid spleen. Noni has a history of use as a topical preparation for joint pain and skin conditions. Fruit juice as a general health tonic, as well as for cancer and chronic conditions such as cardiovascular disease and diabetes
Cautions & Contraindications: Use with caution in cases of deficiency cold
Major Known Ingredients: The roots of this plant contain a number of highly colored anthraquinones substituted in both ring A and ring B. It is reported that anthraquinones are formed via acetate-malonate or shikimate-o-succinyl benzoate routes. Anthraquinones are also produced in tissue (cell) cultures of a number of plants, and there are many reports on the isolation and identification of anthraquinones from plant cultured cells and quite a number of anthraquinones are reported. [460] Contains five known anthraquinones; rubiadin, lucidin, morindone, lucidin-3β-primveroside and morindone-6 β-primveroside and six new quinones; 2-methyl-3,S, 6-trihydroxyanthraquinone, 3-hydroxymorindone, 5, 6-dihydroxylucidin, 2-methyl-3,S,6-trihydroxyanthraquinone- 6 β-prirnveroside, hydroxymorindone-6 β-prirnveroside and 5, 6-dihydroxylucidin-3β-primveroside, respectively.[461]
Pharmacological & Clinical Research: In laboratory research, noni has shown antioxidant, immune-stimulating and tumor-fighting properties.

[460] Bajaj, Yashpal Singh. *Biotechnology in Agriculture and Forestry 4 Medicinal and Aromatic Plants I*, Berlin: Springer-Verlag, 1993; 237.
[461] Bajaj, Yashpal Singh. *Biotechnology in Agriculture and Forestry 4 Medicinal and Aromatic Plants I*, Berlin: Springer-Verlag, 1993; 240.

Chapter 12: Sedatives

Plants Used to Calm or Induce Sleeping

Sedatives are agents used to calm or induce sleeping status. Sleep is a state of rest and repair. It is a conditioned reflex. Tranquilizers imply mental calmness with depression of mental activity or alertness.

This group of plants are divided into two kinds; heavy sedatives and nourishing sedatives. The heavy sedatives are heavy minerals or shells such as oyster shell, cinnabar, magnee and the CNS. They can prolong the sleeping time by barbiturates, reduce activitytite and amber/succinum.

The herbal nourishing sedatives contain protein vitamins and glucosides. They are nourishing to the heart and replenish more yin fluid. They can improve the integrity, mental spirit and thinking process of the brain. They can lower the blood pressure. They can be hypnotic and anti convulsive.

Sour-Sop

The Sedative Plants

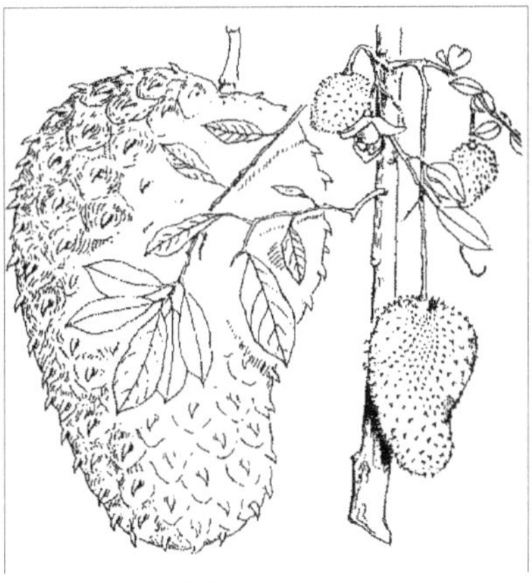

Botanical Name: Annona Muricata .
Family: Annonaceae (Soursop Family).
Region Where Grown: Barima-Waini.
Other Names: Monkey Apple, Sorasaka, Soursop, Wild soursop.
Category: Sedatives.
Properties: Sweet, Hot/Dry.
Esoteric Botanica: Heru.
Governing Organs: Heart, Stomach, Large Intestine .
Actions & Indications: Decoction of dried leaves is used externally to treat rashes and skin diseases and skin infections. Extract of leaves is taken orally for gall bladder trouble. Hot water extract of leaves is used as a tea for asthma sufferer. Decoction of dried leaves is taken orally for grippe, coughs, and asthenia. Fresh fruit juice is taken orally for asthenia. Infusion of hot water: extract of leaves is used as an antispasmodic beverage is prepared as a lactagogue.[462]
Stem: Bark and leaf infusion for a sedative or cardiotonic. Branches contain irritant sap.

---

462 Ross, Ivan A. *Medicinal Plants of the World: Chemical Constituents, Traditional, and Modern Medicinal Uses*. Totowa, NJ: Humana, 1999; 82

Leaf: Narcotic, for antispasmodic infusions and a calmative; in cataplasms to treat whitlow; infusion for fever with a cold, for a sedative, and to relieve overheating; extract calms nervous conditions. Leaves are boiled with water and drunk as a medication for fluttering of the heart.
Fruit: For bedwetting children; decoction for excess foot and hand perspiration; antiscorbutic, febrifuge; for a mild antidysenteric and a good vermifuge. Fruit is used for making a tonic for fever, headache, hypertension and to treat heart problems. Seed: Ingredient in a remedy for convulsions.
ves are boiled with the leaves of avocado and drunk as an anti-hypertensive.
Cautions & Contraindications: Use with caution in cases of severe diarrhea or heat excess.
Major Known Ingredients: Plant contains isoquinoline alkaloids including reticuline, coclaurine, coreximine, antherospermine, stepharine, anomurine and anomuricine. Seed contains galactomannan, sitosterol, stigmasterol and cholesterol. An aqeous extract of decorticated seeds contained glucose, xylose, galactose, mannose, xylopyranosylglucose and ursolic acid.[463]
Pharmacological & Clinical Research:The ethanolic extract of leaves and stem of sugar-apple (a. squamosa) is reported to have anticancer activity. The aporphine alkaloids anonaline, rosemerine, norcorydine, corydine, norisocorydine, isocorydine and glaucine were isolated. [464]
Toxicity: Cancer activity was identified and other comounds found in this species are diazepine, squamolene, friedelin, xylopine, methylarmepavine, languinosine, and a ntrophetheroside.[465]

---

[463] DeFilipps, Robert A., Shirley L. Maina, and Juliette Crepin. *Medicinal Plants of the Guianas (Guyana, Surinam, French Guiana)*. Washington, D.C.: Dept. of Botany, National Museum of Natural History, Smithsonian Institution, 2004; 11.
[464] Lachman-White, D. A., C. D. Adams, and Ulric O'D. Trotz. *A Guide to the Medicinal Plants of Coastal Guyana*. London: Commonwealth Science Council, 1992; 18.
[465] Ibid., p, 18.

Sweet Broom

The Sedative Plants

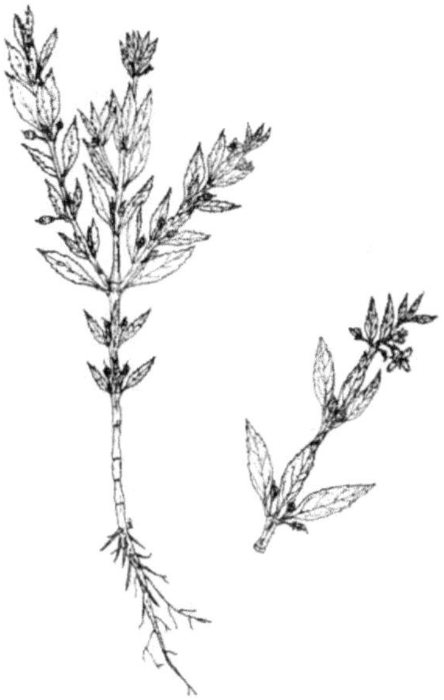

Botanical Name: Scoparia Dulcis.
Family: Scrophulariaceae.
Region Where Grown: Cuyuni-Mazaruni.
Other Names: Sweetbroom.
Category: Sedatives.
Properties: Acrid, Cool/Dry.
Esoteric Botanica: Sebek.
Governing Organs: Lungs, Stomach, Spleen.
Actions & Indications: This plant is used to treat aches and pains, swellings, wounds and as a contraceptive.
The juice of the leaf is used to treat eye problems. Preparations are also used to treat bronchitis and coughs, dysentery, kidney ailments, fever, and hemorrhoids. [466] Traditionally used as a medicament for stomach disorders, bronchitis, diabetes, hypertension, hemorrhoids, hepatosis and as an analgesic and amipyretic.[467]
The plant decoction is taken as a remedy for diabetes, urinary burning, diarrhea and eczema. An infusion is used to bathe infants suffering rash, sores, mange or marasmus.
The expressed juice of the leaves is given as an antidote for jaundice and marasmus and is used as an eyewash, tonic and febrifuge.[468]
Whole plant: Dried for a blood-purifying tea in order to reduce blood sugar levels. Decoction is drunk to treat dizziness. [469]Decoction for children's fever, thrush and mouth sores. Macerated in an infusion or strong decoction for inducing children's vomiting and as an emetic to relieve stomach pain. Used to treat gonorrhoea sores and as a diuretic. Cooked in water and drunk to control bile. Used in treatment of biliousness, as a laxative, for malaria, sores, venereal disease, and for coughs and colds. Plant is boiled and the water drunk as an anti-asthmatic, as an anti-pyretic, as a treatment for back pain, or as a remedy for influenza, for colds and coughing. Macerated plant in water is used for an herbal bath.
Root: Cooked in water which is drunk for a cough remedy. Infused in water for an aphrodisiac.
Stem: Bark decoction used for treating fever.
Stem and Leaf: Juice or a decoction of the leafy branches, when mixed with mother's milk is used as an antivomitive for nursing infants; infusion of aerial parts drunk as a tea for migraine headache or as a

---

[466] Castner, James L., S. Lee. Timme, and James A. Duke. *A Field Guide to Medicinal and Useful Plants of the Upper Amazon.* Gainesville, FL: Feline, 1998 ; 106.
[467] Bajaj, Yashpal Singh. *Biotechnology in Agriculture and Forestry Medicinal and Aromatic Plants IX,* Berlin: Springer-Verlag, 1997; 370.
[468] Morton F. Julia, *Atlas of Medical Plants of Middle America: Bahamas to Yucatan.* Springfield, Illinois: Charles C Thomas Publisher, 1981; 815.
[469] DeFilipps, Robert A., Shirley L. Maina, and Juliette Crepin. *Medicinal Plants of the Guianas (Guyana, Surinam, French Guiana).* Washington, D.C.: Dept. of Botany, National Museum of Natural History, Smithsonian Institution, 2004; 26.

purgative; decoction for febrifuge, dizziness, or wash for headache; plaster for violent and persistent head pain. Infusion for jaundice in mothers of newborn.
Leaf infusion anti diarrheic and emetic. [470]Leaf-juice for coughs, mouth sores, inflammation of gums. Leaves are an ingredient in a bitter tea used to cleanse the blood and skin, and for biliousness. Macerated and applied to treat thrush, sores and ulcers. Macerated and applied to treat thrush, sores and ulcers. Juice from macerated leaves is used as an antibiotic eye-drop. Leaves are boiled and the water used as an eye-wash for infected eyes or as a tonic. l.eaf infusion used for bronchitis, cough, diarrhea, fevers, kidney diseases, and hemorrhoids. [471]
Cautions & Contraindications: Do not use in cases with loose stools or phlegm disorders.
Major Known Ingredients: Contains the toxic alkaloid scoparine, as well as (in root) 6-methoxy-benzoxazolinone (which is hypotensive and antidiabetic), and triterpenoids. Oil from aerial parts contains tritriacontane, dulciol, beta-sitosterol and dulciolone.
Pharmacological & Clinical Research: An oil from the aerial parts yielded tritriacontane, dulciol, beta-sitosterol, dulciolone and two crystalline alcohols. Other compounds that have been found include sitosterol, hexacosanol, D-mannitol, scutellarin, scutellarein, friedelin, glutinol, dulcioic acid and alpha-amyrin. [472]
Pharmacological & Clinical Research: The antidiabetic activity of the Indian *S. dulcis* is attributed to the glycoside ammelin obtained from the fresh plant. The methanolic and water extracts from roots of Formosan S. *dulcis* have been found to exert hypotensive activity, and 6-methoxybenzoxazolinone (MBOA) was isolated as an active principle. MBOA, originally isolated from gramineous plants such as Job's tears *(Coix lacryma johi),* wheat *(Triticum aestivum),* and corn *(Zea mays),* was thereafter reported to show antiinflammatory property. The analgesic and antiinflammatory activities of the ethanolic extract of this plant were recently observed, and a triterpene, glutinol, was detected as a major bioactive component. [473] Biologically active substances isolated include three different types of diterpenoids: (1) labdane type: scoparic acid A, scoparic acid B, scoparic acid C, and scopadiol; (2) scopadulane type: scopadulcic acid A, scopadulcic acid B, and scopaduJciol; (3) aphidicolane type: scopadulin. Among these compounds, scopadulcic acid B was found to possess various biological activities such as inhibitory activities against replication of herpes simplex virus type 1 and gastric H+, K+ -ATPase., antitumor activity and antitumor-promoting activity.[474]
Toxicity: The whole plant contains an unnamed alkaloid, a bitter principle and salicylic acid; also sitosterol, hexacosanol, D~mannitol, tritriacomane, dukiol, scropanol and duldolone. The dried, powdered roots have yielded 6-methoxyben-zoxazolinone betulinic acid and ifflaionic acid. The whole plant has central nervous system activity.[475]

---

470 Duke, James A. *CRC Handbook of Medicinal Herbs*. Boca Raton, FL: CRC, 1985; 154
471 Duke, James A. *CRC Handbook of Medicinal Herbs*. Boca Raton, FL: CRC, 1985; 154.
472 Lachman-White, D. A., C. D. Adams, and Ulric O'D. Trotz. *A Guide to the Medicinal Plants of Coastal Guyana*. London: Commonwealth Science Council, 199; 248.
473 Bajaj, Yashpal Singh. *Biotechnology in Agriculture and Forestry 37 Medicinal and Aromatic Plants I*, Berlin: Springer-Verlag, 1993; 370.
Ibid., p, 371.
475 Morton F. Julia, *Atlas of Medical Plants of Middle America: Bahamas to Yucatan*. Springfield, Illinois: Charles C Thomas Publisher, 1981; 816.

Chapter 13: The Astrigents
Plants that Stop Discharge of Secretions

The astringents contain tannin, organic acids or inorganic salts. The anthelmintic or vermifuge are agents against tapeworms, roundworms, flukeworms and many other parasites.

Fat Pork

Astrigent Plants: **Plants Expel Parasites**

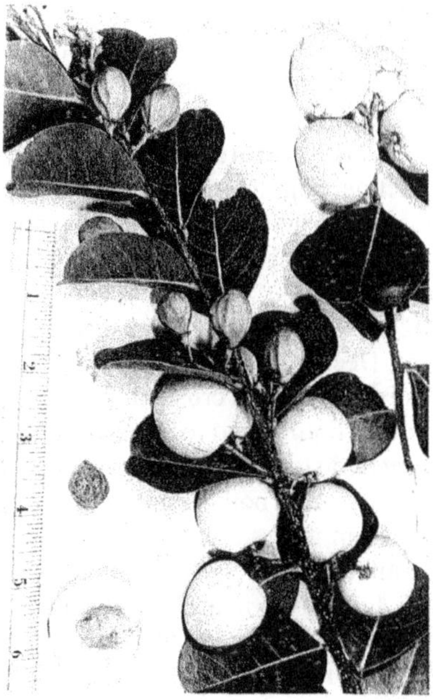

Botanical Name: Chrysobalanus Icaco.
Family: Chryosobalalaceae.
Region Where Grown: Demerara-Mahaica.
Other Names: Caramio, kurimiru.
Category: Astrigents: Plants that Expel parasites (Anthelmintic or Vermifuge).
Properties: Sweet, Cold/Moist.
Esoteric Botanica: Het Heru.
Governing Organs: Kidney, Spleen, Liver.
Actions & Indications: Used for leucorrhoea, anti diarrheic, flaccid scrotum and vulva and dysentery.
Root, Stem-bark and Leaf used as astringent for diarrhoea and leucorrhoea. [476]
Root and Leaf: The juice mixed with oil is used to contract the sphincters of the vulva by women wishing to simulate virginity and the same preparation is used by men for treating flaccid scrotum. [477]
Fruit: Astringent and antidiarrhoeic.
Fruits, leaves, bark or roots in boiling water to overcome chronic diarrhea, hemorrhages and leucorrhea.[478]
The kernel oil has been used as a substitute for almond oil in medical ointments.

---

[476]DeFilipps, Robert A., Shirley L. Maina, and Juliette Crepin. *Medicinal Plants of the Guianas (Guyana, Surinam, French Guiana)*. Washington, D.C.: Dept. of Botany, National Museum of Natural History, Smithsonian Institution, 2004; 82.
[477] Ibid., p, 82.
[478] Morton F. Julia, *Atlas of Medical Plants of Middle America: Bahamas to Yucatan.* Springfield, Illinois: Charles C Thomas Publisher, 1981; 262.

Cautions & Contraindications: If taken with hot tea, the patient may develop diarrhea and belching. Nausea, vomiting and belching are common side effects. It is otherwise a safe herb with low toxicity.
Major Known Ingredients: The fruits and other parts owe their astringency to their tannin content. The kernel contains 20 to *22%* oiJ- 4.4% palmitic acid, 18.7% stearic acid, 1 1. 2 % oleic acid, 6.2% linoleic acid, 1.0% arachidic acid, 0.1% conjugated octadecadienoic acid, 22% ά-eleostearic 1 acid, 10.62% ά - parinaric acid, J 10.0% ά -licanic acid, and 18.0% 4-oxooctadeea-cis-9, *trans-II, tr ans-l3,* cis-15-tetraenoic acid.[479]

Congo Cane

Astrigent Plants: **Plants Expel Parasites**

Botanical Name: Costus Scaber.
Family: Costaceae.
Region Where Grown: Essequibo Isl-W. Demerara.
Other Names: None.
Category: Astrigents: Plants that Expel parasites (Anthelmintic or Vermifuge).
Properties: Astringent, Bitter, Hot/Dry.
Esoteric Botanica: Heru.
Governing Organs: Heart, Stomach, Urinary Bladder.
Actions & Indications: Treatment of internal fever and bronchitis. A deeoction from the root is used to treat stomachaches and snakebites. The juice of crushed flowers and leaves is taken orally as a treatment for worms. Vaginal infections are treated by using a douche made of the flowers. [480]

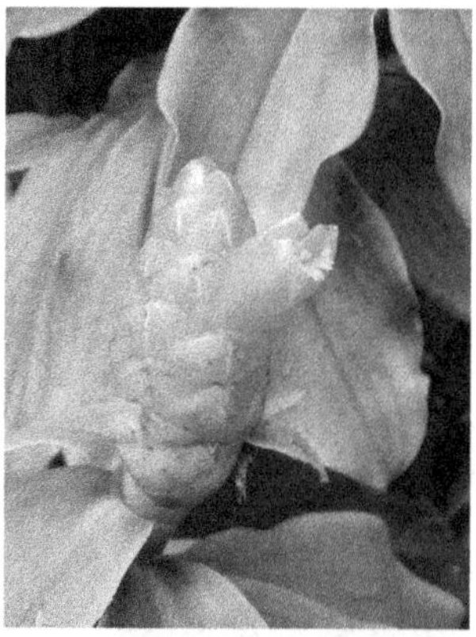

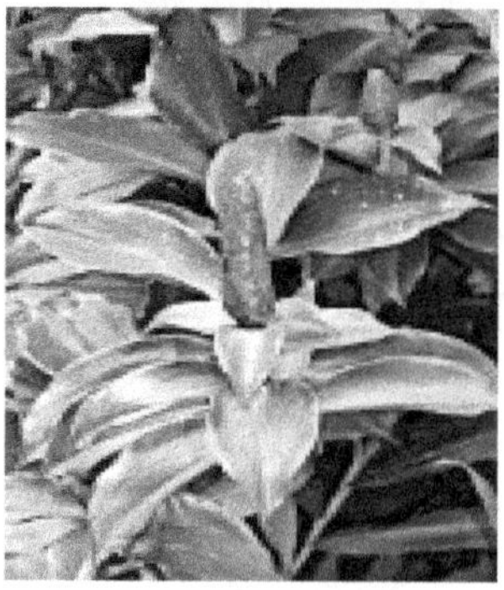

Rhizome: Decoction for leucorrhoea.
Stem: Decoction for leucorrhoea. Infusion to treat blennorrhagia and gonorrhoea. Stems crushed, warmed, added to water and honey, and the resulting liquid used to remedy coughs, grippe and whooping cough. Macerated stems as a laxative, carminative and to treat colic. Stem used to treat sores, and both stem and shoot used to treat colds and coughs. Leaf: Juice from macerated leaves and stem is used as an antibacterial and as an anti-infective.
Leaf: Juice from macerated leaves is warmed and used for treating ear infection, coughs and colds and also pneumonia.
Whole plant: Decoction for high blood pressure and bladder disorders and dysentery; sap for syphilis; infusion of seedling for coughs. Used to treat malaria.
Root: Used to treat groin ruptures and hemorrhoids. Decoction of twigs for remedying syphilis. Both stem and shoot used to treat coughs and colds.
Flower: Used for sore eyes, groin ruptures and hemorrhoids.

---

[479] Ibid., p, 262.

[480] Castner, James L., S. Lee. Timme, and James A. Duke. *A Field Guide to Medicinal and Useful Plants of the Upper Amazon.* Gainesville, FL: Feline, 1998; 43.

Stem and Leaf: The plant for curing stomach ailments.
Stem: Maceration is drunk to remedy colic and as a laxative and carminative. Also used for treating urinogenital tract infections characterized by pus flow. Part of the decoction is drunk and part used to wash the vagina or glans penis.
Cautions & Contraindications: Do not use during pregnancy.

Pumpkin

Astrigent Plants: **Plants Expel Parasites**

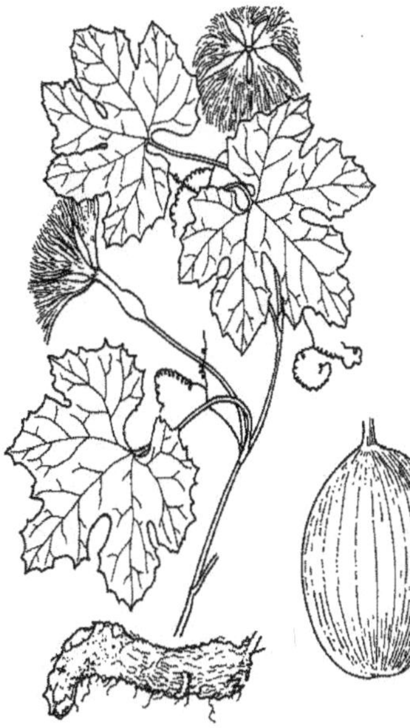

Botanical Name: Cucurbita.
Family: Cucurbitaceae.
Region Where Grown: E. Berbice-Corentyne.
Other Names: None.
Category: Antitussive: Astrigents: Plants that Expel parasites (Anthelmintic or Vermifuge).
Properties: Salty, Cold/Moist.
Esoteric Botanica: Het Heru.
Governing Organs: Kidney, Liver, Stomach.
Actions & Indications: Pumpkin is used to treat jaundice, expel intestinal worms and treatment of prostatic hyperthropy.[481]
Flower: Pumpkin flowers boiled in water with a little salt added after boiling. Used as a remedy for thrush. Remedy for jaundice,[482] treats such biomedically-defined disorders as roundworm, tapeworm, pinworm or fasciolopsis infestations.[483] For phlegm heat, cough with chest pain and thick, difficult-to-expectorate sputum, stifling sensation, pain or diaphragmatic pressure and for dry constipation, especially when it appears in a pattern of lung heat with dry mouth, thirst and irritability. Also promotes healing of sores.[484]

---

[481] Foster Steven, Varro Tyler E. *Tyler's honest Herbal: A Sensible Guide to the Use of Herbs and Related Remedies*. Binghamton, NY: The Haworth Herbal Press, 2000; 406.
[482] DeFilipps, Robert A., Shirley L. Maina, and Juliette Crepin. *Medicinal Plants of the Guianas (Guyana, Surinam, French Guiana)*. Washington, D.C.: Dept. of Botany, National Museum of Natural History, Smithsonian Institution, 2004; 101.
[483] Bensky, Dan, Andrew Gamble, and Ted J. Kaptchuk. *Chinese Herbal Medicine: Materia Medica*. Seattle, WA: Eastland, 1993; 179.
[484] Ibid., p, 180.

Cautions & Contraindications: This herb is used in cooking foods. Contraindicated in cases of diarrhea due to cold from deficiency of the spleen or stomach.
Major Known Ingredients: Saponins, resin and trichosanthic acid.

Sweet-Aloes

Astrigent Plants: **Plants Expel Parasites**

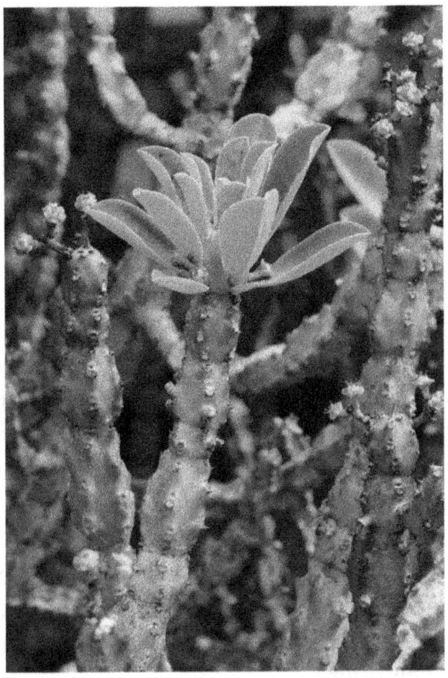

Botanical Name: Euphorbia Neriifolia.
Family: Euphorbiaceae.
Region Where Grown: Mahaica-Berbice.
Other Names: Sahure, Sweet-aloes.
Category: Astrigents: Plants that Expel parasites (Anthelmintic or Vermifuge).
Properties: Sour, Cold/Dry.
Esoteric Botanica: Seker
Governing Organs: Liver, Spleen.
Actions & Indications: Leaf: Leaves are heated, squeezed, and the sap taken with salt to treat wheezing in babies, colds and stomach upset. Used for infected nails, fevers, coughs and colds and for diabetes.
Cautions & Contraindications: Nausea, vomiting and belching are common side effects.
Major Known Ingredients: Contains terpenes, anthocyanins, alcohols and steroids.

Buri

Astrigent Plants: **Plants Expel Parasites**

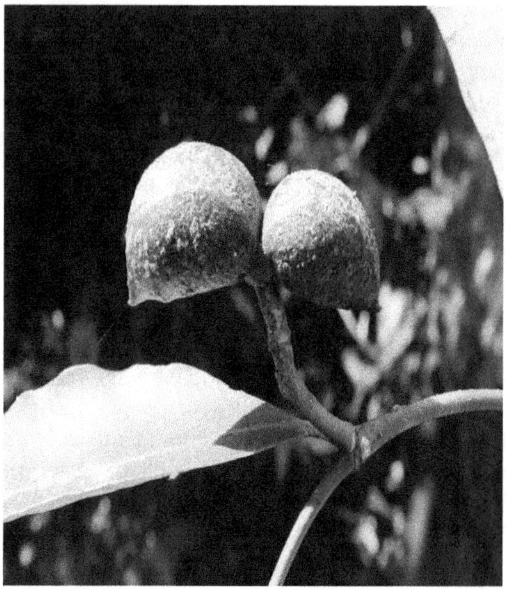

Botanical Name: Tabernaemontana Undulata.
Family: Apocynaceae.
Region Where Grown: Pomeroon-Supenaam.
Other Names: None.
Category: Astrigents: Plants that Expel parasites (Anthelmintic or Vermifuge).
Properties: Sweet, Cold/Moist.
Esoteric Botanica: Het Heru.
Governing Organs: Stomach, Liver, Spleen.
Actions & Indications: Whole plant: Latex used for removing "mosquito worms" from body and placed on cotton plug for toothache. Exudate used to treat munuri ant (Pariponera clavata) bite and sore eyes.
Root: Used to treat headaches.
Stem: Grated bark used in a plaster for headache and as a resolvent for small abscesses; latex extracted from the trunk is placed on absorbent cotton as a tampon for painful dental cavities.
Leaf: Macerated for an eyewash to remedy conjunctivitis. Macerated in rum for swollen feet. Petiole-latex applied to penis for gonorrhoea. Also used to soothe bites, and for skin irritations and snakebite wounds.
Cautions & Contraindications: Do not use during pregnancy.
Major Known Ingredients: Alkaloids in stem-bark include conopharyngine, jollyanine, voacangine, isovoacangine, ibophyllidine, coronaridine and heyneanine. Leaf contains the alkaloids angustine, pleiocarpamine, tubotaiwine, hydroxycoronaridine and hydroxyheyneanine.

Sand Mora

Astrigent Plants: **Plants Expel Parasites**

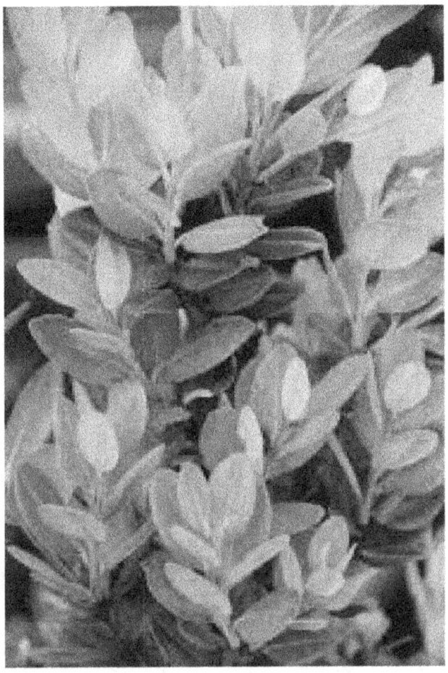

Botanical Name: Mora Excelsa.
Family: Caesalpinaceae.
Region Where Grown: Potaro-Siparuni.
Other Names: Mora. Black Mora, Red Mora. Category: Astrigents: Plants that Expel parasites (Anthelmintic or Vermifuge).
Properties: Sour, Hot/Moist.
Esoteric Botanica: Tehuti.
Governing Organs: Liver, Large Intestines, Lungs.
Actions & Indications: Whole plant: Anthelmintic; for cleaning and healing sores and cuts.
Bark: Bark is either boiled or mixed with water and drunk as an antidiarrheal. Inner bark is scraped, soaked in water overnight and drunk as an antidiarrheal. [485] Bark decoction for an antispasmodic to treat uterine infections, diarrhoea and dysentery. [486] Used to treat diarrhea. Also used for treating skin, worm and urinogenital infections.
Cautions & Contraindications: Use with caution in cases of weakness. Do not use during pregnancy.

---

[485] DeFilipps, Robert A., Shirley L. Maina, and Juliette Crepin. *Medicinal Plants of the Guianas (Guyana, Surinam, French Guiana)*. Washington, D.C.: Dept. of Botany, National Museum of Natural History, Smithsonian Institution, 2004; 71.
[486] Ibid., p. 71.

Worm-Bush

Astrigent Plants: **Plants Expel Parasites**

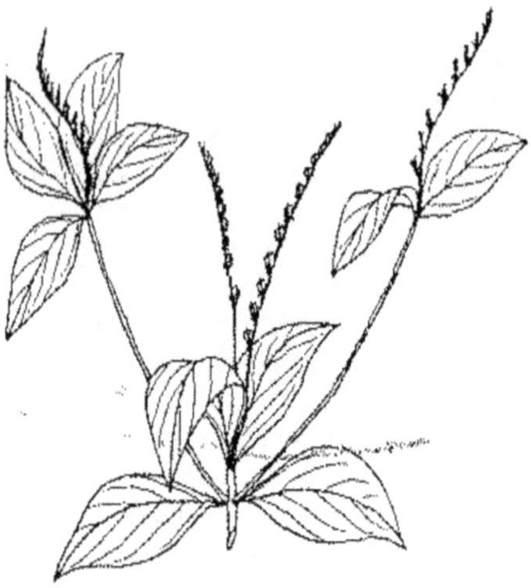

Botanical Name: Spigelia Anthelmia.
Family: Longaniaceae.
Region Where Grown: Potaro-Siparuni.
Other Names: Worm Grass.
Category: Astrigents: Plants that Expel parasites (Anthelmintic or Vermifuge).
Properties: Sweet, Cold/Moist.
Esoteric Botanica: Auset.
Governing Organs: Stomach, Liver, Kidney,Small Intestine.
Actions & Indications: Whole plant: Boiled and the liquid is drunk to treat hypertension and thrush. [487]
Leaf: Vermifuge; Repel cockroaches; anthelmintic.
Sap from leaves used to treat eye infections.
Rhizome: For intestinal problems. Also used in a herbal bath and as an anthelmintic and for stomachache.
Root: Used to bathe children as sedative and tranquilizer.[488]
Cautions & Contraindications: Use with caution in cases of weakness. Do not use during pregnancy.
Major Known Ingredients: Plant is reported to have anthelmintic properties. It is said to cause dimness of vision with dilated pupils, giddiness, spasms of the muscles of the eye and face, and convulsions. It is reported to cause death to domestic animals within 2-3 hours and may be fatal to children. A toxic alkaloid spigeline has been isolted from the leaves.[489]
Pharmacological & Clinical Research: Leaf contains the toxic alkaloid spigeline. Ingestion of plant may cause dimness of vision with dilated pupils, giddiness, spasms of eye and facial muscles, and convulsions; may be fatal to children. Spigeline has affinities with nicotine and lobeline and is used as a vermifuge
Toxicity: Plant is very poisonous (toxic).

[487] DeFilipps, Robert A., Shirley L. Maina, and Juliette Crepin. *Medicinal Plants of the Guianas (Guyana, Surinam, French Guiana)*. Washington, D.C.: Dept. of Botany, National Museum of Natural History, Smithsonian Institution, 2004; 158.
[488] Duke, James A. and Rodolfo Vásquez. *Amazonian Ethnobotanical Dictionary*. Boca Raton, FL: CRC, 1994; 158.
[489] Lachman-White, D. A., C. D. Adams, and Ulric O'D. Trotz. *A Guide to the Medicinal Plants of Coastal Guyana*. London: Commonwealth Science Council, 1992; 264.

Ant Bush

Astringent Plants: **Plants Expel Parasites**

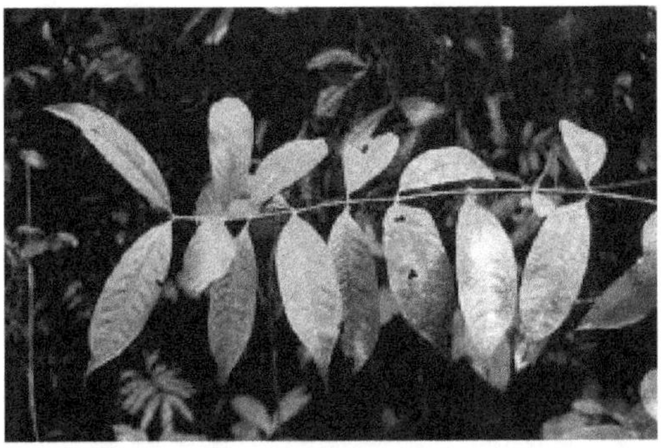

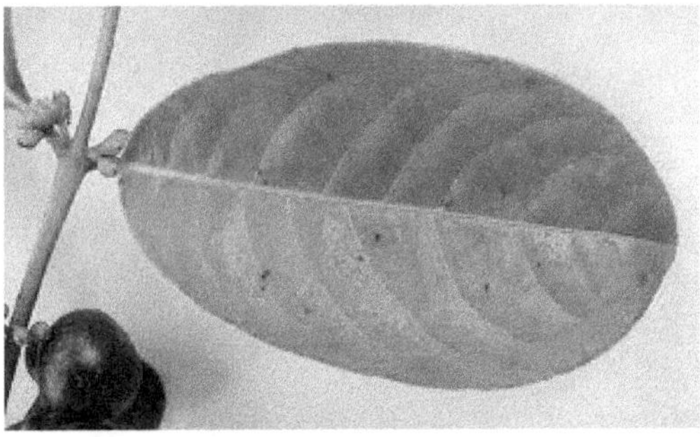

Botanical Name: Siparuna Guianensis.
Family: Monimiaceae.
Region Where Grown: Potaro-Siparuni.
Other Names: Ants bush, Fever Bush, Moonerydany, Nimble Bush. Arawak: Menirie dan Bojaroe, Moeniridan, Muniri-dan, Muniridan. Patamona: tap-ring-yik.
Category: Astrigents: Plants that Expel parasites (Anthelmintic or Vermifuge).
Properties: Sour, Hot/Moist.
Esoteric Botanica: Maat.
Governing Organs: Liver, Spleen, Intestine, Kidney.
Actions & Indications: Considered anodyne, insecticidal and stomachic; for colds, colic, cramps, dermatosis, fever, headache, mange, rbeumatism. [490]
Additionally, this plant has been used in traditional medicine for colds, cramps, skin infections, rheumatism and wounds. [491]
Bark is boiled and the water drunk as an antimalarial, as an anthelmintic (hookw orm) or as an antipyretic. Bark is boiled with water and given to babies for chest colds. [492]
Bark and Leaf: Juice from macerated bark and leaves is used as an anti-fungal. Luke warm mixture of the bark and leaves is used for washing the body to alleviate high temperatures.
Leaf: Infusion for an abortive, aphrodisiac, febrifuge, headache remedy, vulnerary and to aid blood circulation. Infusion given to women convalescing after childbirth. Tincture used for reducing edema and as a vulnerary; decoction is sudorific, hypotensive; decoction in a cataplasm as an anti-inflammatory for bruises during confinement awaiting childbirth. Macerated leaves in cold water are used as an antipyretic. Leaves used to treat wounds and cuts. Leaf and Stem-bark: Decoction as a refresher, febrifuge, especially for grippe. Decoction for diabetes, thrush, hypertension, whooping cough, anthelmintic, ant-bite.
Fruit and Root: Pulp of the fruit and macerated root are used as a medicament for "bush yaws". Also used as an antimalarial and for treating colds. The tea of the leaves and flowers is used as a canninative, in dyspepsia, and pain and spasms.[493]

---

[490] Duke, James A. and Rodolfo Vásquez. *Amazonian Ethnobotanical Dictionary*. Boca Raton, FL: CRC, 1994; 155.
[491] Ibid., p, 116.
[492] DeFilipps, Robert A., Shirley L. Maina, and Juliette Crepin. *Medicinal Plants of the Guianas (Guyana, Surinam, French Guiana)*. Washington, D.C.: Dept. of Botany, National Museum of Natural History, Smithsonian Institution, 2004; 196.
[493] Duke, James A. and Rodolfo Vásquez. *Amazonian Ethnobotanical Dictionary*. Boca Raton, FL: CRC, 1994; 156.

Cautions & Contraindications: Use with caution in cases of extreme weakness. Do not use during pregnancy.
Major Known Ingredients: Contains the oxoaporphine alkaloids liriodenine and cassamedine. The wood contains sitosterol, stigmasterol, liriodenine and cassamedine and the alkaloid fuseine. [494]

[494] Morton F. Julia, *Atlas of Medical Plants of Middle America: Bahamas to Yucatan.* Springfield, Illinois: Charles C Thomas Publisher, 1981; 230

Pomegranate

Astringent Plants: **Plants Expel Parasites**

Botanical Name: Punica Granatum.
Family: Punicaceae.
Region Where Grown: Demerara-Mahaica.
Other Names: Anar.
Category: Astrigents: Plants that Expel parasites (Anthelmintic or Vermifuge).
Properties: Acrid, Astringent, Cool/Dry.
Esoteric Botanica: Sebek.
Governing Organs: Lungs, Kidney, Large Intestine.
Actions & Indications: Pomegranate is one of the oldest drugs known. It is mentioned in the Ebers papyrus of Egypt written in about 1550 BCE and is also included in many Ayurvedic texts.[495] Prescribed as intestinal astringent, anthelmintic. Stabilizes the kidneys and retains the essence; for spermatorrhea and premature ejaculation. Also for excessive uterine bleeding and vaginal discharge due to kidney instability.[496]

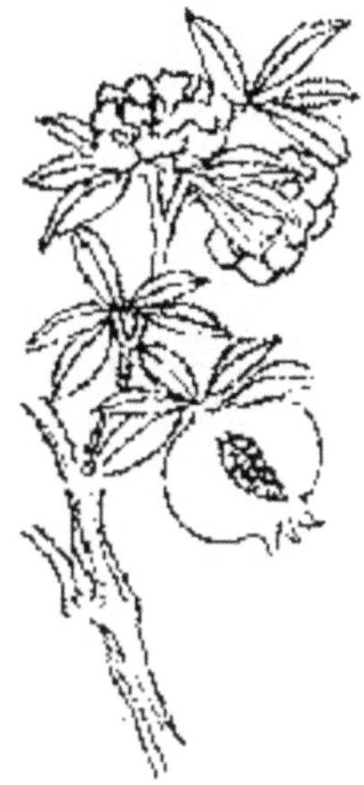

Root: Fresh root-bark for a vermifuge for tapeworms and roundworms.
Stem: A decoction of the boiled bark is drunk to instantly binds up the intestine and relieve diarrhoea.
Fruit: Unripe fruit is employed to relieve diarrhoea, but is less effective than the bark preparation. Rind of fruit in a detersive gargle, or the rind in an infusion drunk for diarrhoea and stomach problems.
Cautions & Contraindications: The bark of *P. granatum* and its contained alkaloids act more powerfully on *Taenia* than on *Ascaris;* but because the large amount of tannin often causes vomiting, the alkaloids alone, in the form of tannates, are preferred; ordinary doses often cause mild toxic symptoms of vertigo, dimmed vision, great weakness and cramps in the legs, formication, convulsive trembling, etc.; toxic doses promptly produce mydriasis, partial blindness, violent headache, vertigo, vomiting and diarrhea, profound prostration, sometimes convulsions. [497]
Major Known Ingredients: Plant contains piperidine alkaloids (in bark, wood and leaf), anthocyanins (in seed coat), and the tannins punicalagin and punicalin (in peel of fruit). The drug contains about 20 % tannin, and 0.5-1.0 % alkaloids consisting of pelletierine ($C_8H_{15}NO$; syrupy liquid, very unstable; b,p. 195; soluble in water, alcohol, chloroform, benzene, ether), methylpelletierine ($C_9H14NO \cdot CH3$; colorless oily liquid; soluble in water, alcohol, chloroform, ether), pseudopelletierine (C9H15NO; orthorhombic prisms; m.p. 54°, b.p. *246*$^{\theta}$ *;* freely soluble in alcohol, chloroform; sparingly soluble in petroleum ether; slightly

[495] Ross, Ivan A. *Medicinal Plants of the World: Chemical Constituents, Traditional, and Modern Medicinal Uses*. Totowa, NJ: Humana, 1999; 274.
[496] Bensky, Dan, Andrew Gamble, and Ted J. Kaptchuk. *Chinese Herbal Medicine: Materia Medica.* Seattle, WA: Eastland, 1993; 384.
[497] Keys, John D. *Chinese Herbs: Their Botany, Chemistry, and Pharmacodynamics*. Rutland, VT: C.E. Tuttle, 1997; 155.

soluble in water, ether), isopelletierine ($C_9H_{15}NO$; oily liquid; soluble in alcohol, chloroform, dilute acids), methylisopelletierine($C_9H_{17}NO$; colorless oily liquid; soluble in water, petroleum ether.[498]

Pharmacological & Clinical Research: The very high tannin content easily explains the antidiarrhoeal effect. The alkaloids interact strongly with nicotinic acetylcholine receptors. They will narcotise tapeworms so that they lose their grip and are expelled. Unfortunately, the alkaloids are absorbed through the intestine and cause undesirable CNS effects.[499] The high tannin and alkaloid content of the skins are possibly responsible for the antidiarrheal effects. An orally administered methanol extract of the seeds, containing steroids, flavonoids and tanmns, has been shown to significantly reduce the frequency of stools and reduce gastrointestinal motility in mice. No clinical studies are available to support the experimental studIes. The alkaloids found in all parts of the plant mean that hIgh doses of P. *granatum* are toxic. Methanol and water extracts of this plant have recently been shown to have significant antimicrobial activity against enteropathogens. [500]

Toxicity: The alkaloids are highly toxic and self medication can be dangerous.

---

[498] Ibid., p, 156.

[499] Van, Wyk Ben-Erik., and Michael Wink. *Medicinal Plants of the World: An Illustrated Scientific Guide to Important Medicinal Plants and Their Uses*. Portland: Timber, 2004; 263.

[500] Ahmad Iqbal, Aqil Farrukh and Owais Mohammad. *Modern Phytomedicine: Turning Medicinal Plants into Drugs.* Germany: Wiley-VCH Verlag GmbH & Co. KGaA, 2006; 259.

Bitter-Gumma

Astringent Plants: **Plants Expel Parasites**

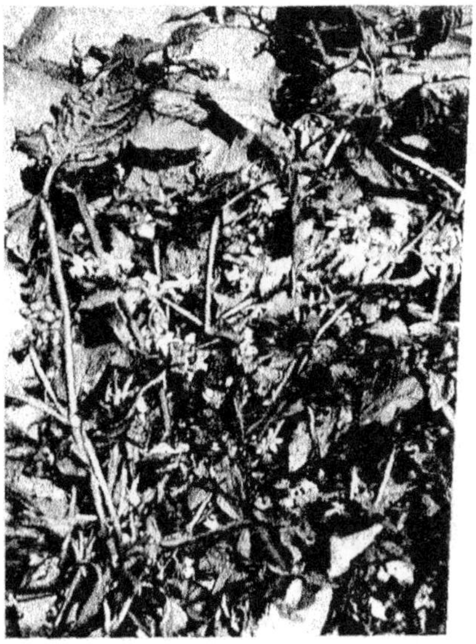

Botanical Name: Solanum Americanum.
Family: Solanacae.
Region Where Grown: U. Takutu-U. Essequibo.
Other Names: Black-calalu, Black nightshade.
Category: Astrigents: Plants that Expel parasites (Anthelmintic or Vermifuge).
Properties:Acrid, Cool/Dry.
Esoteric Botanica: Sebek.
Governing Organs: Lungs, Small Intestine, Heart, Liver.
Actions & Indications: Whole plant: Decoction used as a blood purifier and to expel worms. Used as vermifuge and antispasmodic. Locally recommended for cardialgia, corroding ulcers, suppurating cancers, deep wounds, skin diseases such as dartre and for use in cataplasms for kidney pain. [501]
Stem and Leaf: used in a tea for improved kidney function.
Root: Root is washed clean, boiled with water, mixed with lime juice and a pinch of salt, and is drunk as an anti-malarial. Also used as an ingredient in a curative herbal bath. For tetanus cramps and manic fits of stiffness, contractions of limbs or to clear the head.
Leaf: Decoted is dropped into imflamed eyes and aching cars and is gargled in case of toothache.
Ripe fruits attached, are boiled and the decoction drunk as a bitter tonic and to relieve stomacbache; they also apply it externally on ringworm and other skin afflictions.[502]
Cautions & Contraindications: Do not use during pregnancy.
Major Known Ingredients: The plant has been found high in calcium, iron, riboflavin, thiamine and ascorbic acid.[503]
Pharmacological & Clinical Research: Steroidal alkaloids and sapogenins have been found in many species of solanum. The sapogenin, tigogenin, was reported in the roots of S. Nigrum and acetylcholine-like activity was detected in the fruit.
Toxicity: The green fruit and leaves contain the alkaloid solasodine. Ingestion of the green fruits has caused intoxication in small children.

---

[501] DeFilipps, Robert A., Shirley L. Maina, and Juliette Crepin. *Medicinal Plants of the Guianas (Guyana, Surinam, French Guiana)*. Washington, D.C.: Dept. of Botany, National Museum of Natural History, Smithsonian Institution, 2004; 271.
[502] Morton F. Julia, *Atlas of Medical Plants of Middle America: Bahamas to Yucatan.* Springfield, Illinois: Charles C Thomas Publisher, 1981; 799.
[503] Ibid., p. 800.

Bibliography

Acosta, S.L., L.V. Muro, A.L. Sacrerio, G.L. Monteagudo, A.R. Pena, and S.N. Okwei. "Anti-inflammatory Effects of an Aqueous Extract of *Capraria biflora* L." *Acta Farmaceutica Bonaerense* 22.1 (2003): 53-55. Print.

Ahmad, Iqbal, Farrukh Aqil, and Mohammad Owais. *Modern Phytomedicine: Turning Medical Plants into Drugs*. Weinheim: Wiley-VCH, 2006.

Amen, Ra Un Nefer. *Maat: The 11 Laws of God*. Brooklyn, NY: Khamit Media Trans Visions, 2003.

Amen, Ra Un Nefer. *Qi Gong Success: Prescriptions for Health, Wealth and Happiness.* Brooklyn: Khamit Media Trans Vision, Inc. 2009.

Astschull, S. Von R. *Drugs and Foods from Little-known Plants Notes in Harvard University Herbaria* Cambridge: Harvard University, 1973.

Bajaj, Yashpal Singh. *Medicinal and Aromatic Plants*. Berlin: Springer-Verlag, 1988.

Balandrin, M.F and Klocke, J.A. "Medicinal, Aromatic, and Industrial Materials from Plants, Biotechnology." In Y.P.S. Bajaj (ed.), *Biotechnology in Agriculture and Forestry 4. Medicinal and Aromatic Plant 1.* Berlin: Springer-Verlag, 1988

Balée, William L. *Footprints of the Forest: Ka'apor Ethnobotany-the Historical Ecology of Plant Utilization by an Amazonian People*. New York: Columbia UP, 1994.

Balick, Michael J., Elaine, Elisabetsky, and Sarah, A. Laird. *Medicinal Resources of the Tropical Forest: Biodiversity and Its Importance to Human Health*. New York: Columbia UP, 1996.

Bastien, Joseph William. *Healers of the Andes: Kallawaya Herbalists and Their Medicinal Plants*. Salt Lake City: University of Utah, 1987.

Bensky, Dan, Andrew Gamble, and Ted J. Kaptchuk. *Chinese Herbal Medicine: Materia Medica*. Seattle, WA: Eastland, 1993.

Bhattacharjee, Supriya Kumar. *Handbook of Medicinal Plants*. Jaipur, India: Pointer, 2000.

Bibra, Baron Ernst Von, *Plant Intoxicants: A Classic Text on the Use of Mind Altering Plants*. Vermont: Healing Arts Press, 1995.

Brever, Bep Oliver. *Medical Plants on Tropical West Africa.* London: Cambridge University Press, 1986;

Bryant, D. G., Daniel, Nielsen, and Laura, Tangley. *The Last Frontier Forests: Ecosystems & Economies on the Edge: What Is the Status of the World's Remaining Large, Natural Forest Ecosystems?* Washington, DC: World Resources Institute, Forest Frontiers Initiative, 1997.

Buchman, Dian Dincin. *Ancient Healing Secrets: Practical Herbal Remedies from Around the World That*

Work Today. Avenel, NJ: Crescent, 1996.

"CAB DIRECT." *Phytochemical Resources for Medicine and Agriculture.* N.p., n.d. Web. 27 July 2012. <http://www.cabdirect.org/abstracts/19930320569.html>.

Castner, James L., S. Lee. Timme, and James A. Duke. *A Field Guide to Medicinal and Useful Plants of the Upper Amazon*. Gainesville, FL: Feline, 1998.

Chadwick, Derek, and Joan Marsh. *Bioactive Compounds from Plants: A Wiley-Interscience Publication. Symposium on Bioactive Compounds from Plants Held in Collab. with the Chulabhorn Research Institute at Bangkok, 20-22 February 1990*. Chichester [etc: J. Wiley, 1990.

Clarke, H. D., V. A. Funk, and T. Hollowell. *A Comparative Checklist of the Plant Diversity of the Iwokrama Forest, Guyana*. Fort Worth, TX: Botanical Research Institute of Texas, 2001.

Craker, Lyle E., and James E. Simon. *Herbs, Spices, and Medicinal Plants: Recent Advances in Botany, Horticulture, and Pharmacology*. New York: Food Products.

Cutler, Stephen J., and Horace G. Cutler. *Biologically Active Natural Products: Pharmaceuticals*. Boca Raton, FL: CRC, 2000.

Daniel, M. *Medicinal Plants: Chemistry and Properties*. Enfield, NH: Science, 2006.

DeFilipps, Robert A., Shirley L. Maina, and Juliette, Crepin. *Medicinal Plants of the Guianas (Guyana, Surinam, French Guiana)*. Washington, D.C.: Dept. of Botany, National Museum of Natural History, Smithsonian Institution, 2004.

Dewick, Paul M. *Medicinal Natural Products: A Biosynthetic Approach*. Chichester, West Sussex, England: Wiley, 2002.

Duke, James A., and Rodolfo, Vásquez. *Amazonian Ethnobotanical Dictionary*. Boca Raton, FL: CRC, 1994.

---, *CRC Handbook of Medicinal Herbs*. Boca Raton, FL: CRC, 1985.

Efron, Daniel H., Bo Holmstedt, and Nathan S. Kline. *Ethnopharmacologic Search for Psychoactive Drugs*. Washington, D.C.: U.S. Government Printing Office, 1967.

Foster, Steven, Varro, Tyler E. *Tyler's honest Herbal: A Sensible Guide to the Use of Herbs and Related Remedies*. Binghamton, NY: Haworth Herbal, 1999.

Gehrmann, Beatrice. *Medicinal Herbs: A Compendium*. New York: Haworth Herbal, 2005.

Grieve, M. *A Modern Herbal; the Medicinal, Culinary, Cosmetic and Economic Properties, Cultivation and Folk-lore of Herbs, Grasses, Fungi, Shrubs, & Trees with All Their Modern Scientific Uses*. New York: Dover Publications, 1971.

Gunn, Alan. *Essential Forensic Biology*. Chichester, UK: Wiley-Blackwell, 2009.

Hostettmann, K. *Chemistry, Biological, and Pharmacological Properties of African Medicinal Plants: Proceedings of the First International IOCD-Symposium: Victoria Falls, Zimbabwe, February 25-28, 1996.* Harare: University of Zimbabwe Publications, 1996.

Hou, Joseph P., and Youyu Jin. *The Healing Power of Chinese Herbs and Medicinal Recipes.* New York: Haworth Integrative Healing, 2005.

Jain, Sudhir. *Production of Pharmaceutical Materials from Medicinal and Aromatic Plants, Phase II.* Vienna: United Nations Industrial Development Organization, 1991.

Johnston, Mike, Karen, Davis, and Jeff, Gricar. *The Pharmacy Technician: Foundations and Practices.* Upper Saddle River, NJ: Pearson, 2009.

Kelloff C. L. and V. A. Funk. *Preliminary Checklist of the Plants of the Kaiteur National Park, Guyana.* Washington, DC: Smithsonian Institute, 1997.

Keys, John D. *Chinese Herbs, Their Botany, Chemistry, and Pharmacodynamics.* Rutland, VT: C.E. Tuttle, 1976.

Lachman-White, D. A., C. D. Adams, and Ulric, O'D. Trotz. *A Guide to the Medicinal Plants of Coastal Guyana.* London: Commonwealth Science Council, 1992.

Leeuwenberg, A. J. M. *Medicinal and Poisonous Plants of the Tropics: Proceedings of Symposium 5-35 of the 14th International Botanical Congress, Berlin, 24 July-1 August 1987.* Wageningen: Pudoc, 1987.

Lewis W.E., M. Elvin-Lewis and M.C. Gnerre. "Introduction to the Ethnobotanical Pharmacopoeia of the Amazonian." *Medicinal and Poisonous Plants of the Tropics.* Ed., A. J. M. Leeuwenberg. Wageningen: Pudoc, 1987. 96-103.

McIntyre, A. R. *Curare; Its History, Nature, and Clinical Use.* Chicago: Univ. of Chicago, 1947.

Michel, A. M. *Handbook of Medicinal Plants.* Jaipur: Pointer Pub., 2008.

Miller, Lucinda G., and Wallace, J. Murray. *Herbal Medicinals: A Clinician's Guide.* New York: Pharmaceutical Products, 1998.

Morton F. Julia, *Atlas of Medical Plants of Middle America: Bahamas to Yucatan.* Springfield, Illinois: Charles C. Thomas Publisher, 1981.

Neuwinger, Hans Dieter. *African Ethnobotany: Poisons and Drugs : Chemistry, Pharmacology, Toxicology.* London: Chapman & Hall, 1996.

Nigg, Herbert N., and David S. Seigler. *Phytochemical Resources for Medicine and Agriculture.* New York: Plenum, 1992.

Oksman-Caldentey, Kirsi-Marja, and W. Barz. *Plant Biotechnology and Transgenic Plants.* New York: M. Dekker, 2002.

Pennacchio, Marcello, Lara Vanessa. Jefferson, and Kayri Havens. *Uses and Abuses of Plant-derived*

Bibliography

Smoke: Its Ethnobotany as Hallucinogen, Perfume, Incense, and Medicine. Oxford: Oxford UP, 2010.

Prajapati, Narayan Das, Narayan Das. Prajapati, S. S. Purohit, and Arun K. Sharma. *A Handbook of Medicinal Plants: A Complete Source Book*. Jodhpur: Agrobios, 2003.

PDR for Nonprescription Drugs, Dietary Supplements, and Herbs. Montvale, NJ: PDR Network, 2010.

Robbers, James E. and Tyler, Varro E. Tyler's Herbs of Choice: The Therapeutic Use of Phylomedicinals. London: The Haworth Herbal Press, 1999.

Rodriques RB, Lichtenthaler R., Maria JG, Papagiannopoulous M., Fabricius H., and Marx F. "Total Oxidant Scavenging Capacities of Euterpe Oleracea Mart. (Açaí) Fruits." *Pubmed Abstract PMID:16019315*.

Ross, Ivan A. *Medicinal Plants of the World: Chemical Constituents, Traditional, and Modern Medicinal Uses*. Totowa, NJ: Humana, 1999.

Rutten, A. M. G. *Dutch Transatlantic Medicine Trade in the Eighteenth Century under the Cover of the West India Company*. Rotterdam: Erasmus, 2000.

Schultes, Richard Evans, and Robert F. Raffauf. *The Healing Forest: Medicinal and Toxic Plants of the Northwest Amazonia*. Portland, Or.: Dioscorides, 1990.

Singh, A. P. *Compendia of World's Medicinal Flora*. Enfield, NH: Science, 2006.

Sofowora, Abayomi. *Medicinal Plants and Traditional Medicine in Africa*. Chichester, West Sussex: Wiley, 1982.

Spinella, Marcello. *The Psychopharmacology of Herbal Medicine: Plant Drugs That Alter Mind, Brain, and Behavior*. Cambridge, MA: MIT, 2001.

Steege, Hans Ter. *Plant Diversity in Guyana: With Recommendations for National Protected Area Strategy*. Wageningen: Tropenbos Foundation, 2000.

Stepp, John R., Felice S. Wyndham, and Rebecca K. Zarger. *Ethnobiology and Biocultural Diversity: Proceedings of the Seventh International Congress of Ethnobiology*. Athens, GA: International Society of Ethnobiology, 2002.

Steiner, Richard P. *Folk Medicine: The Art and the Science*. Washington, D.C.: American Chemical Society, 1986.

Tringali, Corrado. *Bioactive Compounds from Natural Sources: Isolation, Characterisation, and Biological Properties*. London: Taylor & Francis, 2001.

Thomson, William A. R. *Herbs That Heal*. New York: Scribner, 1976.

Van, Wyk Ben-Erik, and Michael Wink. *Medicinal Plants of the World: An Illustrated Scientific Guide to Important Medicinal Plants and Their Uses*. Portland: Timber, 2004.

Bibliography

Varela, Alejandro, and Jasiah Ibañez. *Medicinal Plants: Classification, Biosynthesis and Pharmacology*. New York: Nova Biomedical, 2009.

Von, Reis Siri, and Frank J. Lipp. *New Plant Sources for Drugs and Foods from the New York Botanical Garden Herbarium*. Cambridge, MA: Harvard UP, 1982.

Weiner, Michael A., Janet Weiner, and Norman R. Farnsworth. *Weiner's Herbal: The Guide to Herb Medicine*. New York: Stein and Day, 1980.

WHO Monographs on Selected Medicinal Plant: Vol. 1. Geneva: World Health Organization, 1999.

Yaniv, Zohara, and Uriel Bachrach. *Handbook of Medicinal Plants*. New York: Haworth Medical, 2005.

Yeun, Him-che. *Handbook of Chinese Herbs: Chinese Materia Media*. LA: Institute of Chinese Medicine, 1996.

Glossary

Abortifacient. A drug or material that causes the expulsion of the fetus.
Afterbirth. The placenta and fetal membranes expelled from the uterus after childbirth.
Ague. A sharp, intermittent attack of malaria or other fever and chill.
Albuminuria. Presence of albumin in the urine, sometimes indicating kidney disease.
Amen means concealed and corresponds to the essential nature of the Supreme Being which is the same as the essence of Man's being.
Anthelmintic (vermifuge). A drug which causes the destruction and expulsion Of intestinal worms.
Antidiuretic. An agent or mechanism that decreases urinary volume.
Antipyretic. A drug that reduces or prevents fever.
Antisudorific. See antiperspirant.
Antitussive. A drug that reduces or prevents cough.
Anuria. The absence of urine formation.
Aperient. A mild laxative.
Aperitive. An appetite stimulant.
Aphrodisiac – an agent or substance that causes stimulation of sexual passions.
Asthenia. A nonspecific symptom characterized by loss of energy and strength and a Feeling of weakness. It usually accompanies chronic debilitating conditions such As infectious diseases and cancer.
Astringent. A drug that contracts the body tissue to check discharge of secretions, or Arrests capillary bleeding.
Ausar is the indwelling intelligence guiding all of the functions of our spirit and represents the inner drive felt universally by all to unite.
Auset is our intuitive and instinctive faculties governing our ability to care for and nurture others.
Balm. An aromatic, oily resin exuded from various, chiefly tropical, trees and shrubs, And used in medicine.
Balsamic resin. Consisting of or resembling balsam, an oily or gummy oleoresin, Usually containing benzoic or cinnamic acids, obtained from the exudations of Various trees and shrubs, and used as a base for cough syrups, other medicines and Perfumes.
Bechic. A tonic or other remedy that controls coughing.
Biliousness. Popular term used to describe conditions marked by general malaise, Giddiness, vomiting, headache, indigestion, or constipation.
Bright 's disease. Chronic nephritis.
Cardiotonic. Having a tonic affect on the heart.
Caries. Rottenness or ulceration of teeth or bone; dental cavity.
Carminative. S drug or substance which prevents formation of, or promotes Expulsion of, flatus (gas generated in the stomach or bowels).
Catarrh. Mild inflammation of mucous membranes, especially those of the air Passages of the nose and throat.
Cathartic. Drug having a purgative action on the bowls.
Caustic. Capable of eating away tissue by a corrosive or burning effect.
Chancre (canker). A spreading, ulcer-like sore, especially in the mouth.
Cholagogue. A drug which stimulates the flow of bile by the liver; choleretic.
Cicatrisant (cicatrizant). An agent capable of causing scar formation.
Convulsion. Violent irregular motion of limb or body due to involuntary contraction

Of muscles.
Cramp. A sudden, painful involuntary contraction of a muscle or muscles.
Curare. A black resinous substance prepared from the bark of certain south american Plants (mostly loganiaceae and menispermaceae) and used by some amerindians For poisoning arrows. It causes motor paralysis when introduced into the blood Stream and is now used in medicine, such as for heart surgery, to reduce muscular Spasms under certain conditions.
Dandruff. Scurf; dead skin in small scales among the hair.
Demulcent. A substance used for its soothing and protective action which allays Irritation of surfaces, especially mucous membranes.
Depurative. A drug or agent that induces the excretion and removal of waste Material.
Diaphoretic. A drug causing an increase of perspiration as a result of the stimulation Of the sweat glands.
Diuretic. A drug that has the ability to stimulate the kidneys to increase the secretion And flow of urine.
Dropsy. A leakage of the watery part of the blood into any of the tissues or cavities of The body.
Dysentery. A disease caused by bacteria or protozoa, bringing inflammation of the Mucous membrane and glands of the large intestine, accompanied by painful Diarrhoea. The stool is often accompanied by blood and mucus.
Dyspepsia. Indigestion.
Dyspnoea. Difficult breathing.
Dysuria. Difficult or painful urination.
Edema (oedema). A condition in which excessive clear fluid passes from the blood Into the tissues.
Elephantiasis. A condition characterized by chronically thickened and edematous Tissue, especially that of the genitals and legs, due to various causes. Filarial Elephantiasis is also called "mal de cayenne".
Emetic. A drug or agent having the power to empty the stomach by causing vomiting.
Emollient. A substance applied externally to soften the skin, or internally to soothe An inflamed or irritated surface.
Enema. A liquid injected into the rectum either as a purgative or a medicine; clyster.
Epilepsy. A nervous disorder involving temporary loss of consciousness with or Without convulsions and muscular spasms.
Expectorant. A drug that promotes or modifies the ejection of mucous or other Secretions by coughing from the upper respiratory tract, especially the mouth.
Febrifuge. A drug that reduces or prevents fever; antifebrile, antipyretic.
Flatulence. The presence of excessive gas in the stomach and intestines.
Grippe. An epidemic catarrh; an older term for influenza.
Ground itch. Fungal infection between the toes.
Hernia. The abnormal protrusion of an organ through its containing wall.
Heru corresponds to our will which is the freedom to follow or reject divine law and our emotions.
Herukhuti is the divine principle that safeguards our existence from the injustices of others.
Het-Heru is our faculty of visual thinking - the imagination.
Hodgkin's disease. A disease characterized by a progressive enlargement of lymph Glands, spleen and anemia.
Hypertrophy. Enlargement or overgrowth of an organ.
Hypotensive. Abnormally low blood pressure.

Impetigo. A contagious eruption of the skin, either crusted, bullous or pustular, and Caused by streptococci and/or staphylococci.
Impotence. Inability to engage in sexual intercourse.
Latex. A milky liquid produced in certain plants.
Laxative. A drug having the action of loosening the bowels, stimulating defecation.
Leishmaniasis. Any of a group of infectious diseases caused by flagellate protozoan Parasites of the genus *leishmania* and transmitted to man by sandflies of the Genera *phlebotomus* and *lutzomyia.*
Leprosy (hansen's disease). Chronic contagious disease caused by infection With *leprabacillus*, characterized by the formation of nodules on the body surface And, in an advanced stage, often producing deformities.
Leucorrhoea. A white or yellowish mucopurulent discharge from the vagina.
Libido. The sexual urge or instinct.
Lumbago. Muscular rheumatism; a general term for backache in the lumbar region.
Malaria. An acute, usually chronic, disease caused by protozoa of the genus *Plasmodium* and transmitted by the *anopheles* mosquito; characterized by Intermittent fever, anemia and debility, and, in its acute form, by chills, high fever And profuse sweating at regular intervals.
Maat corresponds to the faculty within man wherein is intuited and experienced the urge to live truth.
Measles. An acute infectious viral disease, characterized by skin eruptions, high fever And nasal catarrh, and occurring most frequently in childhood.
Piles. See hemorrhoid.
Pleurisy. Inflammation of the pleura membranes enveloping the lung.
Poultice. A paste of a plant part or drug applied to a sore or inflamed part of the body, To supply moisture or act as a local stimulant; cataplasm.
Prostate. A gland that surrounds the urethra at the bladder in the male.
Pruritus. Severe itching.
Psoriasis. A chronic inflammatory skin disease characterized by reddish patches Covered with white scales.
Puerperal. Pertaining to childbirth.
Pustule. A small elevation filled with pus and situated within or beneath the epidermis Or within a pilosebaceous follicle; pimple.
Pyretic. Referring to fever.
Quinine. The primary alkaloid of *cinchona*, used in treating malaria.
Renal calculi. Kidney stones.
Repellent. An agent that serves to repel pestiferous organisms.
Ringworm. Common contagious disease produced by fungi that affects skin, hair or Nails.
Scabies. Contagious parasitic disease of the skin caused by the mite *sarcoptes scabi.*
Scrofula. Tuberculosis of the lymphatic glands, especially of the neck, in which the Glands become enlarged.
Sebek corresponds to our faculty for thinking verbally.
Sedative. A drug which quiets nervous activity.
Seker is the divine faculty that is in charge of the life-force which is the formative base of all things in the world.
Soporific. A sleep-inducing drug.
Sudorific. A drug or agent causing sweating.
Tehuti represents the inner drive that is universally felt by all men to acquire the knowledge needed for success in all undertakings.

Thrush. A mycotic disease of the upper digestive tract resulting from infection by the Fungus *candida albicans*. It occurs especially in children and is characterized by Small, whitish spots on the tip and sides of the tongue.
Tisane. A herbal infusion used as a beverage for medicinal purposes; a “tea”.
Tonic. A drug that invigorates or generally improves the normal tone of an organ of the Patient.
Unguent. Ointment.
Vermifuge. A drug which causes the destruction and expulsion of intestinal worms; Anthelmintic.
Vitiligo. A disorder of pigmentation in which the melanocytes inhibit melanogenesis And eventually disappear, resulting in a patchy loss of pigmentation.
Yaws. Infectious tropical disease caused by *treponema pertenue* and characterized by An initial lesion, followed by further multiple lesions of the skin; framboesia

Index

D

E

M

N

O

P

Q

R

S

T

U

V

W

Read more about Kazembe at kazembebediako.com.
Or better yet, be his friend on
Facebook.com/kazembebediako1
or follow Kazembe on Twitter at
Twitter.com/kazembebediako.

To Order
Please go to:
KazembeBediako.com
Discount rates are available on the website.

Khianga Publishing

www.ingramcontent.com/pod-product-compliance
Lightning Source LLC
LaVergne TN
LVHW060034210926
848481LV00013B/3857